Home Respiratory Care

Home Respiratory Care

Jeffrey Lucas, RRT
President
North Coast Oxygen Company
Cleveland, Ohio

Joseph A. Golish, MD, FACP, FCCP
Department of Pulmonary Disease
Division of Internal Medicine
Cleveland Clinic Foundation
Cleveland, Ohio

Geoffrey Sleeper, RRT
President
Liberty Respiratory Care, Inc.
Cleveland, Ohio

Jerry A. O'Ryan, BS, RRT
Center Manager
Glasrock Home Health Care
Dayton, Ohio

With a Foreword by David G. Gillespie, MD
Associate Professor of Medicine
Case Western Reserve University
Cleveland, Ohio

APPLETON & LANGE
Norwalk, Connecticut/San Mateo, California

0-8385-3845-2

Copyright © 1988 by Appleton & Lange
A Publishing Division of Prentice Hall
Chapter 2, pages 24–25, from the National Fire Protection Agency. Copyright © National Fire Protection Agency, Quincy, Massachusetts, 1984.
The *O'Ryan Model for Comprehensive Home Care* used in Chapter 11 Copyright © J. O'Ryan, 1985.

88 89 90 91 92 / 10 9 8 7 6 5 4 3 2 1

Prentice-Hall International (UK) Limited, *London*
Prentice-Hall of Australia Pty. Limited, *Sydney*
Prentice-Hall Canada, Inc., *Toronto*
Prentice-Hall Hispanoamericana, S.A., *Mexico*
Prentice-Hall of India Private Limited, *New Delhi*
Prentice-Hall of Japan, Inc., *Tokyo*
Simon & Schuster Asia Pte. Ltd., *Singapore*
Editora Prentice-Hall do Brasil Ltda., *Rio de Janeiro*
Prentice-Hall, *Englewood Cliffs, New Jersey*

Library of Congress Cataloging-in-Publication Data
Home respiratory care / Jeffrey Lucas . . . [et al.]. ; with a foreword
  by David G. Gillespie.
    p. cm.
  Includes index.
  ISBN 0-8385-3845-2
  1. Respiratory therapy. 2. Respiratory organs—Diseases—
Patients—Home care. I. Lucas, Jeffrey.
  [DNLM: 1. Home Care Services. 2. Respiratory Therapy. WF 600
H7655]
  RC735.I5H66 1988
  362.1'962—dc19
  DNLM/DLC
  for Library of Congress   88-16790
                                                                      CIP

Production Editor: Mary Beth Miller
Designer: Kathleen Peters Ceconi
Cover: Michael Kelly

PRINTED IN THE UNITED STATES OF AMERICA

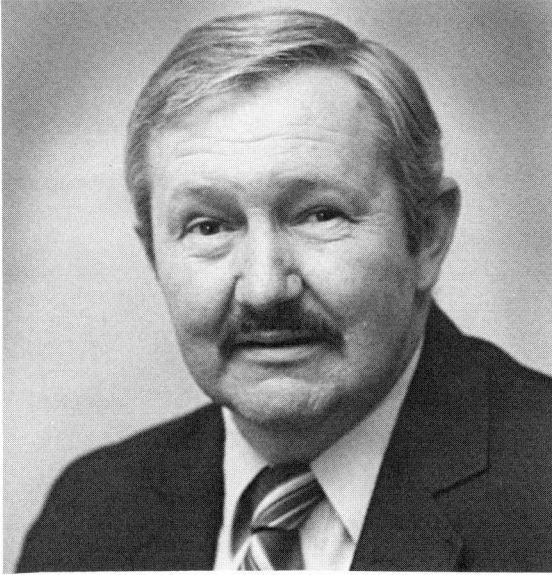

Home respiratory care is beginning to take shape as a cohesive subspecialty attaining scope and direction only within the past decade.

Many fine respiratory therapy clinicians, physicians, and practitioners from all fields of medicine have been involved in providing a substantial foundation for disciplined medical care in the private home.

Ethical practice, the need for industry standards, and a source of reference for home care practices are the major reasons for the production of this text; although the suggestion, guidance, and impetus for this work are directly ascribed to Mr Thomas P. McLeary.

The dedication of this book to Tom McLeary is a tribute to his relentless efforts toward improving patient care standards in the community.

Twenty years ago Tom McLeary, who was Director of Respiratory Care at Fairview General Hospital in Cleveland, Ohio, began formulating methodologies for the home care routines we practice today. At that time he stressed the benefits of early hospital discharge with home-going medical assistance and equipment, the importance of in-home and patient evaluation routines, and the need for development of predischarge planning protocol.

He also substantiated the need and provided the avenue for ventilator-assisted patients and their families to return home. Shortly thereafter, as owner of T & M Oxygen Company, he was responsible for developing one of the largest home ventilator dependent patient populations in the Eastern United States.

More important than Tom McLeary's extensive clinical and business background would certainly be his desire for ethical practice, his work related to improving industry standards, and his benevolence toward peers and patients alike. His instruction always occurs by example. His passion to help all people is exceeded only by his own love for life. Thank you for the lessons, Tom.

Contents

Contributors

David G. Gillespie, MD
Associate Professor of Medicine
Case Western Reserve University
Cleveland, Ohio

Past Medical Director
Respiratory Therapy Technology Program
Cuyahoga Community College
Parma, Ohio

Past Chief of Pulmonary Medicine
Cleveland Metropolitan General Hospital
Cleveland, Ohio

W. Terry Gipson, MD
Director of Psychiatry Residency Training
Department of Psychiatry
Cleveland Clinic Foundation
Cleveland, Ohio

Joseph A. Golish, MD, FACP, FCCP
Department of Pulmonary Disease
Division of Internal Medicine
Cleveland Clinic Foundation
Cleveland, Ohio

Kevin J. Grady, MD
Assistant Director Intensive Care
St John Hospital
Detroit, Michigan

Jeffrey Lucas, RRT
President
North Coast Oxygen Company
Cleveland, Ohio

Glen J. Meden, MD
Clinical Director Intensive Care Unit
Huron Road Hospital
Cleveland, Ohio

Atul C. Mehta, MD, FACP, FCCP
Department of Pulmonary Disease
Division of Internal Medicine
Cleveland Clinic Foundation
Cleveland, Ohio

James P. Orlowski, MD, FAAP, FCCP
Director Pediatric Intensive Care
Cleveland Clinic Foundation
Cleveland, Ohio

Jerry A. O'Ryan, BS, RRT
Center Manager
Glasrock Home Health Care
Dayton, Ohio

Phillip Porte
President
Porte, Stafford and Associates, Inc.
A Washington, DC based government relations/consulting firm
Washington, DC

Linda E. Sinnwell, ACSW
Social Work Continuing Care Department
St Luke's Medical Center
Phoenix, Arizona

Geoffrey Sleeper, RRT
President
Liberty Respiratory Care, Inc.
Cleveland, Ohio

Foreword

During the latter part of the twentieth century we have observed the culmination and convergence of several trends and forces which make the production of this book both relevant and imperative.

Firstly, increased duration of life has been achieved through the conquest of major infectious diseases. With longevity has come a predominance of chronic disorders which are related to our habits or life style. These include cigarette smoking, unhealthful selection of foods, and the use of drugs and alcohol for escape or pleasure. The breathing of air, both outside the home and inside, has become more detrimental to the health of our lungs. Ambient air pollution has paralleled our increasing population density and industrialization. Elevated concentrations of the combustion products of fossil fuels to meet our demands for electric power, transportation, and heat have resulted in additional adverse effects. Modern home construction with low air exchange rates when coupled with the introduction of a variety of noxious substances into our homes has often made the breathing of indoor air more hazardous. However, cigarette smoke, including second-hand smoke, remains the most important factor responsible for chronic lung disease.

Secondly, technical advances of respiratory support have extended the lives of many with chronic disorders. It is not surprising, therefore, that increasing numbers of persons are requiring respiratory care.

Thirdly, the development of Social Security's entitlements, Medicare and Medicaid, has permitted many more people to utilize these benefits. It is hardly surprising that the delivery of complex respiratory care to this large number of eligible patients would be accompanied by rising care cost. This combined with increased costs of other medical care so alarmed the federal government that it shifted to a system of total payment pegged to the patient's diagnosis. This is commonly known as diagnostic related groups (DRGs). This new system of payment encouraged reduction of the hospital stay and thereby heightened the importance of early predischarge planning which hopefully would provide the patient with effective home care. Based on their experience, the authors have presented a well-thought-out team approach for such planning which is found in Chapter 11. Not every medical community will want to adopt the entire plan, but most will find much to adapt to their situation.

Most physicians, nurses, and respiratory therapists receive training focused on, if not limited to, in-hospital care. When only few, if any, of these health care givers have been exposed to home visits in training or practice they can scarcely be expected to grasp the full reality of the patient's problems and their possible solutions. The absence of this extra-hospital experience incompletely prepares one for effective involvement in current respiratory care as influenced by DRGs. Furthermore, the accumulated costs of prolonged institutional care, especially when the costs of such care exceed the coverage, may leave the patient and family little option except home care.

With the current trend in shorter hospitalization and more care outside the hospital, it would be important that didactic training of health care professionals include the subjects discussed in Chapters 2, 3, 7, and 8. Further, the employment of home visits would identify and emphasize the importance of resolving the little problems of home care and would improve the quality of life for these patients. For example, a modest increase of a patient's mobility occasions large gains in daily participation with significant improvement in the patient's ability to cope.

I am impressed with the book's quality, relevance, and scope. I was particularly gratified to observe the authors' sensitivity to their patients. If I had any reservations about my time committed to the founding and nurturing of the Schools of Respiratory Therapy and Respiratory Technology at Cuyahoga Community College, these are dispelled, and I am amply rewarded by this work.

David G. Gillespie, MD
Associate Professor of Medicine
Case Western Reserve University
Cleveland, Ohio

Preface

The rapid growth of the home care industry within the past decade has, by necessity, attracted medical professionals from every segment of the health care team. By trial and error, clinicians have modified existing treatments and developed new techniques to serve the needs of patients and their families in an environment untried by the clinician.

This book is intended to be utilized as a guide into that environment by interested students, respiratory therapists, nurses, home care personnel, discharge planners, social workers, and physicians.

This text is the first source of practical information offering a foundation and reference for the sound application of respiratory care in the private home. A very large segment of home respiratory care lies in the appropriate administration of oxygen. Therefore this text begins with a review of the physiologic basis supporting oxygen therapy. Information relating to the decision making process in choosing the appropriate oxygen delivery system and comparisons of equipment design and function then follow. Technology has entered the home care market place and has offered a variety of useful accessory equipment for the patient. Respiratory equipment enhancements have been outlined as a reference to what is presently available. A compendium on travel specifications with oxygen is a valuable guide for clinician and patient. The section on ventilator care at home is a concise orientation not only to the methodology of returning the patient to his or her home, but also an acknowledgment of the related psychosocial problems associated with this type of care. Adult and newborn sleep disorders are described from pathogenesis through treatment. The final chapters cover the psychologic aspects of chronic pulmonary disease, discharge planning, and legal issues surrounding home care. These are subject areas designed to be useful to the practitioner.

Home care is a broad field and is in its infancy. This text has outlined only the segment of home respiratory care. Many books will follow and many will be needed, as this area of care continues to flourish.

Government statistics anticipate Americans over the age of 65 will more than double in number in 50 years. Individual life expectancy will continue to increase dramatically within the same time period. Coincidently, the working-age class in this country, that taxable segment of our population presently funding a majority of our elderly's health care, is shrinking. Coupled with the government's attitude toward reductions in health-care funding, serious problems may soon arise.

Home health care will inevitably continue to grow, for a number of reasons: (1) the continued growth of our aged population; (2) subacute maintenance care for individuals is less costly at home; (3) skilled nursing facilities remain extremely expensive; (4) most individuals would prefer to recuperate at home; (5) many types of care required at home are easily learned and implemented by patients and their families; and (6) technological advances in equipment allow for enhanced mobility, compactness, and simplicity in providing care routines at home.

As the field grows so will the number of clinicians entering it. We must continue to guide each other and to communicate, thereby improving the standards of care and helping others to benefit from others' trials and errors.

Jeffrey Lucas
Joseph A. Golish
Geoffrey Sleeper
Jerry A. O'Ryan

Acknowledgments

The emergence of home respiratory care as it is practiced today did not happen by itself. Many interested, dedicated people left positions in hospitals and unrelated businesses to come together and work toward the common goal of providing comfortable, assisted care in the private home.

The development of this text did not occur without the help and guidance of many individuals who also believed in the need for the development of both home respiratory care, and a text to guide those entering the field—*The Authors*.

I would like to first thank the employees at North Coast Oxygen Company for their continued support and friendship, specifically: Randy Light for his unflagging commitment to our company's goals, his strength, and his dedication to our patients; and Joyce Rising, LPN, for her unmatched ability to meet challenges and her talent for always finding a way to get the job done. I would like to extend a hearty thanks to Rick Murrell, EMT. North Coast Oxygen could not have accomplished our community based goals without him. Mark Brochetti, RRT, Sharon Updegrove—you are both so important to our continued strength—and my partner Mr John Bauer, MBA, RRT—who always looked the other way when it was necessary—also deserve my thanks. A special thank you to my parents who consistently said "no" when I wanted "yes." I am grateful to my very good friend, Mr Kim Richmond, MS, RRT, who taught me the value of knowledge, for without it personal growth ceases. I want to thank Sharlene Stevens for her patience during this project. A special heartfelt thanks to Miss Barb Shrum, RRT, for her long-term support in all my endeavors. And last, but certainly not least, I would like to thank my children, Nicole and Daniel, for being so understanding and supportive throughout. I love you both very much—*Jeffrey Lucas*.

I would like to thank everyone at Liberty Respiratory Care for their devotion to excellence in patient care: Barbara, Nancy, Joe, and Dave. And of course, I want to thank our Vice President, Don Sleeper, my advisor, best friend, and (coincidently) my father. Special thanks also go to Valerie Dennison for her unwavering support and love. And finally, I want to extend a special dedication to the memory of my mother, Lillian, for just about everything—*Geoffrey Sleeper*.

I would like to dedicate my contribution to this book to the memory of M.P.D., a truly great lady and a dear patient, whose courage and devotion to family were without limit; and to her beloved husband, who is proof that heroes <u>still</u> exist . . . —*Joseph A. Golish*.

SCIENTIFIC BASIS AND PRACTICAL APPLICATION OF HOME CARE

The Physiologic Basis for Long-Term Oxygen Therapy

JOSEPH A. GOLISH, MD
GLENN MEDEN, MD

INTRODUCTION

Chronic obstructive pulmonary disease (COPD) is a nonhomogeneous disease entity that in its later stages leads to chronic hypoxemia. Numerous diseases may lead to acute and chronic hypoxemia, but none has been studied so extensively as COPD as to the effects of a low partial pressure of oxygen. The components of COPD that make it nonhomogeneous are bronchitis, emphysema, and bronchospasm. A history of chronic sputum production is sufficient to document the presence of bronchitis, with the stricter definition being near daily sputum production for 3 months in each of 2 consecutive years. Emphysema classically has been a pathologic diagnosis requiring biopsy or postmortem examination. Pulmonary function testing showing air-flow obstruction and a diminished diffusing capacity is the most sensitive premortem test for an emphysematous component. The bronchospastic (or asthmatic) component can be determined in the pulmonary function laboratory with simple spirometry by showing a significant improvement in the forced expiratory volume in one second (FEV_1) either acutely or chronically after administration of bronchodilators. The determination of each component is important in therapeutic decisions, but most patients have mixed chronic obstructive bronchitis and emphysema. The concept that unifies all components is obstruction to air flow, leading to ventilation–perfusion mismatching and eventual hypoxemia on room air, occurring sooner in patients with a major bronchitic component ("the blue bloater") than in those with a primary emphysematous component ("the pink puffer").

The natural history of severe obstruction is deterioration of lung function over time, with prognosis related to the FEV_1. When the FEV_1 is between 20% and 29% of the predicted value, the 5-year mortality rate is 70% to 90%. The most frequent causes of death are respiratory insufficiency, pneumonia, and cor pulmonale. Bronchodilators, antibiotics, steroids, chest physiotherapy, and patient education have been useful in reducing symptoms of cough, sputum production, and breathlessness, but none have been shown to have an impact on survival. The use of screening spirometry and special tests of small-airway dysfunction (closing volumes, frequency dependence of dynamic compliance, volume of isoflow), in hope of detecting earlier those patients more likely to develop significant lung disease, has not stood the test of time. To date only two methods of reducing mortality have been shown to be significant: the first is smoking cessation and the second is low-flow continuous oxygen.

Oxygen is an element, which in its molecular form makes up 20% of the ambient air; when delivered in higher concentrations, however, it is best described as a drug requiring a physician's prescription. It has been used medically since the 1930s, when it was first provided for patients with pneumonia and shortness of breath. The next step involved home use, pioneered by Alvin Barach. Through the 1960s and 1970s, progress was made in providing home systems at a reasonable cost, and studies proliferated on oxygen's ability to subjectively improve the patients' quality of life. Also, numerous physiologic benefits were found, but most importantly, two large multicenter studies, published in the 1980s, provided conclusive evidence that survival was improved in patients with severe COPD and that low-flow near-continuous delivery was the preferred method (*see* Fig 1–1).

One of these two studies was sponsored by the British Medical Research Council and was published in *Lancet* in 1981. It compared the use of oxygen only during sleep and no oxygen at all in a total of 90 patients. The criteria for entrance into the study were a Pao_2 of between 40 and 60 torr and severe obstructive lung disease with an FEV_1 of less than 1.2 L. Their patients had an average Pao_2 of 50 torr and an average $Paco_2$ of 55 torr. After 1½ years there was a statistically significant difference in survival between the group using nocturnal oxygen (averaging 15 hours per day) and those using no oxygen. The 5-year mortality rate of the oxygen users was 42%, whereas in those not using oxygen, it was 67%. At the 1½-year mark, the yearly risk of death for those not on oxygen was 29%, and for those receiving nocturnal oxygen it was 12%.

The second important study was sponsored by the National Heart, Lung, and Blood Institute. It was published in the *Annals of Internal Medicine* in 1980. Its goal was to compare continuous oxygen therapy (COT) to nocturnal oxygen therapy (NOT), and this landmark paper has come to be known as the NOT–COT study. The total number of patients evaluated was an impressive 203, and more than one center was involved. Criteria for admission into the study were severe obstructive lung disease with a Pao_2 of less than or equal to 55 torr, or 50 to 59 torr and evidence of end-organ damage. The average Pao_2 was 55 torr, and the average Pco_2

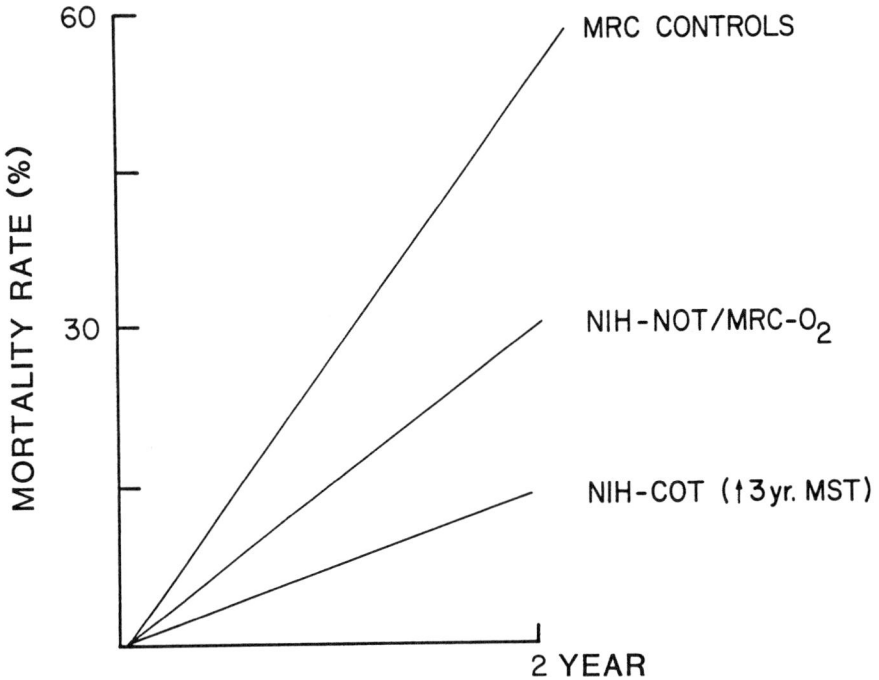

Figure 1–1. Effect of long term O_2 therapy on mortality MRC and NIH composite survival data. *(Adapted from* Lancet *1981; 1:681;* Ann Intern Med *1980; 93:391.)* COT = continuous oxygen therapy; MRC = (British) Medical Research Council; MST = mean survival time; NIH = National Institutes of Health; NOT = nocturnal oxygen therapy.

was 44 torr. The average FEV_1 was 30% of the predicted value. At 1 year, the mortality of the group using near-continuous oxygen was only 12%, and they averaged 20 hours per day of use. Those using nocturnal oxygen had a significantly higher mortality at 21%. They used their oxygen for an average of 12 hours. At 2 years, mortality for the continuous users of oxygen was 22%; that of the nocturnal-only users was nearly double at 41%.

The striking conclusion afforded by these two studies is that in patients with severe obstructive lung disease and hypoxemia, survival is improved by the use of oxygen and that maximum benefit is obtained when it is used nearly continuously. Another way to look at this is that continuous oxygen "buys" 3¼ years of additional life.

The reasons for improved survival are only conjectural at this time, but it is clear from the above empirical evidence that survival *is* improved, and this is the final common denominator for improved overall

Pathophysiologic
mechanisms of → Low PaO₂ →
hypoxemia

Pulmonary Circulation
Right Ventricle
Central Nervous System
Bone Marrow
Kidneys

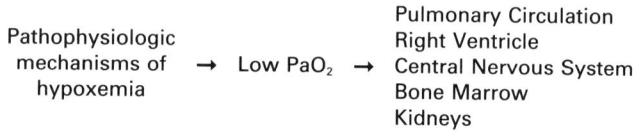

Figure 1–2. The physiologic consequences of hypoxemia.

physiologic function of key organs. The physiologic basis for oxygen supplementation, therefore, can best be reviewed by looking at the pathophysiologic consequences of hypoxemia evidenced by end-organ damage. The key organs that will be reviewed are the lungs, heart, brain, hematopoietic system, and kidneys (*see* Fig 1–2).

The physiologic mechanisms that cause hypoxemia are listed in Table 1–1. Of these, the most common is ventilation–perfusion mismatching, and it is the most common mechanism seen in COPD. Ventilation–perfusion mismatching also happens to be the most responsive to supplemental oxygen.

THE LUNGS

The effect of hypoxemia on the lungs is primarily seen on the pulmonary vasculature (*see* Table 1–1). This is reflected by an increase in pulmonary artery pressure (PAP), which is the most common and most important effect of hypoxemia in COPD. The normal pulmonary artery pressures are 25 mmHg systolic, with a varying diastolic value of 5 to 10 mmHg. The mean PAP is 9 to 15 mmHg. The pressure within the pulmonary vasculature is directly proportional to flow and resistance. The increase in PAP during hypoxemia is secondary to an increase in the resistance of the pulmonary vascular system. There are three mechanisms of increased resistance in hypoxemia caused by COPD (*see* Fig 1–3).

The first of these is a reduced capillary cross-sectional surface area resulting from destruction of capillary vasculature bed, seen in pathologic studies. This is not well correlated to PAP or resistance.

The second mechanism is the most important for acute increases in PAP. Arteriolar smooth muscle contraction (vasospasm) can occur; hypoxemia is the most potent stimulus for this. It is felt to be due to a local vasoconstriction (as opposed to the systemic vascular response to hypoxemia, which is due to carotid body afferents). The existence of a single mediator cannot be postulated at this time; multiple stimuli have been suggested. These stimuli include chemical mediators released from effector cells, such as histamine or serotonin from mast cells. Direct smooth-muscle depolarization also occurs. Another set of mediators that have

TABLE 1–1. HYPOXEMIA: PHYSIOLOGIC MECHANISMS AND ADVERSE EFFECTS

Physiologic Mechanisms	Adverse Effects	
	Pulmonary Circulation	*Heart*
Ventilation–perfusion mismatching	Increased pulmonary artery pressure	Right ventricular hypertrophy
Right-to-left intracardiac or intrapulmonary shunt	Increased pulmonary artery resistance	Right heart failure
Hypoventilation	Arteriolar smooth-muscle contraction	Premature atrial and ventricular contractions
Changing cardiac output	Smooth-muscle hypertrophy	ST-T wave depression
Diffusion impairment		Prolongation of QT interval
Low fraction of inspired oxygen		Right bundle branch block
	Central Nervous System	*Bone Marrow*
	Impaired cognitive function	Polycythemia
	Impaired motor function	
	Memory deficits	
	Fitful sleep	
	Morning headaches	
	Kidneys	
	Reduced blood flow	
	Reduced glomerular filtration rate	
	Increased sodium retention	

7

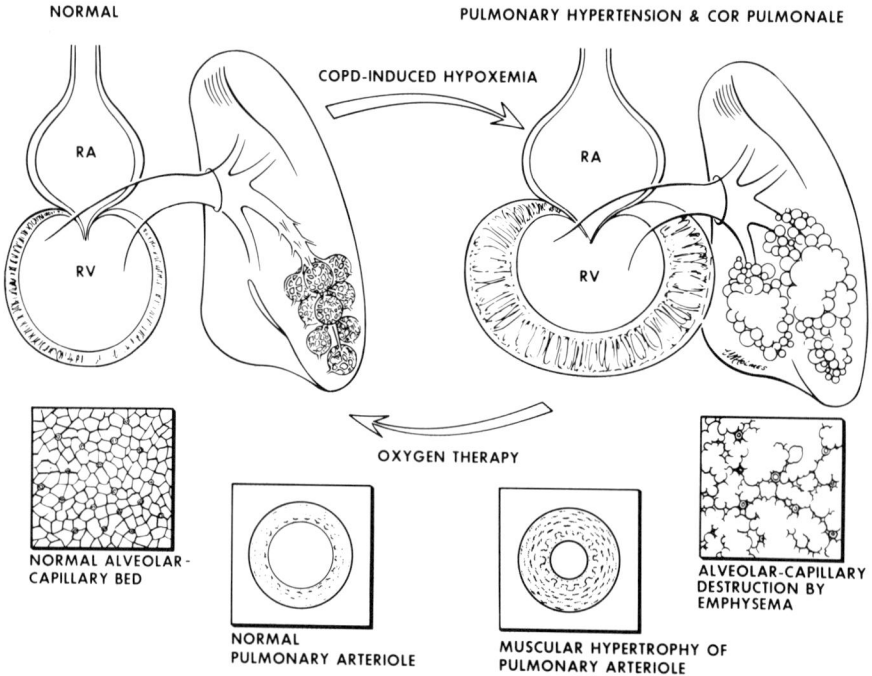

Figure 1–3. Effect of COPD, hypoxemia, and O_2 therapy on PVR and the right heart.

been implicated are the prostaglandins. The actual trigger is probably a low alveolar Po_2. The walls of small vessels are in close proximity to the alveolar gas at the precapillary or muscular-arteriolar level. The level of alveolar Po_2 that leads to vasoconstriction is within the range of 30 to 150 torr, with the most potent vasoconstriction occurring between 30 and 60 torr. When the Pao_2 is less than 30, vasodilation may result. Hydrogen ions also act as a vasoconstrictor, and they enhance the hypoxic event. In patients with severe COPD, hypercarbia magnifies the effect of hypoxemia. This vasospasm serves the purpose of matching local perfusion to local ventilation and, like many local organ-protecting features within the human body, may lead to significant secondary deleterious effects.

The third mechanism of increased resistance is smooth-muscle hypertrophy resulting from chronic hypoxemia. A chronic hypoxemic stimulus is more prominent in bronchitic than in emphysematous patients. It has been best studied in idiopathic pulmonary fibrosis and congenital heart disease, but it has been reported to occur in COPD. Anatomically, the muscular layer has been shown to extend out into the smaller arterioles. There also is proliferation of longitudinal smooth muscle internal to the internal elastic lamina. In addition, pericytes and intermediate cells transform into smooth-muscle cells at the level of the smaller arterioles. The medial hypertrophy of the muscular pulmonary arteries is not seen as it is with other disorders related to chronic hypoxemia, such as primary pulmonary hypertension. There may be a reduction in the number of small arterioles as a result of obliteration from endothelial cells swelling along with the medial hypertrophy.

Although an at-rest PAP may be found to be normal in early disease, during exercise the increased flows of a higher cardiac output and increased alveolar pressures can lead to pulmonary artery hypertension.

Many of the earlier studies on low-flow oxygen showed significant improvements both in PAP and pulmonary artery resistance. There has been some evidence that reduction of pulmonary hypertension can occur with just 15 hours of supplemental oxygen per day. The NOT–COT study did not find a statistically significant reduction in the PAP, but there was an 11% reduction in the pulmonary vascular resistance (PVR), which was statistically significant after 6 months. In addition, the decrease in mortality in patients using near-continuous oxygen was not associated with pulmonary hemodynamics. The reduction in PAP that has been reported in prior studies takes a matter of months to occur. Others have shown that even though PVR and PAP may not change, the progression of pulmonary hypertension is slowed with chronic low-flow oxygen. It appears that COPD patients vary as to their pulmonary artery hypertension response to oxygen.

THE RIGHT HEART

One of the leading causes of death in COPD is cor pulmonale. Cor pulmonale is defined as hypertrophy of the right ventricle resulting from primary lung disease. In the case of COPD, right ventricular hypertrophy and failure are secondary to the increasing pulmonary artery resistance and PAP (*see* Table 1–1). The clinical criteria for the diagnosis of cor pulmonale include dependent edema, jugular venous distension, a right ventricular gallop heard loudest at the subxiphoid area and increased during inspiration, a new tricuspid murmur of regurgitation, and the pulmonic valve sound of the second heart sound becoming louder than the aortic valve closing sound. Electrocardiographic criteria (*see* Fig 1–4) include an S_1–Q_3 pattern, an axis of greater than 110 degrees and S_1–S_2–S_3 pattern, and an R:S ratio in lead V_6 of less than 1.0. P pulmonale is defined as the presence of a P wave greater than 3 mm in leads II, III, or aV_F. The ECG sensitivity for cor pulmonale is low; it is specific when present. Radiographic criteria of pulmonary artery hypertension can be obtained with good posteroanterior (PA) and lateral radiographs. On the

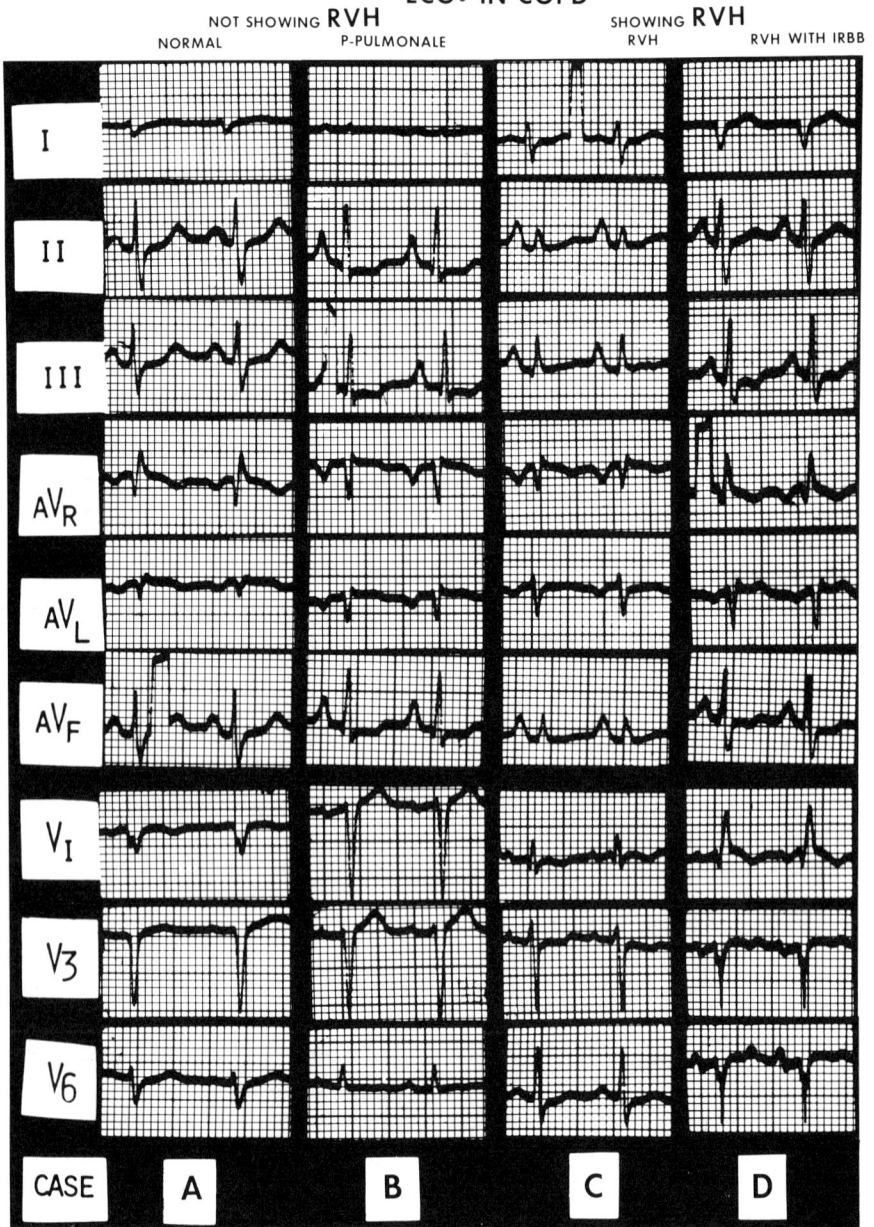

Figure 1–4. ECG in COPD: **(A)** Normal ECG in a COPD patient. **(B)** Right atrial enlargement is manifested as P pulmonale with tall, peaked P waves >3 mm in height in leads II, III, aV_F. **(C)** Early right ventricular hypertrophy is demonstrated as mild right-axis deviation, tall R relative to small S in V_1, low frontal QRS voltage, and P pulmonale. **(D)** Severe right ventricular hypertrophy is manifested as marked right-axis deviation; large S in I, II, and III; large R waves in V_1, deep S waves in V_3 through V_6, and incomplete right bundle branch block (RSR^1) in V_1.

PA view, if the right pulmonary artery is greater than 16 mm in diameter, or on the lateral view, if the left pulmonary artery is greater than 18 mm, pulmonary artery hypertension is said to be present. Radionuclide studies include a right ventricular ejection fraction that is insensitive to the presence of right ventricular dysfunction; however, sensitivity may be improved when a right atrial emptying rate is added to the right heart ejection fraction.

Cardiac arrhythmias have been shown to be due to chronic hypoxemia, especially sleep hypoxemia, when a low basal oxygen saturation has been shown to correlate with ECG recordings of premature atrial and premature ventricular contractions. There also is a relationship between sleep hypoxemia and an increased resting heart rate, right bundle branch block, prolonged QT interval, and ST-T wave depression in some patients. Multifocal atrial tachycardia is often a manifestation of acute hypoxemia. Oxygen is the therapy of choice when these abnormalities are present.

CENTRAL NERVOUS SYSTEM FUNCTION

It is clear that patients with severe COPD have a high incidence of measurable deficits in central nervous system (CNS) function. The higher cognitive functions, such as abstraction and complex perceptual motor integration, are impaired at least to a moderate degree in up to 40% of patients. Motor speed, strength, and coordination decrements are seen in nearly half. Overall, the incidence of CNS impairment is 77%. It is frequently noted by patients or their families that with progression to severe disease, there are behavioral disturbances, memory deficits, fitful sleeping, and headaches upon awakening in the morning (*see* Table 1–1).

Research done in the study of altitude sickness has shown that mild acute hypoxemia can lead to impaired ability to concentrate, make complex tasks difficult to learn, and reduce short-term memory. When hypoxemia is more severe, cognitive functions are impaired, euphoria may be present, lethargy has been described, and muscular incoordination also occurs.

It is no wonder that the brain may actually be one of the most sensitive organs to hypoxemia, as it is one of the most metabolically active organs. The oxygen needs of brain tissue are nearly constant. In the awake human being, the brain requires 3.5 ml of oxygen per 100 g of brain every minute. The weight of the brain in an average 70-kg man is approximately 1400 g. It takes 50 ml of oxygen every minute to maintain its function. With a total oxygen consumption of approximately 250 ml per minute for the total body, that means 20% of minute-to-minute oxygen needs are for brain metabolism.

The NOT–COT results are the best documented for large numbers of patients requiring low-flow continuous oxygen. The studies showed a modest measurable improvement in approximately half the patients when they were given neuropsychologic testing both before and after chronic low-flow oxygen. The actual testing both times was done on room air. The improvements were selective—not across the board. Particularly good improvement was seen in cognitive functions. It was clear that continuous oxygen was better than nocturnal oxygen. Much of the neurologic testing showed that 12 months was required in order to see a benefit. It was also noted that benefits were not related to the drop in hematocrit that can be seen with improvement of hypoxemia. There was no change in quality of life or emotional state.

The reasons for improved cognitive functions with low-flow oxygen are conjectural at this time. In general, cellular metabolism revolves around adenosine 5'-triphosphate (ATP), but animal studies have shown no change in the concentration of ATP with mild to moderate hypoxemia. However, neurotransmitter turnover can be altered by even mild degrees of hypoxemia. Many of the neurotransmitters depend on oxygen for synthesis. These include catecholamines and serotonin as well as the amino-acid neurotransmitters: glycine, serine, alanine, glutamate, and aspartate. The most likely explanation at this time is that acetylcholine, whose synthesis is also oxygen-dependent, may be the key player in the neuropsychiatric changes. The cholinergic system is important for the reticular activating system. A reduction in acetylcholine synthesis may theoretically lead to those changes seen in chronically hypoxic COPD patients.

BONE MARROW

It is well recognized that arterial hypoxemia is a stimulus for bone marrow production of red cells. Patients with severe COPD may have hypoxemia, but the carboxyhemoglobin from cigarette smoke can also lead to a similar sequence. Tissue hypoxemia seems to be the primary stimulus, with erythropoietin secretion from the kidney being the inciting event. Erythropoietin increases the incorporation of iron into hemoglobin and increases the rate of maturation of red blood cells, leading to the increased red blood cell mass. Unlike the situation in altitude-induced hypoxemia, there is no predictable response between the degree of hypoxemia and the increase in red blood cells, nor is there a predictable relation to severity of air-flow obstruction. It is thought that this is due to a relative decrease in the responsiveness of the bone marrow rather than a deficiency in erythropoietin release. When the hematocrit is about 50%, the organism loses any advantages of increased oxygen-carrying capacity because of the increased blood viscosity (see Table 1–1).

There is a significant improvement after the use of low-flow continuous oxygen in patients who are hypoxemic, with the hematocrit falling in most, if not all, patients. It takes approximately 4 to 6 weeks for this to occur; however, it will not help if the patient continues to smoke. It was also shown by the NOT–COT study that continuous oxygen was better than nocturnal oxygen. In the former group, there was a fall in the hematocrit by 9.2% at 18 months.

THE KIDNEYS

The effect of hypoxemia on the kidneys includes a reduction in blood flow and glomerular filtration rate and an increase in sodium retention (*see* Table 1–1). These lead to an increased blood volume and fluid retention, which can exacerbate the cardiovascular derangements seen with cor pulmonale.

CRITERIA FOR LOW-FLOW CONTINUOUS HOME OXYGEN

One requires adequate evidence of hypoxemia. This can be in the form of an arterial blood gas or ear oximeter determination. The "absolute criteria" are a PaO_2 of less than or equal to 55 torr or saturation of less than or equal to 85% (*see* Table 1–2). Failing the absolute criteria, there is one other set of criteria that may make the patient eligible for low-flow continuous home oxygen. These include a PaO_2 of between 56 and 59 torr or a saturation of 86% to 89%, plus evidence for end-organ damage as documented by one of the following:

1. Dependent edema.
2. P pulmonale on ECG defined as a P wave greater than 3 mm in leads II, III, or aV_F.
3. A hematocrit of greater than 56%.
4. Evidence of pulmonary hypertension.
5. Impairment of cognitive processes.
6. Nocturnal restlessness.
7. Morning headache.

Nocturnal oxygen may be indicated in those patients with normal resting daytime PaO_2 or SaO_2 if during sleep the PaO_2 drops below 55 torr or the saturation drops below 85%. This can be determined with an ear or pulse oximeter, and one needs to have the associated signs of end-organ damage to fulfill this set of criteria. Oxygen used during exercise may be of benefit for increasing a patient's exercise tolerance. This should be thoroughly evaluated with an exercise test plus blood gas determinations or oximetry, in which the patient and physician are ignorant as to whether oxygen or compressed air is being delivered. Significant im-

TABLE 1–2. MEDICARE REIMBURSEMENT GUIDELINES FOR HOME OXYGEN THERAPY

Chronic lung disease, such as COPD, interstitial fibrosis, bronchiectasis, cystic fibrosis, or cancer

    Severe

    Stable

    Optimally treated

Hypoxemia at rest, with exercise, or during sleep

$PaO_2 \leq 55$ mmHg (or O_2 saturation $\leq 85\%$ by ear oximetry)

OR

PaO_2 56–59 mmHg (or O_2 saturation 86–89%)

AND

edema, hematocrit > 56%, P wave > 3 mm in II, III, or aV_F

---

provement in duration of exercise or maximum work attained while using oxygen is a prerequisite. The patients who need this test have been well characterized. They are individuals with COPD in whom all of the above basic criteria for continuous low-flow home oxygen are absent and on pulmonary function testing show a diffusing capacity of less than 55% of predicted. It has been shown that when the diffusing capacity of the lung for carbon monoxide (DLCO) is greater than 55% of predicted, exercise desaturation rarely occurs.

NECESSITY FOR MEASUREMENT OF ARTERIAL BLOOD GAS OR OXIMETRY

The symptoms of hypoxemia include breathlessness, palpitations, mental confusion, agitation, dependent edema, and morning headaches. These are all very nonspecific. Signs of hypoxemia include hypertension, hypotension, lower extremity pitting edema, tachycardia, bradycardia, and the heart tones noted earlier indicating the presence of pulmonary artery hypertension. Cyanosis is included, but this requires that 5 g/dl of hemoglobin be desaturated. All of these symptoms and physical signs are nonspecific and are insensitive to the presence of hypoxemia. Even cyanosis can be misleading insofar as it is insensitive in patients with anemia, and interobserver error has been described, suggesting a lack of specificity.

THE OXYGEN PRESCRIPTION

It is imperative that the prescription written for home oxygen be detailed because of the expense involved in setting up and maintaining low-flow systems. It should include the flow rate and concentration, the frequency of use, the duration of need, the specific diagnosis, indications of end-organ damage, and the specific laboratory evidence of hypoxemia. It is important to note here that of the patients initially registered for the

NOT–COT study, after 3 weeks of intense therapeutic endeavors that included bronchodilators and chest physiotherapy, 20% no longer required low-flow continuous oxygen because of an improvement in their PaO$_2$ and in physical signs of end-organ damage. Along with writing out the prescription, it is a key task for the respiratory therapist, nurse, or physician involved with the patient's education to stress that oxygen prescribed in this fashion is intended to improve that patient's survival. Many patients are still under the misconception that oxygen is to be used only during periods of shortness of breath, and it may take many repetitions by numerous individuals to make the patient understand that just like undetected hypertension, chronic hypoxemia can be a silent killer.

COMPLICATIONS

A potential problem from the use of oxygen can be seen in the patient with coexisting hypercarbia who requires a hypoxic drive for respiratory drive. The quantity of oxygen and the flow rate of oxygen must therefore be carefully determined by measurement of arterial blood gases with serial changes in the flow rate, the goal being a PaO$_2$ between 58 and 62 torr and a saturation between 88% and 92%.

Although oxygen may be a fire hazard, this is exceedingly rare.

Of some concern is the psychologic dependency that a patient may acquire for oxygen, although more often the patient is adverse to using low-flow continuous oxygen, feeling that he or she has become a respiratory cripple.

Another real complication is that of cost. The cost includes that of the patient evaluation as well as the cost of the oxygen itself.

Finally, there is a theoretical concern over lung toxicity. Oxygen toxicity has been described in patients who have been given high concentrations over long periods of time, usually because of other very severe diseases of the lungs. Postmortem studies of patients who died during the NOT–COT study showed varying degrees of pulmonary fibrosis and hyperplasia near areas of scarring. These were felt to be minimal and very unlikely to have clinical or physiologic significance.

SUMMARY

Long-term low-flow oxygen has been shown to improve the survival of patients with severe COPD when certain criteria have been met. Significant improvements in physiologic function of the brain, heart, pulmonary vasculature, and bone marrow have been shown, but none have been clearly shown to be the explanation for the improved survival. The British Medical Research Council study and the NOT–COT study have shown that some oxygen is good, and more is better in terms of length of time used per day. The effects of low-flow oxygen are both acute, as in reversal of hypoxic vasoconstriction, and chronic, as in the measurable changes by neuropsychiatric testing that may not be seen for as long as 12 months.

REFERENCES

Abraham AS, Cole RB, Bishop JM: Reversal of pulmonary hypertension of prolonged oxygen administration to patients with chronic bronchitis. *Circ Res* 1968;*23*:147.

Boysen PG: Nocturnal oxygen therapy and hemodynamic changes in COPD. *Chest* 1984;*85*:2.

Fleetham J, West P, Mezon B, et al: Sleep, arousals, and oxygen desaturation in chronic obstructive pulmonary disease: The effect of oxygen therapy. *Am Rev Respir Dis* 1982;*126*:429.

Fletcher EC, Levin DC: Cardiopulmonary hemodynamics during sleep in subjects with chronic obstructive pulmonary disease: The effect of short- and long-term oxygen. *Chest* 1984;*85*:6.

Gibson GE, Pulsinelli W, Blass JP, et al: Brain dysfunction in mild to moderate hypoxia. *Am J Med* 1981;*70*:1247.

Heaton RK, Grant I, McSweeny AJ, et al: Psychologic effects of continuous and nocturnal oxygen therapy in hypoxemic chronic obstructive pulmonary disease. *Arch Intern Med* 1983;*143*:1941.

Jacques J, Cooney JP, Silvers GW, et al: The lungs and causes of death in the nocturnal oxygen therapy trial. *Chest* 1984;*86*:230.

Meyrick B, Reid L: Pulmonary hypertension. *Clin Chest Med* 1983;*4*:199.

Murphy ML, Hutcheson F: The electrocardiographic diagnosis of right ventricular hypertrophy in chronic obstructive pulmonary disease. *Chest* 1974;*65*:622.

Nocturnal Oxygen Therapy Trial Group: Continuous or nocturnal oxygen therapy in hypoxemic chronic obstructive lung disease. *Ann Intern Med* 1980;*93*:391.

Owens GR, Rogers RM, Pennock BE, et al: The diffusing capacity as a predictor of arterial oxygen desaturation during exercise in patients with chronic obstructive pulmonary disease. *N Engl J Med* 1984;*310*:1218.

Petty TL: *Prescribing Home Oxygen for COPD*. New York, Thiene-Stratton, 1982.

Report of the Medical Research Council Working Party: Long-term domiciliary oxygen therapy in chronic cor pulmonale complicating chronic bronchitis and emphysema. *Lancet* 1981;*1*:681.

Timms RM, Khaja FU, Williams GW, et al: Hemodynamic response to oxygen therapy in chronic obstructive pulmonary disease. *Ann Intern Med* 1985;*102*:29.

Tirlapur VG, Mir MA: Nocturnal hypoxemia and associated electrocardiographic changes in patients with chronic obstructive airways disease. *N Engl J Med* 1982;*306*:125.

Weitzenblum E, Sautegau A, Ehrhart M, et al: Long-term oxygen therapy can reverse the progression of pulmonary hypertension in patients with chronic obstructive pulmonary disease. *Am Rev Respir Dis* 1985;*131*:493.

2

Home Oxygen Therapy Equipment

G. SLEEPER, RRT

There are three systems commonly used to deliver home medical oxygen: high-pressure cylinders, liquid oxygen systems, and oxygen concentrators. This chapter will closely examine the workings of these systems, beginning with oxygen cylinders.

HIGH-PRESSURE CYLINDERS

Medical oxygen is available in a number of different-sized compressed gas cylinders. The Department of Transportion (DOT), a federal regulatory agency, defines the term *compressed gas* as ". . . any material or mixture having in the container an absolute pressure exceeding 40 psi at 70°F or, regardless of the pressure at 70°F, having an absolute pressure exceeding 104 psi at 130°F . . . (Compressed Gas Association [CGA], 1981, p 5)." Medical oxygen is commonly available in cylinders filled to about 2200 psi.

Because such high pressures can present safety hazards if not handled correctly, a myriad of regulations and standards have evolved as the use of these cylinders has increased.

Regulatory Agencies

DOT. The first medical oxygen cylinder was manufactured in 1888 by Liquid Carbonics, now a division of General Dynamics. By the turn of the century, the federal government charged the Interstate Commerce Commission (ICC) to regulate cylinder specifications for safe transportation in conjunction with the Bureau of Explosives, which is not a federal agency but an agency of the Association of American Railroads. In 1967, this responsibility was transferred to the DOT, which continues to work with the Bureau of Explosives. Currently, the DOT is the most influential federal agency regulating the manufacture, marking, testing, and transportation of cylinders. The various subdivisions of DOT regulate different means of cylinder transport as follows:

1. The Federal Highway Administration (FHA) regulates transportation by highway.
2. The United States Coast Guard (USCG) regulates transportation by water.
3. The Federal Railroad Association (FRA) regulates transportation by railroad.
4. The Federal Aviation Agency (FAA) regulates transportation by air.

FDA and OSHA. The federal Food and Drug Administration (FDA) regulates the labeling and purity of medical oxygen by enforcing the federal Food, Drug, and Cosmetic act. This act mandates the standards for medical gases as established by the United States Pharmacopeia (USP) or the National Formulary (NF). The labeling requirements include identifying the manufacturer, packer, or distributor, and the content, which is usually the content volume at 70°F. The purity of medical oxygen must meet or exceed 99%. The FDA also regulates the repackaging of drugs, which means that home care companies that transfill cylinders must comply with these regulations by registering with the FDA as a repacker and complying with certain sections of the good manufacturing practice (GMP) regulations for drug products. The FDA has published the *Compressed Medical Gases Guideline* for manufacturers and dealers to describe acceptable transfilling practices and procedures.

The Occupational Safety and Health Administration (OSHA) was developed by the federal government to regulate matters concerning occupational health and safety. Many standards and regulations from various industry groups have been incorporated by OSHA. Compliance officers inspect all aspects of industry to ensure employee safety.

TABLE 2-1. COMMONLY USED OXYGEN CYLINDERS*

Cylinder Style	Dimensions O.D. × Length (inches)	Nominal Volume (L)	Oxygen Capacity (L)
B	3 × 15	1.5	200
D	4 × 17	3.0	400
E	4.2 × 29	4.9	680
M	7 × 45	22.0	3450
H	9 × 55	45.0	6700

*All specifications are averages derived from various manufacturers.

Components of an Oxygen Cylinder System

A high-pressure oxygen cylinder consists of a seamless cylinder of alloy steel, carbon steel, or aluminum; a pressure-relief device; and a cylinder valve. The cylinders have internal volumes, known as nominal or water volumes, ranging from about 1 to 45 L. The more common sizes are identified with the letters B (or M9), D, E, M, G, and H (or K). Table 2–1 lists these oxygen cylinders and their capacities.

Common Oxygen Cylinder Types. Cylinders are identified by DOT symbols that indicate the material used in manufacture. The most common types of cylinders used for medical oxygen are

- DOT–3A: These are seamless carbon-steel cylinders and are not heat-treated.
- DOT–3AA: These are seamless alloy-steel cylinders that are heat-treated for greater hardness, allowing a lighter weight than a comparable 3A cylinder.
- DOT–AL: These are seamless aluminum cylinders. This is the most recently established type, first being published in the Federal Register in 1981.

Pressure-Relief Devices. Medical oxygen cylinders are fitted with a mechanism that allows the gas to escape if the pressure increases as a result of adverse conditions, such as extreme heat. The Compressed Gas Association (CGA), a nonprofit service organization, has developed standards for these mechanisms and defines the term *pressure-relief device* as "a device designed to prevent rupture of a normally charged cylinder when it is placed in a fire as required by . . . DOT regulations . . . (CGA, 1981, p 67)." The CGA also states that the terms "pressure-relief device" and "safety-relief device" are synonymous. There are basically two types of pressure-relief devices used in high-pressure medical cylinders:

1. Type CG–1: rupture disk, which is nonreclosing and works by bursting a pressure-containing disk. This is the most common type (*see* Fig 2–1).
2. Type CG–4: combination rupture disk and fusible plug, which is also nonreclosing and works with both the disk and a fusible plug, which will melt at a particular temperature. These devices are usually part of the cylinder valve assembly.

Cylinder Valves. High-pressure medical oxygen cylinders use a direct-acting valve, as seen in Figure 2–2. This is a type of needle valve, a one-piece mechanism in which the rotation of the handwheel directly seats or unseats the threaded valve. The inlet of the cylinder valve assembly is threaded into the cylinder neck. These inlet threads have been standard-

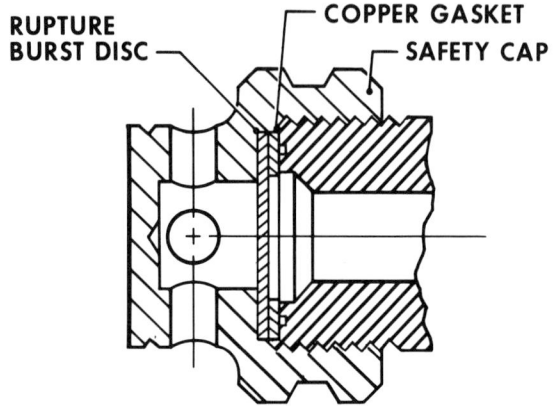

Figure 2–1. Rupture disc safety relief device.

ized by the CGA; the most common of these valve-to-cylinder connections is the national gas taper thread (National Pipe Thread [NPT]).

The outlet of the cylinder valve assembly is threaded and is the means of attaching the regulator, which reduces the cylinder pressure to working pressure. These threads are also standardized by the CGA so that regulators for different gases may not be interchanged. The American National Standards Institute (ANSI) has adopted these standards. For oxygen cylinders of size E and below, the Pin-Index Safety System (PISS) was developed; this uses a yoke-type connection and a mating pin-and-hole

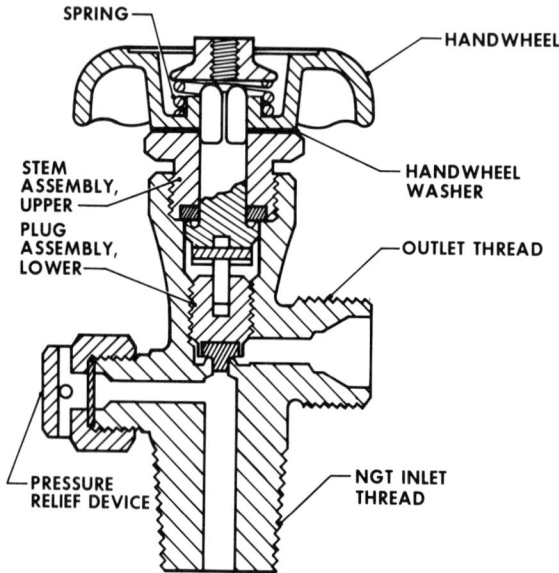

Figure 2–2. Cylinder valve.

STEM NUT

CGA OUTLET

PIN INDEX

NGT
INLET THREAD

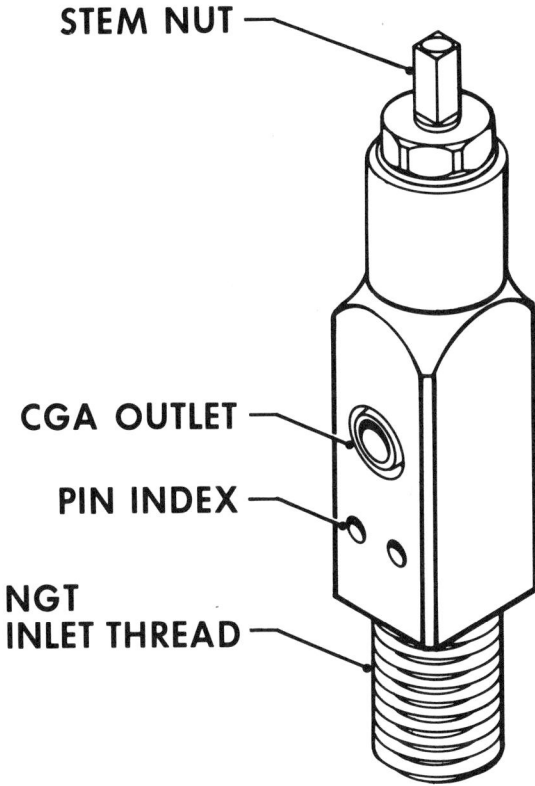

Figure 2–3. Cylinder valve with pin index holes.

arrangement (Fig 2–3). Oxygen cylinders sized M and above use the American-Canadian standard valve outlet connection number 540, which is a nipple-and-nut arrangement.

Required Cylinder Markings.   There are two categories of markings that are required to appear on oxygen cylinders by the DOT. The first relates to the construction of the cylinder itself, whereas the second relates to the oxygen contents.

Specification Markings.   The DOT requires a number of specifications to be indicated on the cylinder. They are generally found stamped on the neck of the cylinder (Fig 2–4). The required specifications are as follows:

1. The type of cylinder manufactured.
2. The service pressure in psig.
3. The word SPUN or PLUG when the end was sealed by either of these methods.
4. A serial number.
5. The manufacturer's registered name or identifying symbol.

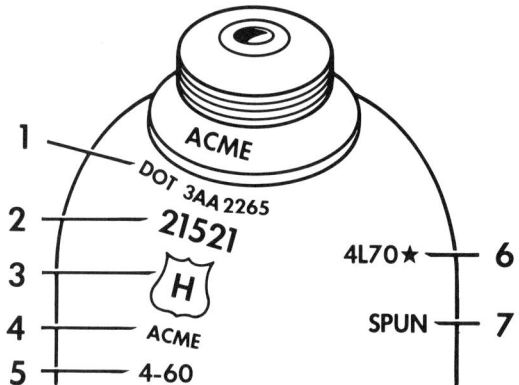

Figure 2–4. E-cylinder markings. (1) DOT 3AA—Type of Cylinder 2265—Service pressure; (2) 21521—Serial number; (3) H—Manufacturer's inspection mark; (4) ACME—Owner's registered identifying symbol; (5) 4–60—Date of manufacture and original hydrostatic test; (6) 4L70*—First retest; (7) SPUN—Method of manufacture.

6. The month and year of the final inspection after manufacture, followed by retest dates. If required, the inspector's initial or symbol may appear between the month and year; for example: 4-DS-83. A plus sign (+) after the test date indicates that the cylinder may be filled up to 10% higher than the service pressure, a common practice for cylinders size M and larger. A star (*) after the test date on DOT–3A and DOT–3AA cylinders indicates that retesting is to be performed every 10 years. If there is no star indicated, or the cylinder is DOT–3AL, the retest date is every 5 years. Aluminum cylinders designated 3E do not require retesting.

Content Markings. This category may be subdivided into two subcategories: marking the cylinder to identify the gaseous contents and labeling the cylinder to identify the principal hazards of the gaseous contents.

The first subcategory is detailed in the American industrial safety standard entitled "American National Standard Method of Marking Portable Compressed Gas Containers to Identify the Material Contained," which has been adopted by the CGA. It states that "compressed gas containers shall be legibly marked with at least the chemical name or a commonly accepted name of the material contained . . . (CGA, 1981, p 113)" and then specifies the details of this marking. In addition to the marking of the gas contents, the CGA has devised a color code to aid in the identification of medical gas cylinders. CGA pamphlet C–9 establishes a color for the cylinder of each medical gas in current use. Oxygen cylinders are to be green for use in the United States, white for Canada.

The second subcategory is detailed in a statement by the CGA that presents guidelines for labeling cylinders to warn of the principle hazards of each compressed gas. Proper labeling should include a "signal word" such as DANGER!, WARNING!, and CAUTION!, to identify both the presence and degree of the hazard; a "statement of hazard" identifying hazards that may be anticipated with normal use; and "precautionary measures and instructions in case of contact or exposure," if necessary.

Under this system, the name of the content is OXYGEN, the signal word is WARNING, the statement of hazard is VIGOROUSLY ACCELERATES COMBUSTION, and the precautionary measures are KEEP OIL AND GREASE AWAY. USE ONLY WITH EQUIPMENT CONDITIONED FOR OXYGEN SERVICE.

In 1976, the CGA combined the cylinder marking for content and the labeling of the hazard class in an appendix so as to be consistent with labeling requirements of the DOT Hazardous Materials Regulations published in the Federal Register in the same year. This system is called the CGA Basic Marking System, which includes the "basic marking" and additional information relating to cylinder and contents. The "basic marking" (Fig 2–5) consists of a panel on the left containing the name of the content and a diamond to the right containing the hazard class. For medical oxygen, the content is labeled OXYGEN USP and the hazard class is labeled OXIDIZER or OXYGEN. Additional material may appear above, below, or beside the "basic marking."

Inspection and Testing

The DOT requires periodic hydrostatic testing and retesting of most medical oxygen cylinders. The most common method of hydrostatic testing is the water-jacket volumetric method. This test, as well as others, is approved by the Bureau of Explosives. Detailed information on hydrostatic testing methods may be found in CGA pamphlet C–1.

The DOT also requires that interior and exterior inspections be performed when the cylinder is retested. The guidelines for visual inspection may be found in CGA pamphlet C–6, "Standards for Visual Inspection of Compressed Gas Cylinders."

Safe Handling, Storage, and Use

Medical oxygen cylinders that are manufactured in accordance with DOT specifications and maintained in accordance with DOT Hazardous Materials Regulations are safe when handled correctly. In addition to the

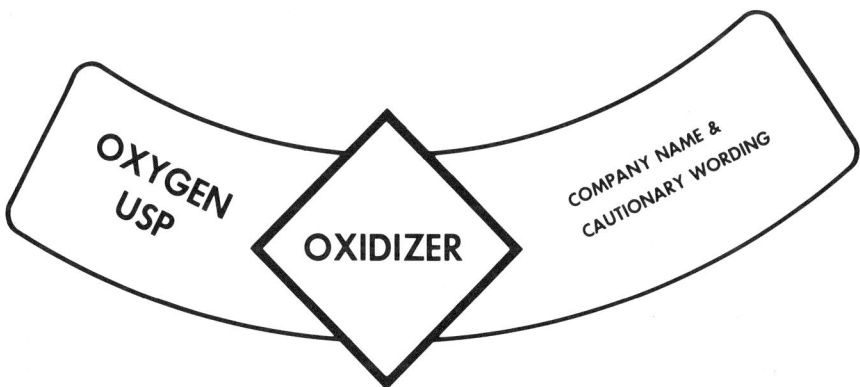

Figure 2–5. Basic markings.

DOT and CGA regulations and recommendations, the National Fire Protection Agency (NFPA), a nongovernmental organization, has issued recommendations for safe handling, storage, transportation, and use of medical oxygen cylinders in the home. The following section lists recommendations for home use of oxygen combined from the NFPA and the CGA.

Handling

1. Patients and members of the patient's family should familiarize themselves with the proper handling of cylinders and containers and proper use of carts, if employed (NFPA, F–6–4.1).*
2. Never permit oil, grease, or other readily combustible substances to come in contact with cylinders, valves, regulators, gauges, hoses, and fittings. Oil and certain gases such as oxygen or nitrous oxide may combine with explosive violence (CGA, 4.1.1).
3. Never lubricate valves, regulators, gauges, or fittings with oil or any other combustible substance (CGA, 4.1.2).
4. Cylinders or containers should not be handled with hands, gloves, or other clothing that contain grease or oil (NFPA, F–6–4.8).*
5. Very cold cylinders and containers should be handled with care to avoid frostbite on the bare skin (NFPA, F–6–4.7).

Storage

1. When tank valve protection caps are supplied, they should be secured tightly in place at all times except when the tank is in use (CGA, 6.4.2).
2. Freestanding cylinders should be properly chained or supported in an appropriate cylinder cart or base (NFPA, F–6–4.6).*
3. Cylinders and containers should not be supported by or in the proximity of radiators, steam pipes, or heat ducts. *Note:* Cylinder container pressure will rise if heated. Pressure-relief devices are sensitive to pressure. If the relief device breaks, the contents will be discharged into the room, and a severe fire hazard will be created (NFPA, F–6–4.6.2).*

Transportation

1. Never drop cylinders or permit them to strike each other violently (CGA, 4.2.2).
2. Avoid dragging or sliding cylinders. It is safer to move large cylinders even short distances by using a suitable truck, making sure

that the cylinder-retaining chain or strap is fastened in place (CGA, 4.2.3).

Use

1. Do not remove valve protection cap until ready to withdraw contents or to connect to a manifold (CGA, 4.2.2).
2. After removing the valve protection cap, slightly open the valve for an instant to clear the opening of possible dust and dirt. This should not be done with a cylinder containing flammable gas (CGA, 4.4.4).
3. When opening the valve, point the outlet away from you. Never use wrenches or tools except those provided or approved by the gas supplier. Never hammer the valve wheel in attempting to open or to close the valve (CGA, 4.4.5).
4. Regulators, pressure gauges, and manifolds provided for use with a particular gas or group of gases must not be used with cylinders containing other gases (CGA, 4.4.6).
5. Never permit gas to enter the regulating device suddenly. Always open the cylinder valve slowly (CGA, 4.4.9).

Transfilling. Transferring by supplier of gaseous oxygen to be used for respiratory therapy in the home is to be performed using equipment designed to comply with the performance requirements of CGA pamphlet P–2.5, *Transfilling of High-Pressure Gaseous Oxygen to Be Used for Respiration* and adhering to those procedures.

Note: Accidents involving the transfilling of cylinders have been reported. Because of the high risks involved and the lack of technical expertise that can be expected on the part of home users, the Committee believes strongly that transfilling cannot be condoned in the home (NFPA, F–6–8.1).*

LIQUID OXYGEN SYSTEMS

There are several liquid oxygen systems currently on the market today. Their popularity is primarily due to the portability these systems afford the oxygen-dependent patient. Liquid systems also provide economical and convenient sources of high-volume oxygen. These systems, while having important differences in design and mechanical configuration, are similar in principle.

---

*Reprinted with permission from NFPA 99-1984, Health Care Facilities, Copyright © 1984, National Fire Protection Association, Quincy, Mass 02269. This reprinted material is not the complete and official position of the NFPA on the referenced subject, which is represented only by the standard in its entirety.

Liquid Oxygen

Oxygen enters the liquid state at or below $-297.3°F$ at 1 atmosphere (14.7 psia), where it acquires a light-blue color. The usefulness of liquid oxygen comes from its characteristic compactness. Oxygen in the liquid state occupies 862 times less volume than does gaseous oxygen. This allows relatively small volumes of liquid oxygen to provide high flow rates of gaseous oxygen to a patient.

Storage. Liquid oxygen is stored in the home in a reservoir unit known generically as a Dewar. A Dewar is essentially a very efficient thermos bottle. It consists of a stainless steel inner vessel, which contains the liquid, and an outer vessel; the two are separated by a partial vacuum. The inner vessel is generally wrapped in a reflective material to reduce heat transfer by thermal radiation. The vacuum helps maintain the low temperatures by reducing convection, and the separation of the inner and outer vessels reduces heat transfer by conduction. To help maintain this relative vacuum, special materials, known as "getters," are added to help remove stray molecules. One such material is a form of zeolite, a molecular sieve that adsorbs stray nitrogen molecules in the same manner as an oxygen concentrator.

Saturation. After a liquid vessel has been filled, there is a separation of liquid and gaseous oxygen (Fig 2–6). This results in a balanced state, in

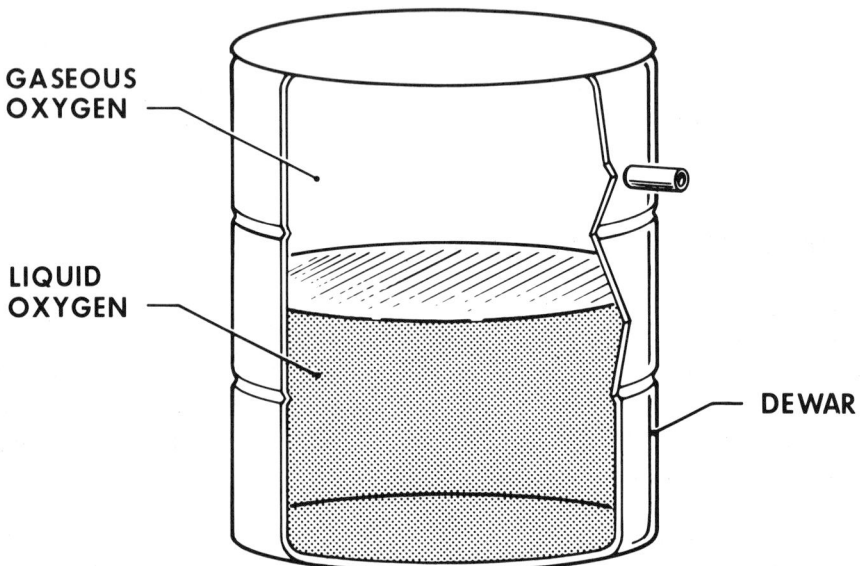

Figure 2–6. Saturated oxygen.

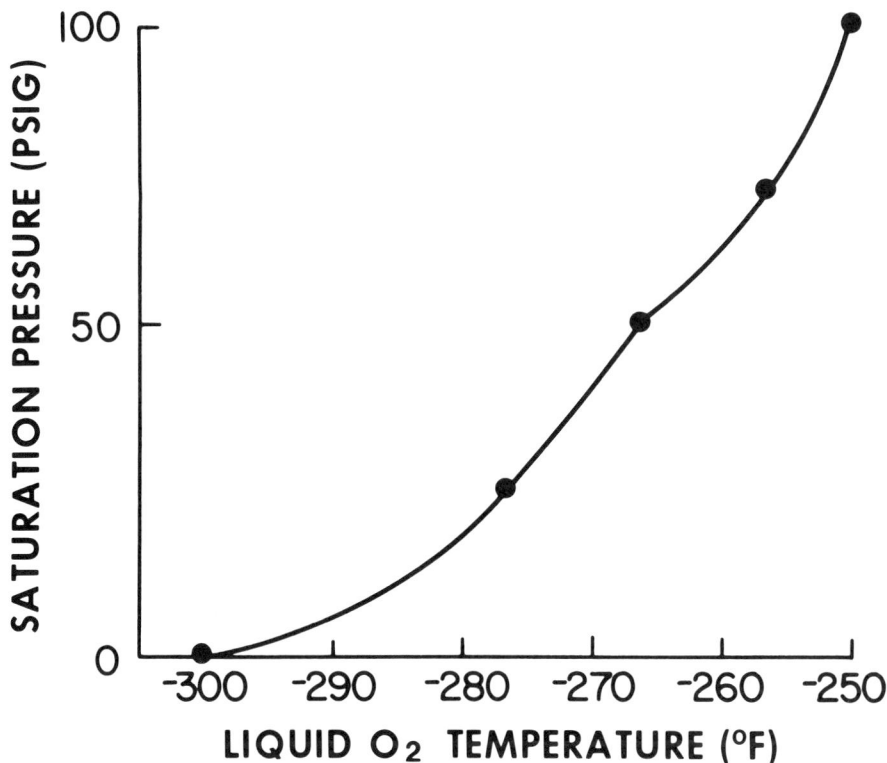

Figure 2–7. Liquid oxygen saturation pressure versus temperature.

which the liquid is not evaporating into a gas and the gas is not condensing into a liquid. This state, which depends on temperature and pressure, is termed the saturation point. If the temperature is increased or the pressure is decreased, the liquid oxygen will boil. If these conditions are reversed, the gaseous oxygen will condense. There is a range of saturation points (Fig 2–7). If the saturation temperature changes, the saturation pressure must change proportionally to maintain this balance.

A "Typical" Reservoir

The following section discusses a hypothetical generic reservoir unit that employs the components common to most commercially available units. Refer to Figure 2–8 for the following discussion.

Filling. Liquid oxygen transfer occurs in response to a pressure gradient established between the supply vessel and the reservoir unit. The supply vessel is typically pressurized between 50% and 100% higher than the reservoir pressure. All manufacturers offer units in the 20 to 22 psig range. The liquid is introduced to the reservoir unit by means of a supply line

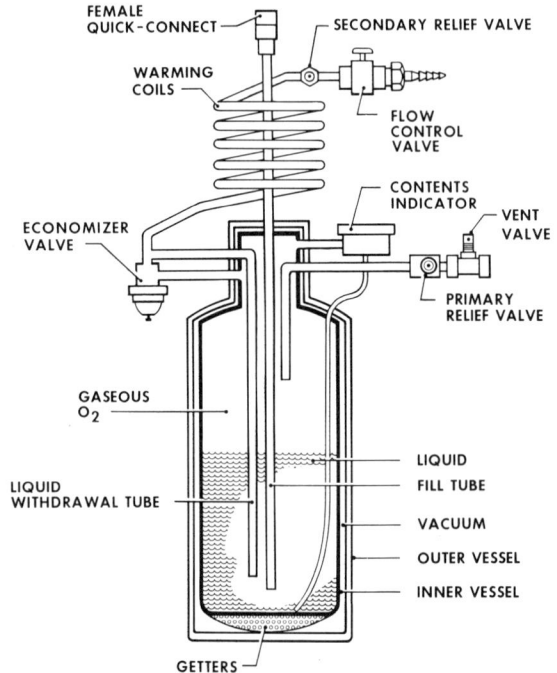

Figure 2-8. Liquid oxygen reservoir.

that mates with the female quick-connect adapter on the reservoir. The liquid flows through the quick-connect and fill tube into the inner vessel. This flow will only occur when the vent valve is opened. Initially, a good deal of the liquid entering the unit evaporates and escapes from the unit through the vent valve because the internal components are warm. As the filling procedes, these internal components cool, and more liquid remains in the unit. There will be additional oxygen loss at this point as a result of the liquid displacing the gaseous oxygen. When the inner vessel is full, liquid oxygen spurts out the vent valve. At this point, closing the vent valve will end the filling process.

Two factors that will adversely affect the fill process are oversaturation and undersaturation. Oversaturation refers to the condition resulting from filling a unit from a source vessel with a much higher saturation pressure. The supply liquid must desaturate by boiling, resulting in high losses of gas through the vent valve. Undersaturation refers to the condition resulting from filling with a low saturation pressure. The reservoir unit might require hours to build pressure up to the normal saturation pressure, making the unit unavailable for patient use during this time.

Normal Use. When the flowmeter is set at the prescribed flow rate, a pressure gradient is created between the flowmeter outlet (atmospheric pressure) and the gas-filled upper section of the inner vessel (head pressure).

This pressure differential causes the gas to flow from the inner vessel, through the economizer valve to the warming coils, where ambient temperatures warm the gas on the way out through the flowmeter to the patient.

As the gas flow continues, the head pressure begins to drop. When the pressure drops 0.5 psig or so, the economizer valve closes, causing liquid oxygen to flow up the withdrawal tube, through the warming coils, where it becomes a gas on the way to the flow-rate controller. This type of economizer system, as well as other variations of this system, maintains a constant flow of oxygen to the patient.

Nonusage. When a liquid reservoir is filled but not used, the ambient heat will cause the head pressure to increase until the primary relief valve opens, typically about 2 psig above the working pressure. This venting will continue until the unit empties. Should the primary relief valve fail, the secondary valve, which acts as a safety backup, will open at about 10 psig above the working pressure.

This is an obvious limitation to liquid oxygen systems; unlike other systems, liquid oxygen will eventually empty whether it has been used or not.

Condensation. Water from the atmosphere will tend to condense on the warming coils because of the intense cold. The water is collected and directed through a condensation tube into a collection container, which must periodically be emptied by the patient.

Contents Indicator. Each manufacturer has a contents indicator on the reservoir unit to measure the level of the liquid oxygen. Electrical capacitance and pressure differential are two methods used to indicate liquid levels. Some of these gauges require batteries to function.

The "Typical" Portable Unit

The liquid portable unit is a lightweight Dewar or cryogenic container. These units weigh in the range of 5 to 14 lb, are filled from the reservoir unit, and are designed to be carried or towed by the patient. The design and operation of the portable unit are virtually identical to the reservoir unit (Fig 2–9).

Filling. The portable unit is filled from the reservoir unit by mating with the female quick-connect on the reservoir unit. This is generally the same connector that is used to fill the reservoir from the supply vessel.

The connector may be mounted either on the top or side of the reservoir unit. The mating connector on the portable unit fills in one of two positions. With top-mounted connectors, the portable unit is inverted, filling top to top. Side-mounted connectors fill with the portable

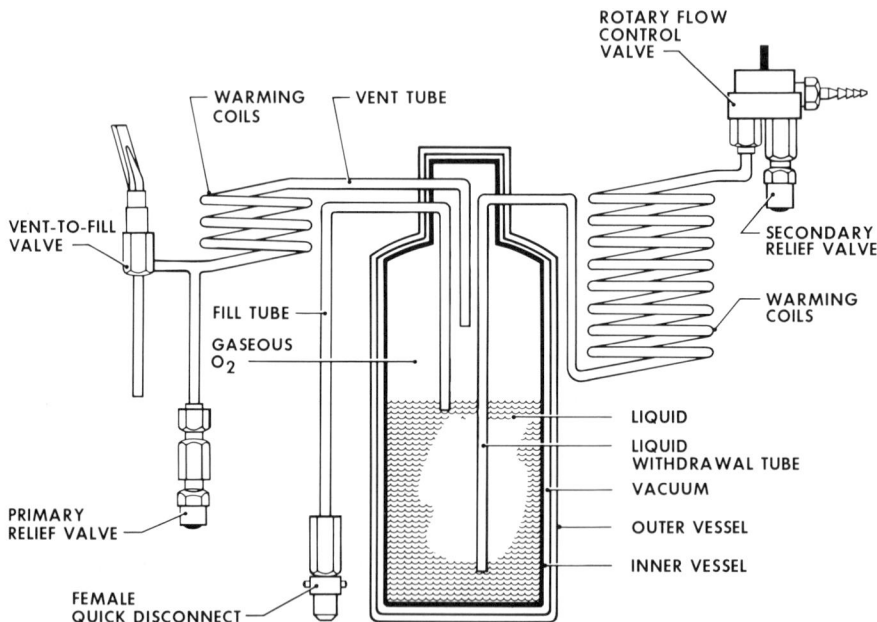

Figure 2-9. Liquid oxygen portable unit.

unit in an upright position. Oversaturation is seldom a problem, because the portable unit is normally filled from the reservoir unit. Undersaturation may occur, however, if the reservoir is itself undersaturated. This condition would cause the patient to receive lower flow rates.

The patient or family should be taught these basic steps to fill the portable unit:

1. Make sure there is enough liquid oxygen in the reservoir to fill the portable unit.
2. Check the connectors on both units to make sure that they are clean and dry. Moisture on these connectors could cause the connectors to freeze together.
3. Connect the portable unit to the reservoir according to the manufacturer's instructions. The flow-rate controller should be turned off.
4. Open the portable unit vent. Allow the portable unit to fill until the vent valve begins to pass liquid oxygen instead of gas. Close the vent valve.
5. Disengage the portable unit according to the manufacturer's instructions.

Safety Precautions

There are a number of safety considerations for both the home care company and the patient using liquid oxygen. The CGA has issued safety bulletins describing recommended practice for liquid oxygen transportation, transfilling, and use.

Transportation. The vehicles used by the home care companies to transport liquid oxygen to the patient homes must have the driving compartment separated from the cargo department by a bulkhead. The cargo department must be well ventilated to prevent the buildup of vented oxygen, and permanently mounted vessels must be vented to the outside. Signs must be prominently displayed prohibiting smoking and open flames. For more detailed requirements, consult the CGA safety bulletin CGA, SB–9.

Transfilling and Use. The safety hazards involved in transfilling liquid oxygen include the potential for severe thermal "burns," the chance of contaminating the oxygen during the fill, and the combustion-supporting properties of oxygen.

    If the manufacturer's directions are followed, there is very little chance that either the patient or the home care workers will come in contact with the liquid oxygen. In the unlikely event that someone is exposed to the liquid, appropriate first aid measures, including gradually warming the affected body part, should be employed.

    Home care companies must comply with the same regulations when transfilling liquid oxygen as when transfilling a gas. This means that the company must comply with the applicable regulations and standards set forth by the DOT, FDA, CGA, OSHA, and any state or local ordinances. These regulations are not applicable to patients filling portable systems at home; however, these patients should be carefully instructed in all aspects of the use of their system.

    Liquid oxygen presents the same oxidizing hazards as does gaseous oxygen. Hazardous conditions exist if the oxygen system becomes contaminated with grease, oils, or other hydrocarbons. For more detailed requirements and standards for transfilling liquid oxygen, refer to the CGA pamphlet CGA, P–2.6.

Manufacturers of Liquid Oxygen Systems

The John Bunn Company. The John Bunn Company manufactures a liquid oxygen system consisting of a 30-L capacity reservoir unit and a 1.2 L portable unit (Fig 2–10). The portable unit fills from the top of the reservoir. The John Bunn Company merged with Inspiron, another manufacturer of liquid oxygen systems, in April of 1986.

Bunn Reservoir. The Bunn reservoir unit has a self-contained back-pressure-compensated Thorpe-type flowmeter. Just upstream of the flowmeter is a 10-psi pressure regulator to ensure accurate flowmeter readings in the face of head-pressure fluctuations. The available flow rates range

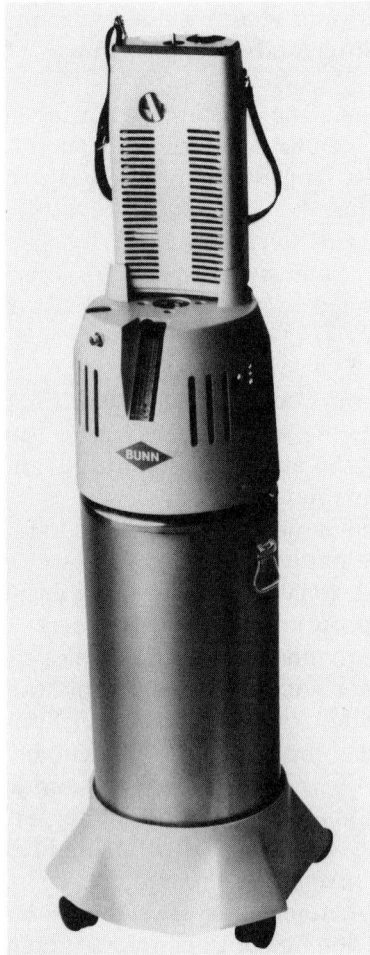

Figure 2–10. The John Bunn liquid system. *(Courtesy of the John Bunn Company.)*

from 0 to 6 lpm in one-half-lpm increments. A unique feature of the flowmeter system is a toggle switch that allows the patient to set the flowmeter at the prescribed flow rate and then turn the unit off and on without resetting the flowmeter. This feature, as well as the physical layout of the switch, is intended to aid the visually-impaired patient. Another unique feature is that the side-mounted quick-connector used to fill the unit is separate from the top-mounted quick-connector that mates with the portable. This allows the system to fill a portable unit immediately after the reservoir has been filled without the chance of the connectors freezing. The contents indicator is a mechanical gauge consisting of a float inside the manifold, which rides on the liquid's surface. The height of the float, and therefore of the liquid, is transmitted to a meter by torque linkage. The Bunn reservoir unit features a roller base to permit easy movement around the home (*see* Table 2–2 for specifications).

TABLE 2–2. SPECIFICATIONS OF THE BUNN RESERVOIR

Specifications	Reservoir
Dimensions (in)	40 H × 12.25 D
Weight full (lb)	130
Capacity (liquid L)	30 (75 lb)
Gaseous equivalent (L, NPT)	25,000
Duration at 1 lpm (h)	416
Operating pressure (psig)	20
Primary relief valve pressure (psig)	22
Secondary relief valve pressure (psig)	30
Normal evaporation rate (lb/day)	1 ± 5%
Fill time (cold, min)	5–8

Courtesy of The John Bunn Company.

Bunn Portable. The Bunn portable employs a self-contained rotary valve flow-rate control device. The available flow rates range from 0 to 6 lpm in 1/2-lpm increments. The contents indicator is an internal spring scale that measures the total weight of the unit while it is suspended by the carrying straps. The contents level is indicated on a meter mounted in the top of the unit. Unlike the reservoir, the portable unit does not have an economizer valve. The Bunn portable unit has partial-fill capacity, so the patient may fill the unit with the appropriate amount of oxygen for each activity (*see* Table 2–3 for specifications).

Cryogenics Associates. The Liberator/Stroller is the liquid oxygen system manufactured by Cryogenics Associates. There are three reservoir units available, the Liberator 20, Liberator 30, and the Liberator 45; and two portable units, the Stroller and the Stroller Sprint (Fig 2–11). These portable units fill from the side of the reservoir unit.

Liberator 20, 30, and 45. The Liberator series has a standard self-contained rotary valve flow-rate control device, which offers 1/4, 1/2, 3/4,

TABLE 2–3. SPECIFICATIONS OF THE BUNN PORTABLE

Specifications	Portable
Dimensions (in)	14.5 H × 7.25 D
Weight full (lb)	10.2
Capacity (liquid L)	1.2 (3 lb)
Gaseous equivalent (L, NPT)	950
Duration at 1 lpm (h)	16
Operating pressure (psig)	20
Primary relief valve pressure (psig)	22
Secondary relief valve pressure (psig)	30
Normal evaporation rate (lb/day)	1
Fill time (cold, min)	1 1/2–2

Courtesy of The John Bunn Company.

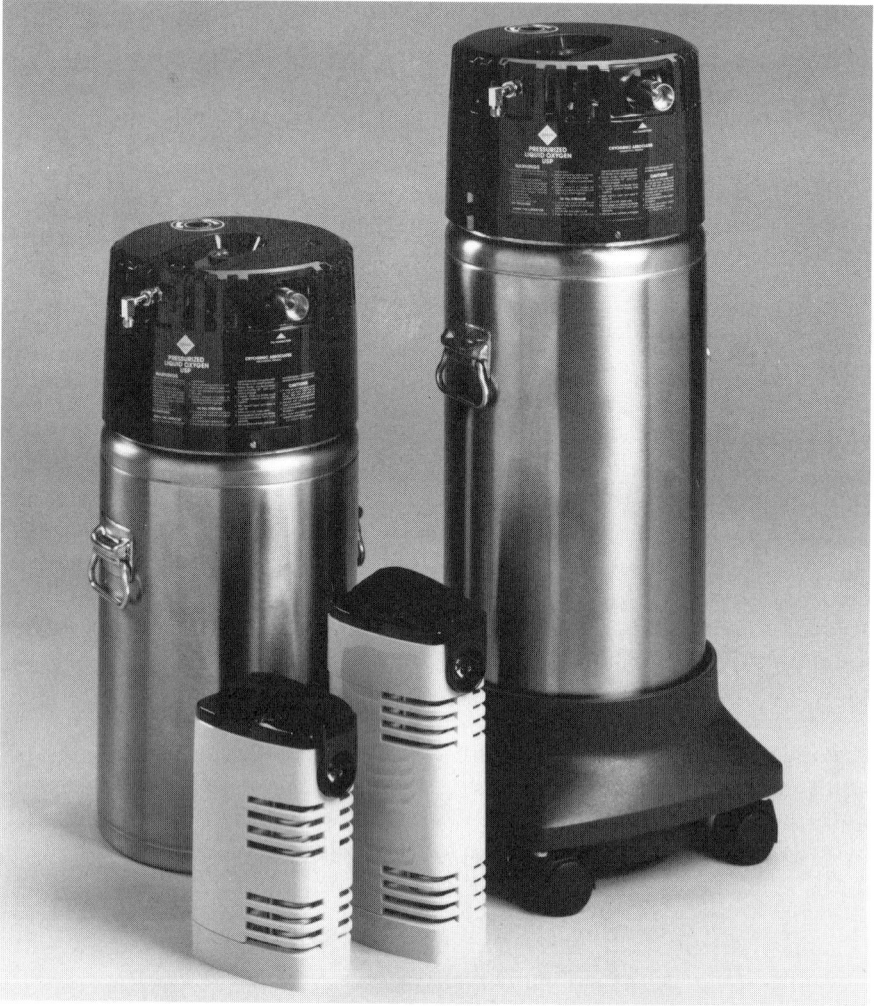

Figure 2–11. The Liberator/Stroller liquid oxygen system. *(Courtesy of Cryogenics Associates.)*

1, 1 1/2, 2, 2 1/2, 3, 4, 5, and 6 lpm. The contents indicator is a capacitance-type mechanism, with a meter of either a needle (old style) or LED type. Both meters require a 9-volt transistor battery, which must be periodically replaced. The Liberator is available with a roller base to allow movement around the home (*see* Table 2–4 for specifications).

Stroller and Stroller Sprint. The Stroller series also employs a rotary valve flow-rate control. With the standard flow-rate valve, the Stroller has a flow

TABLE 2–4. CRYOGENICS RESERVOIRS

Specifications	Liberator 20	Liberator 30
Dimensions (in)	27.5 H × 12 D	35 H × 12 D
Weight full (lb)	85.5	121.5
Capacity (liquid L)	20 (50 lb)	30 (75 lb)
Gaseous equivalent (L, NPT)	17,200	25,800
Duration at 1 lpm (h)	286	430
Operating pressure (psig)	20	20
Primary relief valve pressure (psig)	22	22
Secondary relief valve pressure (psig)	30	30
Normal evaporation rate (lb/day)	1.0	1.0
Fill time (cold, min)	8	8

Courtesy of Cryogenics Associates.

range of 0.25 to 6 lpm. The Sprint has a 0.25 to 3 lpm range. The Stroller series features a standard flow-locking device, which permits the dealer to preset the liter flow to ensure that the prescribed flow rate is not exceeded. Like the Liberator, the Strollers incorporate a capacitance-type contents indicator, with both needle (old style) and light emitting diode (LED) meters. The Stroller series also has partial-fill capability, so the patient may fill the unit with the appropriate amount of oxygen for each activity. Unlike the Liberator reservoir series, the Stroller portable series does not have an economizer valve (*see* Table 2–5 for specifications).

Cryo₂ Corporation. The $Cryo_2$ Corporation produces two reservoir units, the Grandeair and the Stationair, and two series of portable units, the Travelair/Wanderair series and the Pulsair series (Fig 2–12). These portables fill after connecting to a reservoir unit from either the top or side

TABLE 2–5. CRYOGENICS PORTABLES

Specifications	Stroller Sprint	Stroller
Dimensions (in)	10.5 H × 4.5 W × 7.8 D	13.5 H × 4.5 W × 7.8 D
Weight full (lb)	6.9	9.6
Capacity (liquid L)	0.60 (1.5 lb)	1.23 (3.1 lb)
Gaseous equivalent (L, NPT)	516	1058
Duration at 1 lpm (h)	8	17
Operating pressure (psig)	20	20
Primary relief valve pressure (psig)	21	21
Secondary relief valve pressure (psig)	30	30
Normal evaporation rate (lb/day)	1	1
Fill time (cold, min)	0.75	0.75

Courtesy of Cryogenics Associates.

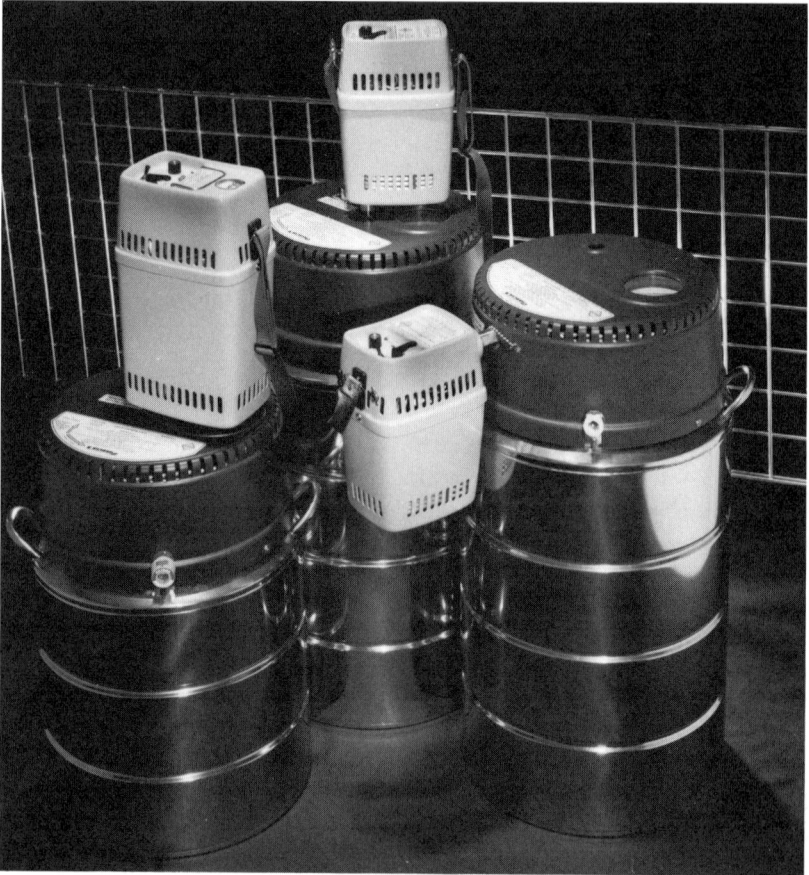

Figure 2–12. The reservoir and portable units of Cryo$_2$ Corporation. *(Courtesy of Cryo$_2$ Corporation.)*

of the reservoir unit, depending upon which type of transfilling config-uration has been selected.

Grandeair/Stationair Series. The original Grandeair/Stationair series has been updated and designated as the Concept II. All of the specifications listed in Table 2–6 are approximately the same as for the original series. The Grandeair/Stationair units have a Thorpe tube-type (rotameter) flow-meter, which connects to the units with a quick-connect coupler. These flowmeters are calibrated from 0 to 8 lpm. The content indicator is a differential pressure gauge, which operates by measuring the difference between the gas pressure directly above the liquid and the pressure at the bottom of the Dewar. Since the pressure at the bottom of the Dewar equals the pressure above the liquid plus the liquid hydrostatic head, the content gauge indicates the difference between the two pressures, or the hydrostatic head. No batteries are required for operation.

TABLE 2–6. CRYO₂ RESERVOIRS

Specifications	Grandeair II	Stationair II
Dimensions (in)	33.7 H × 16 D	26 H × 16 D
Weight full (lb)	142.6	98.9
Capacity (liquid L)	39.8 (96 lb)	25.5 (61.5 lb)
Gaseous equivalent (L, NPT)	32,852	21,049
Duration at 1 lpm (h)	548	350
Operating pressure (psig)	20	20
Primary relief valve pressure (psig)	22	22
Secondary relief valve pressure (psig)	30	30
Normal evaporation rates (lb/day)	1.5	1.3
Fill time (cold, min)	4	4

Courtesy of Cryo₂ Corporation.

Travelair/Wanderair Series. Like the Grandeair/Stationair, the Travelair/ Wanderair series has been updated and designated Concept II. Most of the specifications of Concept II are the same as the original series. Improvements incorporated in the Concept II include greater capacity with less unit weight, the addition of an economizer valve, and a patented purge cup, which directs dry gas vented during portable filling to the cryogenic coupler area to prevent frost formation by keeping airborne moisture away from the couplings during transfilling. Both units have orifice-type rotary-valve flow controls with 1, 1 1/2, 2, 2 1/2, 3, 4, and 5 lpm flow-rate settings. The content indicator differs from unit to unit. The Wanderair IID employs an external-tare suppressed-spring scale calibrated to indicate total weight of the liquid. The Travelair II employs a patented counterbalanced internal spring, known as a "tare-spring," in conjunction with a hydraulic load cell coupled to a pressure gauge to indicate liquid remaining. The Travelair/Wanderair series has partial-fill capacity (*see* Table 2–7 for specifications on these portable units).

Pulsair I and II. The second series of portable units offered by Cryo₂ consists of the Pulsair I and II. The distinguishing feature of these units is the "pulsed" mode, which is designed to deliver a dose of oxygen only at the beginning of inspiration. This is achieved by a mechanism called a *demand oxygen controller* (DOC), which senses the slight negative pressures generated on inspiration through a conventional nasal cannula. This signal is boosted by a fluidic amplifier, which triggers a pressure switch, which in turn triggers a solenoid valve that releases a given volume of oxygen to the patient. This volume is approximately 16.5 ml per each lpm set on the flow-rate selector. The sensitivity of the unit to inspiratory efforts is as low as 0.01 cm H_2O, and the response time is a maximum of 20 ms. The duration of the pulse is approximately 0.1 seconds per each lpm. This system is powered by a rechargeable battery and requires eight hours to fully charge for one filling of oxygen for the Pulsair II and four hours for the Pulsair I.

TABLE 2–7. CRYO$_2$ PORTABLES

Specifications	Travelair II	Wanderair II
Dimensions (in)	14.6 H × 10.5 W × 8.5 D	10.4 H × 7.2 W × 5.5 D
Weight full (lb)	14	6.6
Capacity (liquid L)	1.81 (4.6 lb)	0.49 (1.2 lb)
Gaseous equivalent (L, NPT)	1560	401
Duration at 1 lpm (h)	26	6.7
Operating pressure (psig)	20	20
Primary relief valve pressure (psig)	22	22
Secondary relief valve pressure (psig)	30	30
Normal evaporation rate (lb/day)	1.5	1.3
Fill time (cold, min)	1	1

Courtesy of Cryo$_2$ Corporation.

There are two basic advantages to a pulsed system. The first is efficiency. Since expiration is normally twice as long as inspiration, continuous oxygen is wasted for two thirds of the cycle. Further, oxygen that actually goes toward increasing the Po_2 can only be delivered during the first 40% of the inspiratory phase. The net savings of oxygen delivered by a pulsatile flow system can be more than three times that of a continuous system.

The second advantage to a pulsed system is the ability to provide a relatively constant Fio_2 within a range of respiratory rates, up to 40 breaths per minute. A continuous system will cause a drop in Fio_2 with an increase in rate because of the increase in entrained room air in relation to a constant oxygen flow.

Both Pulsair units have a flow rate selector with 1, 1 1/2, 2, 2 1/2, 3, 4, and 5 lpm settings and can deliver those rates in either continuous or pulsatile mode. The content indicator of the Pulsair I is an external-tare suppressed-spring scale that is calibrated to indicate the weight of the liquid content, like the Wanderair IID. The Pulsair II employs the internal-load-cell, tare-suppressed arrangement of the Travelair II, which measures the weight of the liquid oxygen only. Like the Travelair/Wanderair series, the Pulsair units offer an economizer valve and partial-fill capacity (*see* Table 2–8 for Pulsair specifications).

CSI. Cryogenic Services Incorparated, known as CSI, has been a manufacturer of liquid oxygen systems for Puritan-Bennett and Inspiron and has recently introduced its own system called Care-Ease (Fig 2–13). The Care-Ease system consists of a 30-L reservoir and a 1.2-L portable, which fills from the side.

Care-Ease Reservoir. The reservoir unit has a fixed-orifice rotary-valve flow-rate control with 12 positions from 1/4 to 6 lpm. The contents indicator

TABLE 2–8. CRYO₂ PULSAIR

Specifications	Pulsair I	Pulsair II
Dimensions (in)	10 H × 7.2 W × 5 D	13.5 H × 8.2 W × 5.5 D
Weight full (lb)	7.1	10.4
Capacity (liquid L)	0.49 (1.2 lb)	1.09 (2.6 lb)
Gaseous equivalent (L, NPT)	400	865
Duration at 1 lpm (h)	21.3 (pulsed)	45.4 (pulsed)
Operating pressure (psig)	20	20
Primary relief valve pressure (psig)	22	22
Secondary relief valve pressure (psig)	30	30
Normal evaporation rate (lb/day)	1.3	1.3
Fill time (cold, min)	0.6	1.0

Courtesy of Cryo₂ Corporation.

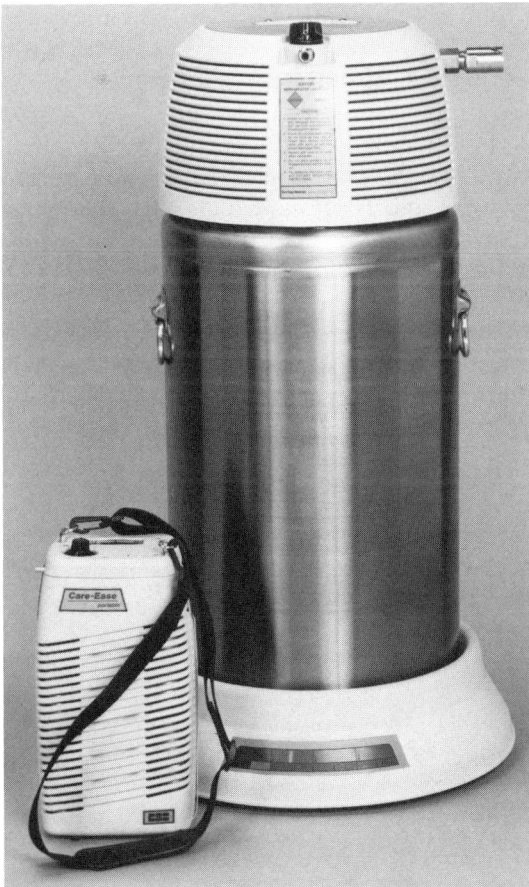

Figure 2–13. The Care-Ease Reservoir and The Care-Ease Portable. *(Courtesy of Cryogenic Services, Incorporated.)*

TABLE 2–9. CRYOGENIC SERVICES CARE-EASE RESERVOIR

Specifications	Reservoir
Dimensions (in)	31 H × 14 D
Weight full (lb)	121
Capacity (liquid L)	30
Gaseous equivalent (L, NPT)	25,800
Duration at 1 lpm (h)	430
Operating pressure (psig)	22
Primary relief valve pressure (psig)	25 ± 1.25
Secondary relief valve pressure (psig)	30 ± 1.5
Normal evaporation rate (lb/day)	1.5
Fill time (cold/min)	7

Courtesy of Cryogenic Services, Incorporated.

is a mechanical spring scale on the base of the reservoir. A roller base is an optional accessory (*see* Table 2–9 for specifications).

Care-Ease Portable. The portable unit also has a fixed-orifice rotary-valve flow-rate control from 1/4 to 6 lpm. The contents indicator is an integrally mounted spring mechanism. This lightweight portable is available with an optional clip-on handle (*see* Table 2–10 for specifications).

Inspiron Company. Inspiron manufactures a liquid oxygen system consisting of two reservoir units and one portable unit, termed the A series (Fig 2–14). Also available are the H and S series, which have the same specifications with slight feature differances. The Inspiron portable fills from the side of the reservoir unit. The Inspiron Company has merged with the John Bunn Company, another manufacturer of liquid oxygen systems.

8530A/8520A Reservoirs. The series A reservoirs have a rotary-valve flow-rate control that can be set at 1, 1 1/2, 2, 2 1/2, 3, 4, and 6 lpm. A 10-

TABLE 2–10. CRYOGENIC SERVICES CARE-EASE PORTABLE

Specifications	Portable
Dimensions (lb)	12.5 H × 7.3 W × 5.3 D
Weight (lb)	8.25
Capacity (liquid L)	1.2 (3 lb)
Gaseous Equivalent (L, NPT)	1034
Duration at 1 lpm (h)	17
Operating pressure (psig)	22
Primary relief valve pressure (psig)	22 ± 1.1
Secondary relief valve pressure (psig)	30 ± 1.1
Normal evaporation rate (lb/day)	1.25
Fill time (cold, s)	90, or less

Courtesy of Cryogenic Services, Incorporated.

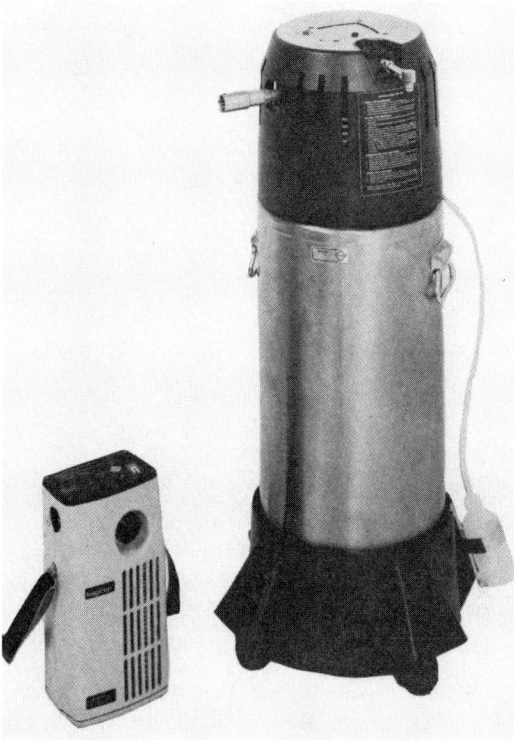

Figure 2–14. Inspiron liquid system. *(Courtesy of Inspiron Company).*

psig-pressure regulator is positioned between the warming coils and the flow-rate selector to ensure accurate flows in the face of head-pressure fluctuations. The contents indicator is a capacitance-type mechanism with a needle-type meter readout. This indicator system requires a 9-volt battery, which must be periodically replaced. The Inspiron reservoirs come with a standard roller base (*see* Table 2–11 for specifications for the A series).

TABLE 2–11. INSPIRON RESERVOIRS

Specifications	8530A	8520A
Dimensions (in)	36 H × 12.25 D	29 H × 12.25 D
Weight full (lb)	128	87
Capacity (liquid L)	30 (75 lb)	20 (50 lb)
Gaseous equivalent (L, NPT)	25,800	17,200
Duration at 1 lpm (h)	430	286
Operating pressure (psig)	20	22
Primary relief valve pressure (psig)	22	22
Secondary relief valve pressure (psig)	30	30
Normal evaporation rate (lb/day)	1	1
Fill time (cold, min)	6	2

Courtesy of Inspiron Corporation.

TABLE 2–12. INSPIRON PORTABLE

Specifications	8510
Dimensions (in)	13.5 H × 5 W × 6.8 D
Weight full (lb)	10.5
Capacity (liquid L)	1.2 (3 lb)
Gaseous equivalent (L, NPT)	1034
Duration at 1 lpm (h)	17
Operating pressure (psig)	20
Primary relief valve pressure (psig)	22
Secondary relief valve pressure (psig)	30
Normal evaporation rate (lb/day)	1
Fill time (cold, min)	1

Courtesy of the Inspiron Corporation.

The series H reservoir has same specifications as the 8530A with the addition of 1/4, 1/2, and 8 lpm settings on the flow-rate selector.

The series S is also identical in specifications to the 8530A, but without the 10-psig regulator. This provides a 20-psig delivery pressure to the patient instead of 10 psig like the A series.

8510 Portable. Like the reservoir series, the series A portable unit has a rotary-valve flow-rate control that can be set at 1, 1 1/2, 2, 2 1/2, 3, 4, and 6 lpm. Unlike the reservoir series, there is no 10-psig pressure regulator or economizer valve. The contents indicator is a capacitance-type mechanism with a content-meter readout. This indicator system requires a 9-volt battery, which must be periodically replaced. The 8510 portable has partial-fill capacity (*see* Table 2–12 for the series A portable specifications).

The series H portable has nearly identical specifications as the series A but with the addition of 1/4, 1/2, and 8 lpm settings of the flow-rate selector.

The series S portable is identical in all specifications with the series A.

Penox Technologies, Inc. Penox manufactures three reservoirs and four portables (Fig 2–15). The reservoirs are identified as the 40-L, 28-L, and 18-L base units. The original three portables are identified as 1, 2, and 3, and the most recent addition to the line is the Penox Lightweight. The portable units fill from the top of the base-unit reservoir.

Base Units. The Penox base units have a back-pressure-compensated Thorpe-type flowmeter, which connects to the units with a quick-connect coupler. An optional locking flowmeter is available. These flowmeters are

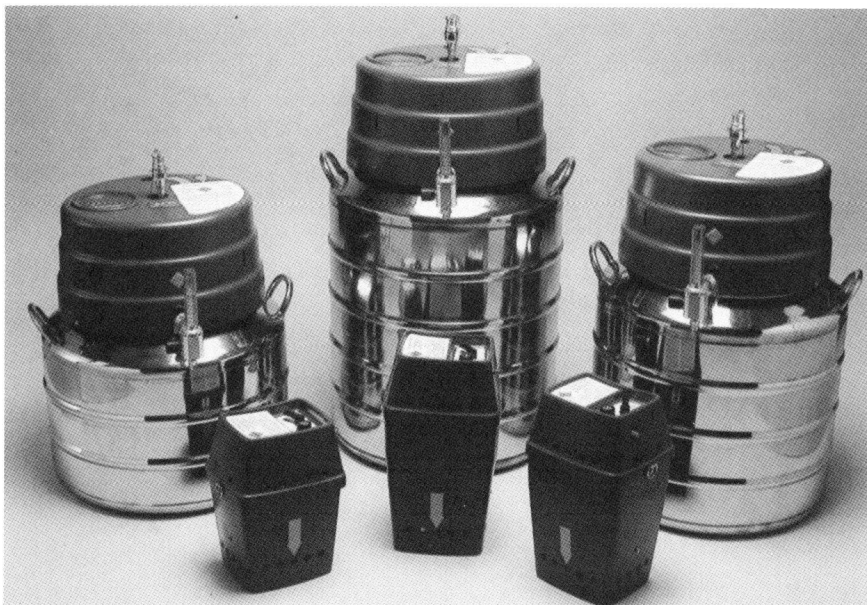

Figure 2–15. Penox liquid system. *(Courtesy of Penox Technologies, Incorporated.)*

calibrated from 0 to 8 lpm. The contents indicator is a magnehelic gauge, which is a differential pressure gauge. This indicator operates by measuring the difference between the head pressure and the pressure at the bottom of the Dewar and then indicates the content with a needle meter readout. No batteries are required for operation. An optional roller base is available (*see* Table 2–13 for specifications).

TABLE 2–13. PENOX RESERVOIRS

Specifications	18-Liter	28-Liter	40-Liter
Dimensions (in)	23 H × 18 D	27 H × 18 D	33 H × 18 D
Weight full (lb)	91	122	160.5
Capacity (liquid L)	18 (45 lb)	28 (73 lb)	40 (100 lb)
Gaseous equivalent (L, NPT)	15,480	24,097	34,186
Duration at 1 lpm (h)	252	396	570
Operating pressure (psig)	22	22	22
Primary relief valve pressure (psig)	22	22	22
Secondary relief valve pressure (psig)	30	30	30
Normal evaporation rate (lb/day)	1	1	1
Fill time (cold, min)	4	6	7

Courtesy of Penox Technologies, Incorporated.

TABLE 2–14. PENOX PORTABLES

Specifications	One	Two	Three
Dimensions (in)	10.75 H × 7 W × 6 D	13 H × 7 W × 6.5 D	13.75 H × 7 W × 6 D
Weight full, with straps (lb)	7.08	9.08	11.88
Capacity (liquid L)	0.5 (1.25 lb)	1 (2.5 lb)	2 (5 lb)
Gaseous equivalent (L, NPT)	430	860	1721
Duration at 1 lpm (h)	5.5	12.3	21.4
Operating pressure (psig)	21	21	21
Primary relief valve pressure (psig)	22	22	22
Secondary relief valve pressure (psig)	30	30	30
Normal evaporation rate (lb/day)	N/A	N/A	N/A
Fill time (cold, s)	30	45	65

Courtesy of Penox Technologies, Incorporated.

1, 2, and 3 Portable. The 1, 2, and 3 portable series employs a rotary-valve flow-rate control with 1, 1 1/2, 2, 2 1/2, 3, 4, and 5 lpm flow-rate settings. A pediatric flow-rate selector is available with a 1/4-to-2 lpm range with 1/4 lpm intervals, as well as a high flow-rate selector with 1, 2, 3, 4, 5, 6, and 8 lpm flow-rate settings. The content indicator is an external-spring scale, which hooks to the carrying straps. These portable units have no economizer valve and have partial-fill capacities (*see* Table 2–14 for specifications).

Lightweight Portable. Weighing just over 4 lb full, the Penox Lightweight portable is the lightest portable unit available. Like the other Penox portables, the Penox Lightweight employs a rotary-valve flow-rate control with 1, 1 1/2, 2, 2 1/2, 3, 4, and 5 lpm flow-rate settings, and it has an economizer valve. The content indicator is an external-spring scale, and the unit has partial-fill capacity (*see* Table 2–15 for specifications).

Puritan–Bennett Corporation. The Puritan–Bennett Corporation produces two lines of liquid oxygen systems, the Companion and the Mark 4 (*see* Figs 2–16A and B). The Companion series, a low-pressure system, has been marketed since 1983 and consists of three stationary units, the Companion 21, 31, and 41, and one portable unit, the Companion 1000. In December of 1985, Puritan–Bennett purchased Union Carbide Corporation's Cryogenic Medical Division and began manufacture and distribution of the Mark 4 system. Like the Companion system, the Mark 4 reservoir is available in three sizes, 40-lb, 70-lb, and 90-lb. This system includes a lightweight portable that is filled from the top of the reservoir. The Mark 4 system is available in both standard pressure (50 psig) and low pressure (20 psig).

TABLE 2–15. PENOX LIGHTWEIGHT PORTABLE

Specifications	Lightweight Portable
Dimensions (in)	8.5 H × 8.5 W × 6.25 D
Weight full (lb)	4.1
Capacity (liquid L)	0.35 (0.9 lb)
Gaseous equivalent (L, NPT)	302
Duration at 1 lpm (h)	5.5
Operating pressure (psig)	21
Primary relief valve pressure (psig)	22
Secondary relief valve pressure (psig)	30
Normal evaporation rate (lb/day)	1
Fill time (cold, min)	1

Courtesy of Penox Technologies, Incorporated.

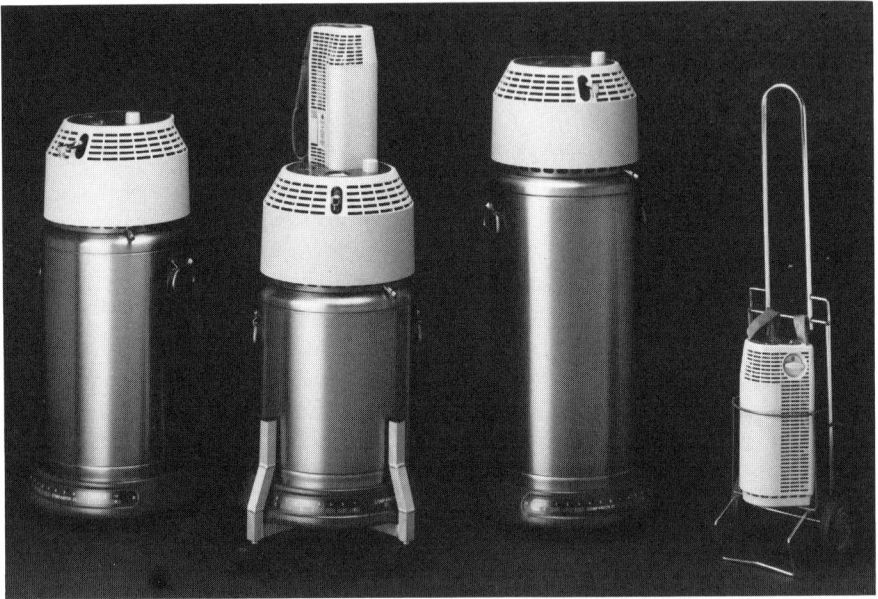

Figure 2–16. (A) The Companion liquid system. *(Courtesy of Puritan–Bennett Corporation.)*

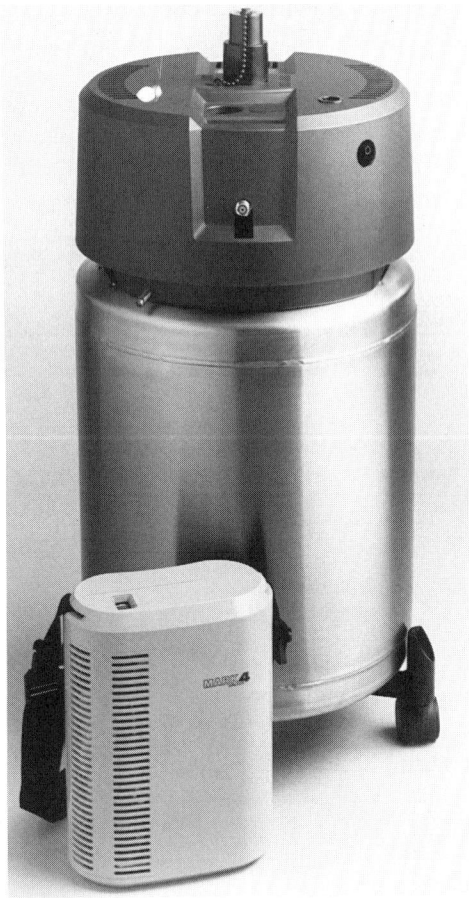

Figure 2–16. (B): The Mark 4 liquid system. *(Courtesy of Puritan–Bennett Corporation.)*

Companion Reservoir. The Companion reservoirs have a self-contained rotary flow-control valve with a device allowing the home care company to lock the flow control at the maximum desired flow rate. The standard 12-position flow-control valve includes flows ranging from 1/4 to 6 lpm. Two optional flow-control valves are available and provide a range of flows from 1/8 to 10 lpm. The amount of liquid oxygen in the unit is measured by means of an integral differential-pressure indicator, which displays a constant reading that is visible through the top of the unit (*see* Table 2–16 for specifications).

Companion 1000 Portable. The Companion portable also features a self-contained rotary flow-control valve, which includes flows ranging from 1/4 to 6 lpm. One optional flow-control valve is available that will extend the range of flows to include 1/8 lpm as well as other low flows not included in the standard valve. The Companion T, a unit especially designed for high-liter flows, is capable of 15 lpm flow rates. The contents indicator is an internal-spring scale with a top-mounted needle meter, which is read while suspending the unit by the carrying strap. A unique feature is that if the unit is tipped over, the patient has 60 seconds to return the portable to an upright position before liquid escapes through the primary relief valve. The unit is lightweight, body contoured, and has partial-fill capability (*see* Table 2–17 for specifications).

Mark 4 Reservoir. The Mark 4 Reservoir system has a diameter index safety system (DISS) outlet, which allows the use of any standard flowmeter or standard flow-control valve. The amount of liquid oxygen in the reservoir is measured by means of an integral differential-pressure indicator, which displays a constant reading that is visible through the top of the unit. This system is listed by Underwriters Laboratory (*see* Table 2–18 for specifications).

Mark 4 Walker. The Walker features a self-contained flow-control valve, which includes flows ranging from 1/4 to 6 lpm. There is one optional flow-control valve available that will extend the range of flows to include 1/8 lpm as well as other low flows not included in the standard valve. The amount of liquid oxygen in the Walker is measured by means of an integral differential-pressure indicator, which displays a constant reading that is visible through the top of the unit. A unique feature of the Walker is that it will not vent liquid when placed on its side, because of the design of the primary relief valve. The Walker also features an automatic fill-termination system that allows the patient to select either a full or half full condition (*see* Table 2–19 for specifications).

TABLE 2–16. PURITAN-BENNETT COMPANION RESERVOIRS

Specifications	Companion 21	Companion 31	Companion 41
Dimensions (in)	26.5 H × 14.25 D	32 H × 14.25 D	37.75 H × 14.25 D
Weight full (lb)	92	125	160
Capacity (liquid L)	21 (50 lb)	31 (75 lb)	41 (100 lb)
Gaseous equivalent (L, NPT)	17,290	25,523	33,756
Duration at 1 lpm (h)	288	426	562
Operating pressure (psig)	19.5	19.5	19.5
Primary relief valve pressure (psig)	22	22	22
Secondary relief valve pressure (psig)	30	30	30
Normal evaporation rate (lb/day)	1.6	1.6	1.6
Fill time (cold, min)	7	8	10

Courtesy of the Puritan-Bennett Corporation.

TABLE 2–17. PURITAN-BENNETT COMPANION PORTABLE

Specifications	Companion 1000
Dimensions (in)	13.8 H*
Weight full (lb)	7.5
Capacity (liquid L)	1.2 (3 lb)
Gaseous equivalent (L, NPT)	1058
Duration at 1 lpm (h)	17
Operating pressure (psig)	22
Primary relief valve pressure (psig)	22
Secondary relief valve pressure (psig)	30
Normal evaporation rate (lb/day)	1
Fill time (cold, min)	0.75

*Irregular cross-section
Courtesy of the Puritan-Bennett Corporation.

TABLE 2–18. PURITAN-BENNETT MARK 4 RESERVOIRS

Specifications	R50/40	R20/40	R50/70	R20/70	R50/90	R20/90
Dimensions (in)	24.6 H × 15.5 D	24.6 H × 15.5 D	30.0 H × 15.5 D	30.0 H × 15.5 D	33.6 H × 15.5 D	33.6 H × 15.5 D
Weight full (lb)	78	79	115	117	140	143
Capacity (liquid L)	17.3 (40 lb)	17.3 (41 lb)	30.3 (70 lb)	30.3 (72 lb)	38.9 (90 lb)	38.9 (93 lb)
Gaseous equivalent (L, NPT)	13,800	14,300	23,900	24,800	30,800	31,900
Duration at 1 lpm (h)	230	238	398	412	513	530
Operating pressure (psig)	50	19.5	50	19.5	50	19.5
Primary relief valve pressure (psig)	55	22.5	55	22.5	55	22.5
Secondary relief valve pressure (psig)	N/A*	N/A*	N/A*	N/A*	N/A*	N/A*
Normal evaporation rate (lb/day)	1.4	1.4	1.5	1.5	1.9	1.9
Fill time (cold, min)	3.5	3.5	4.2	4.2	6.0	6.0

*Uses 175 psig bursting disk.
Courtesy of the Puritan-Bennett Corporation.

TABLE 2–19. PURITAN-BENNETT MARK 4 WALKERS

Specifications	W 50	W 20
Dimensions (in)	12 H	12 H
Weight full (lb)	8.3	8.4
Capacity (liquid L)	1.2 (2.8 lb)	1.2 (2.9 lb)
Gaseous equivalent (L, NPT)	960	1000
Duration at 1 lpm (h)	16	16.6
Operating pressure (psig)	50	19.5
Primary relief valve pressure (psig)	55	22.5
Secondary relief valve pressure (psig)	150	150
Normal evaporation rate (lb/day)	1	1
Fill time (cold, min)	2.0	2.0

Courtesy of the Puritan-Bennett Corporation.

CONCENTRATORS

Oxygen concentrators are electrical devices that separate oxygen from the other gaseous elements in the atmosphere, collect this separated oxygen into a tank, and then deliver the oxygen to the patient via a flow-rate control device (Fig 2–17). The advantage of this system of oxygen delivery is that the frequent visits by the home care company necessitated by other systems are not required. Of course, oxygen delivery is dependent on a continuous supply of electricity; backup oxygen cylinders are required by Medicare and are a matter of course with most home care companies. Concentrators have been commercially available since 1974.

There are two types of oxygen concentrators available. The most common uses a molecular sieve material to separate the oxygen from the rest of the air by the process of adsorption. There are currently about 20 manufacturers of this type of concentrator. The second system, more properly termed an oxygen enricher, uses a permeable plastic membrane to separate oxygen and water vapor from the rest of the air by differences in gas diffusion rates. This type of system is manufactured by the Oxygen Enrichment Company.

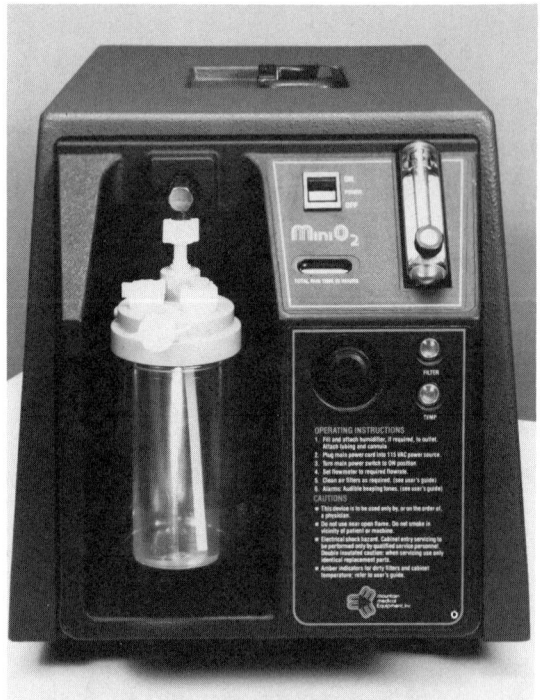

Figure 2–17. Oxygen concentrator. *(Courtesy of Mountain Medical Equipment, Incorporated.)*

Principles of Operation

Oxygen Concentrators. The following discussion describes a hypothetical pressure-swing-cycle oxygen concentrator that uses the components common to most commercially available units. The variations among manufacturers include the number of sieve beds, the number and location of valves, the molecular sieve bed specifications, and the percentage of oxygen delivered at a given liter flow. The concentrator in this description has two sieve beds, as do the majority of units currently manufactured. The other common design uses a single sieve bed.

The two molecular sieve beds are the heart of the oxygen concentrator. The term *pressure swing cycle* refers to the operating phases in which one bed is pressurized to produce oxygen while the other is depressurized to purge the unwanted waste gases. The molecular sieve material itself is a granular zeolite crystal, which has the unique ability to separate gases from each other according to the gases' molecular size and polarity. This is because zeolite crystals contain a precisely arrayed network of small, uniform holes. These holes are about 5 Å in diameter, and together they form the molecular sieve. The particular zeolite in an oxygen concentrator has a preferential affinity for nitrogen, water, carbon dioxide, carbon monoxide, and all hydrocarbons, whereas oxygen and minute quantities of argon pass through. In addition to molecular size and polarity, the amount of any particular gas adsorbed is proportional to the partial pressure of that gas, which is why the molecular sieve beds are pressurized. These system pressures currently range from 10 to 30 psig.

For the following sequence of operation see Figure 2–18. Room air enters the machine through a gross-particle inlet filter and a fine-particle filter and then enters the compressor. The air exits the compressor through another fine filter and a relief valve maintains the system pressure. The air flows through a heat exchanger, which removes the heat added from the compressor, and enters a solenoid valving system, which directs the flow to the sieve beds. This solenoid is controlled by an electronic logic device, such as a printed circuit (pc) board or microprocessor that governs the timing of the pressure-swing cycle. As a result of this electronically controlled valving, each sieve bed has two distinct operating phases, the pressurizing interval and the depressurizing interval. When the first sieve bed enters the pressurizing interval, the solenoid directs the air into that cylinder, and a restrictor downstream of the bed builds the air pressure to increase the adsorption of nitrogen as the oxygen passes through. The crossover assembly passes the first small portion of this oxygen flow to the product tank for storage and patient use. The remainder of the oxygen is diverted to the second sieve bed to purge the nitrogen adsorbed from the previous cycle. As the first sieve bed is becoming saturated with ni-

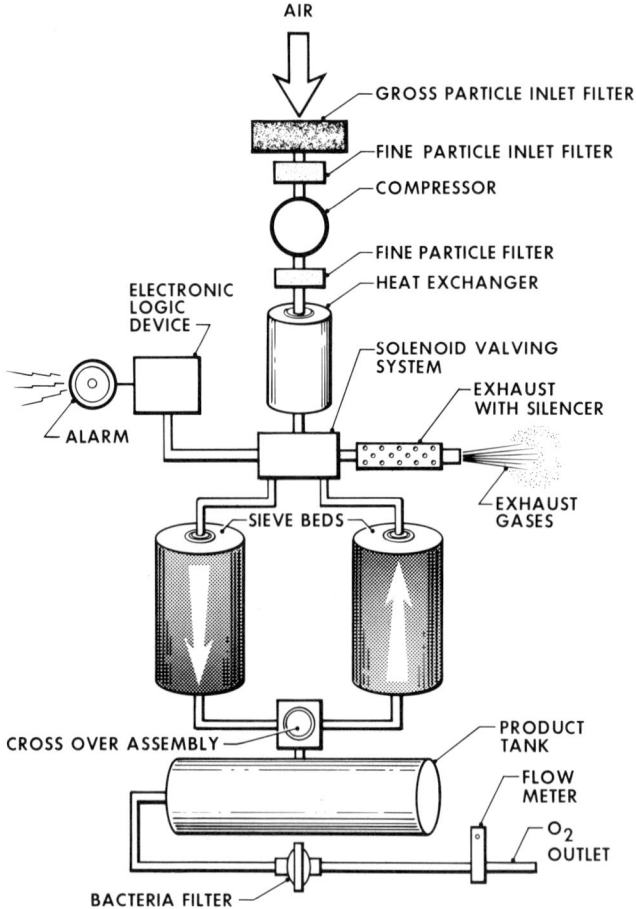

Figure 2–18. Oxygen concentrator schematic.

trogen, the electronic logic device switches the solenoid to the depressurizing interval by opening the exhaust to the first sieve bed, allowing backflow to occur in this bed. This reduces the partial pressure of the nitrogen, promoting desorption. This backflow also draws oxygen from the second bed, which is now pressurizing, further promoting desorption. This bed is now regenerated and ready for the next cycle.

These cycles are typically timed in the range of 10 to 30 seconds, depending on the manufacturer. It is interesting to note that the majority of oxygen produced by this process is used for regeneration. The net oxygen available for patient use is the difference between production and regeneration.

There is a silencer located after the exhaust to muffle the sound of the nitrogen as it discharged into the room air. The noise generated by these units is caused by this exhaust and the compressor, and range from about 40 to 50 dB. The oxygen in the product tank is regulated down to the range of 3 to 10 psig, where it flows through a bacteria filter and into a flowmeter for patient use. Most flowmeters are backflow compensated. An alarm system will sound an audible alarm if the power to the unit is interrupted or if the electronic logic device senses low system pressures or overheating. Alarm systems vary among manufacturers, and most require a 9-volt battery, which itself will trigger the alarm when running down.

The single sieve bed concentrators work in a similar fashion. The compressed air is introduced into the sieve bed by a solenoid valving system, the bed is pressurized, and nitrogen is adsorbed. After a timed interval, the bed is depressurized, the oxygen is stored in the product tank, and the nitrogen is removed from the bed by means of a partial vacuum. Surge reservoirs may be added to the system to buffer the surges that occur with the operation of a single sieve bed. The Bunn 3001 is an example of a single-sieve-bed concentrator.

Oxygen concentrators are decreasingly efficient as the flow rates increase. Most will produce about 95% at 2 lpm, but as the liter flow increases, the percentage drops off (*see* Table 2–20 for specifications of concentrators and enrichers).

The Oxygen Enricher. The Oxygen Enrichment Company (OECO) manufactures two membrane oxygen enrichers, the OECO high-humidity system and the OE Junior. Both models employ a plastic membrane less than 1 μm thick, which separates gases primarily on the basis of gas diffusion rates. Oxygen and water vapor will diffuse most readily, so that the units deliver a constant 40% oxygen with three times the ambient relative humidity, while delivering subambient levels of carbon monoxide and other pollutants at all flow rates. The membrane also acts as a filter against all bacteria, viruses, and particulates. A pressure gradient is established across the membrane by a diaphragm vacuum pump (*see* Fig 2–19 for a schematic diagram).

To deliver an Fio_2 to the patient comparable to a 100% source, the enricher, delivering 40%, must be operated at a higher flow rate. According to the manufacturers' recommendation, the flow rates should be three times the flow rate used with a 100% oxygen source. For example, to achieve 28% with an oxygen cylinder, the flow rate would be set at 2 lpm. The OECO units would be set at 6 lpm to achieve the comparable Fio_2.

High-humidity System. The OECO High-Humidity Membrane Oxygen Enricher (Model OE-4A) has a built-in inlet humidifier, which allows adjustable levels of absolute humidity up to 38 mg H_2O/L. A heated tube is used to deliver the saturated water vapor at body temperature to a conventional cannula. The system is designed to prevent airway dehy-

TABLE 2-20. OXYGEN CONCENTRATOR COMPARISON

Manufacturer (Model)	Weight (Pounds)	Dimensions (Inches)	Power Consumption (Watts)	Output (%, ± 3% at 1-3 lpm)
AirSep				
MDI	50	13 × 12 × 25	320	90 ± 3% at 4 lpm / 95% at 3 lpm
Briox Tech				
Briox 4 Plus	55	15 × 15½ × 20	280	93% at 3 lpm
Briox 6 Plus	60	15 × 15½ × 28	340	93% at 3 lpm
John Bunn Company				
Bunn Natural	29	18¾ × 9½ × 13½	250	90% at 5 lpm
Bunn Lite	28	18½ × 12 × 13¾	250	90% at 2 lpm
Bunn 3001	43	18½ × 13¾ × 13½	280	90% at 3 lpm
Bunn 5001	50	17½ × 14½ × 11½	375	95% at 3 lpm
Baby Bunn	28	18¾ × 9½ × 13½	250	94% at 1¼ lpm
Cryogenics Association				
Roomate III	55	27 × 14 × 10	290	92% at 3 lpm
DeVilbiss				
DeVo/44	44	23¾ × 15½ × 13	390	95% at 3 lpm
DeVo/MC29	29	21½ × 12½ × 14	265	90% at 3 lpm
Erie Medical				
Eriette	57	16 × 15 × 17	420	95% at 2 lpm
Healthdyne				
BX–3000	55	17½ × 16½ × 22	340	95% at 3 lpm
Hospitak 7000	35	10 × 16 × 11	330	92% at 1–2 lpm / 86% at 3–1 lpm
Hudson				
6400	59	23¾ × 16¾ × 13½	330	93% at 3 lpm

Inspiron				
7500	57	18½ × 14 × 19¾	350	95% at 2 lpm
3500	45	19¾ × 13¾ × 18½	350	90% at 4 lpm
Invacare				
PrimeAir–PA_{O_2}	95	24 × 14½ × 20½	490	95% at 2 lpm
Mobilaire III	64	18 × 23¼ × 14½	320	95% at 2 lpm
Mada Medical				
Resp O_2	44	15¼ × 15½ × 17½	400	90 ± 3% at 1–3 lpm 95% at 2 lpm
Mountain Medical				
Aspen	42	21½ × 16½ × 12½	200	93% at 2 lpm
Sage	48	25 × 17 × 13	420	95% at 2 lpm
Summit	59	25 × 17 × 13	430	95% at 3 lpm
Nidek Mark 4	61	16 × 21 × 15	380	93% at 3 lpm
Oeco				
OE Junior	58	30 × 14 × 14½	200	40% at 1–6 lpm
High Humidity	110	30 × 14 × 16	225	40% at 1–6 lpm
OXYCON				
SF–230	51	14 × 14⅛ × 21⅛	350	94% at 2 lpm
Penox				
Mini O_2	52	14¾ × 15⅝ × 23	325	95% at 2 lpm
BX–5000	55	22 × 16 × 12	345	90% at 4 lpm
Puritan-Bennett				
Companion 492	50	24 × 12 × 16	330	95% at 3 lpm
Roman Labs				
Freedom O_2	32	16 × 21 × 20¾	218	90% at 3 lpm
Smith & Davis				
Oxycon Gemini	56	14 × 14⅛ × 21⅛	350	94% at 4 lpm
Oxycon Polaris	51	14 × 14⅛ × 21⅛	350	90% at 4 lpm
Timeter				
Criterion II	51	25¼ × 17¼ × 14¼	400	93% at 2 lpm

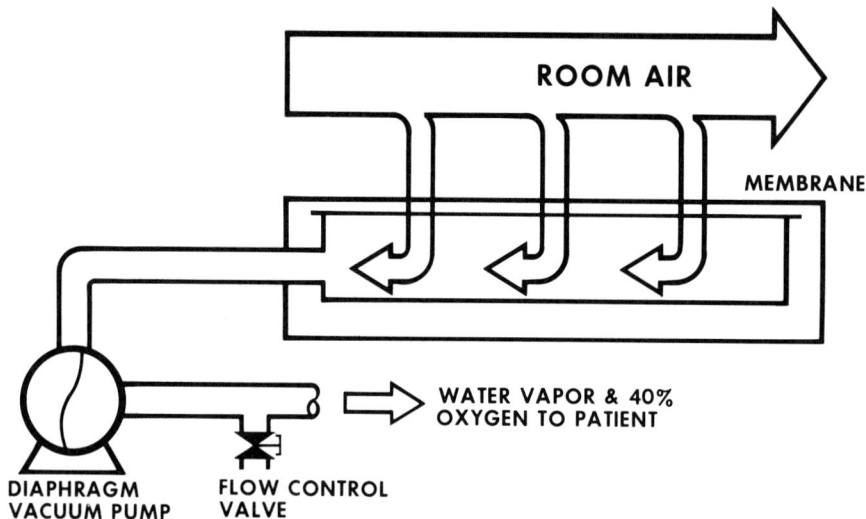

Figure 2–19. OECO oxygen enricher, schematic

dration and promote mucus clearance in patients with pulmonary disease.

REFERENCES

High-Pressure Cylinders

Bureau of Drugs; Food and Drug Administration (HFD-320): *Compressed Medical Gases Guidline*. Rockville, Md, Food and Drug Administration, 1981.

Burton GG, & Hodgkin JE: *Respiratory Care: A Guide to Clinical Practice*, ed 2. Philadelphia, Lippincott, 1984.

Compressed Gas Association: *Handbook of Compressed Gases*, ed 2. New York, Van Nostrand Reinhold, 1981.

Federal Register: *Specification and Usage Requirements for 3AL Seamless, Aluminum Cylinders*. Dec 24, 1981.

McPherson SP: *Respiratory Therapy Equipment*, ed 3. St Louis, Mosby, 1985.

National Fire Protection Agency: *NFPA 99 Health Care Facilities 1984*. Quincy, Mass, NFPA, 1984.

Liquid Oxygen Systems

Compressed Gas Association: *Recommended Practice for the Outfitting and Operation of Vehicles Used in the Transportation and Transfilling of Liquid Oxygen to Be Used for Respiration, CGA SB–9*. Arlington, Va, CGA, 1983.

Compressed Gas Association: *Transfilling of Liquid Oxygen to be Used for Respiration, CGA P–2.6*. Arlington, Va, CGA, 1983.

John Bunn Company: *Bunn Service Manual for Liquid Oxygen System.* Tonawanda, NY, The John Bunn Company.

Cryogenic Associates: *Liberator Stroller Service Manual.* Indianapolis, Cryogenics Associates.

$Cryo_2$ Corporation: *Service Manual.* Fort Pierce, Fla, $Cryo_2$ Corporation.

Inspiron Corporation: *Inspiron 8500 Liquid Oxygen System Service Manual.* Cucamonga, CA, Inspiron Corporation.

Penox Technologies: *Liquid Oxygen Manual.* Pittston, PA, Penox Technologies.

Puritan-Bennett Corporation: *Technical Manual.* Indianapolis, Puritan-Bennett Corporation.

Union Carbide Corporation: *Medical Products Technical.* Indianapolis, Union Carbide Corporation.

Oxygen Concentrators

Invacare Respiratory Corporation: *Prime Air O_2 Service Manual.* Elyria, Ohio, Invacare Respiratory Corporation.

Mountain Medical Equipment, Inc: *Service Manual.* Littleton, Colo, Mountain Medical Equipment, Inc.

Union Carbide Corporation: *Medical Products Technical.* Indianapolis, Union Carbide Corporation.

3

Selecting the Optimal Oxygen System

JEFFREY LUCAS, RRT

Long-term domiciliary oxygen therapy (LTDO$_2$) is now a well-documented and accepted practice in treating the selected patient with chronic obstructive pulmonary disease (COPD) and contributing cor pulmonale, pulmonary hypertension, and neuropsychiatric disturbances (Ashutosh, Mead, Dunsky, 1983; Flasterstein & Klocke, 1982; Krop, Block, & Cohen, 1973; Levine, Bigelow, Hainstra, et al, 1967; Nocturnal Oxygen Therapy Trial Group, 1980).

Often, however, oxygen therapy in the home is viewed as very basic therapy or routine care by many health-care professionals not experienced with home care protocol, and with oxygen therapy in particular. It should not be so viewed, and the information presented in this chapter on how to determine the proper oxygen system may help provide the reader with a new, enlightened clinical perspective.

Therefore, this chapter will focus on the many factors involved in determining the oxygen system most appropriate for an individual within his or her environment, one that will complement the patient's life style and also meet the goals of the physician's prescription. In discussing how to best administer and distribute oxygen to the patient, the following objectives will be considered:

1. The types of oxygen systems available for use in the home.
2. What factors must be considered when choosing the appropriate oxygen system for the patient's use.
3. Management of patient and oxygen system to attain optimal benefit.
4. Methods of improving compliance and oxygen-economizing devices.
5. Future outlooks and concerns regarding long-term oxygen therapy.

OXYGEN SYSTEMS

Fundamentally, there are three types of oxygen systems that can be placed in the patient's home. They are

1. Compressed gas cylinders (CGC).
2. Oxygen concentrators (OC).
3. Liquid oxygen (LOX).

Each of these systems has inherent advantages and disadvantages, depending upon the situation it is applied to in the home.

Compressed Gas Cylinders

Advantages. The advantages to using CGCs in the home are outlined in Table 3–1.

Oxygen cylinders can be the economical system of choice for the low-volume and the intermittent user of oxygen at home.

Low-volume use refers to the total amount of gas consumed by the user. Oxygen use is usually described as low- or high-liter-flow usage.

Use of oxygen in the home requires evaluation of the oxygen system being used and thus the specific gas volume limitations within that system. Table 3–2 shows how to determine gas usage of an H-cylinder, a commonly used size of oxygen cylinder.

Below are two useful examples of patients who might be using oxygen by cylinder.

> *Example A:*
> The nocturnal user of oxygen at a flow rate of 2 lpm (assuming use of ten hours a night) will consume 1200 L or 42.4 cu ft in one "use day."

TABLE 3–1. ADVANTAGES AND DISADVANTAGES ASSOCIATED WITH CGC* USE IN THE HOME

Advantages	Disadvantages
1. The economical system of choice for the *low-volume* and the intermittent oxygen user	1. Some form of securing mechanism needed
2. Allows for long-term storage of oxygen	2. Additional expense as a result of waste if patient is not instructed in proper use
3. Can be applied as a 50-psi presssure source for application to certain mechanical ventilators in the home	3. Regular replacement required
	4. Large size and weight eliminate its portability within the home
4. Does not require electrical operation	5. Difficulty of operation imposed on the blind or handicapped patient
	6. Unsightly appearance in the home

*CGC = compressed gas cylinder.

TABLE 3–2. GAS USAGE DETERMINATIONS

Total Liter Use per Day:
Equation A:
Liter flow per minute (lpm) × minutes per hour (60) × hours of use (?) =
Total liters of oxygen used per "use day"

Total Cubic Feet Used per Day:
Equation B:

$$\frac{\text{Total liters of oxygen used}}{28.3 \text{ (factor to convert liters to cubic feet)}} = \text{Total number of cubic feet used}$$

Total Number of "Use Days" per H-cylinder:
Equation C:

$$\frac{282 \text{ cu ft per each H cylinder}}{\text{Total number of cubic feet consumed per "use day"}} = \frac{\text{Number of use days}}{\text{per H-cylinder}}$$

Example B:
The pediatric patient at home requiring one quarter liter per minute on a continuous (20 hour) basis will consume 300 L or 10.6 cu ft per one "use day."

Example A is that of an intermittent user and Example B is that of a low-volume continuous user. In both cases these patients consume relatively small amounts of oxygen. (For practical purposes throughout this chapter, the H-size cylinder, pressurized at 2400 psi and containing 7980 L [282 cu ft] of gas will be used.)

The patient in Example A would consume 4.5 H-cylinders of oxygen per month according to the calculations in Table 3–2. In actuality, six H-cylinders would have to be delivered to this patient's home per month to allow for variable factors encountered in oxygen use at home.

The pediatric patient in Example B is very well situated for oxygen administration by a CGC. By calculation one H-cylinder will last 26 "use days." This patient is not only a low-flow user but also a low-volume user. CGC in this instance would be the most economical oxygen system. A general industry rule-of-thumb states that when oxygen consumption via CGC meets or exceeds six H-cylinders per month, the oxygen concentrator then becomes most economical for the payor of services.

Factors to be considered when figuring a proper and safe level of oxygen in the home include:

1. Delivering another cylinder before the initial cylinder is com-
pletely empty. On the basis of personal experience, we recommend replenishing the cylinder while there is a volume of at least 1.5 "use days" remaining.

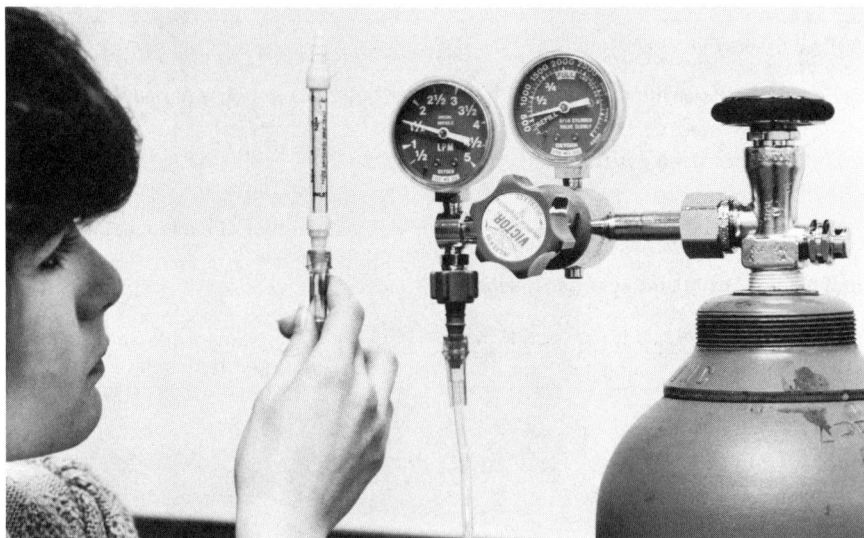

Figure 3–1. Regulator being checked for accuracy with simple flow-checker device before being sent to patient's home.

2. Not all flow-metering devices are accurate as to the exact liter flow. All flowmeters should be checked and calibrated before leaving the service center (Fig 3–1). Even new regulators and flow-metering devices can be severely off calibration right out of the box.
3. There will be some measurable difference in the liter-flow setting every time the flowmeter is used and readjusted by the patient. It cannot be assumed that every individual manipulating the flowmeter will return to the exact setting every time. This will result in varying durations of cylinder use and should be allowed for.
4. Delivery schedules are not etched in stone, and many things can occur on any given delivery day. Leeway should be allowed for these unforeseen occurrences, so the patient is never without oxygen.

The above factors influencing the duration of cylinder use and delivery schedule must be calculated into the initial month's usage. By calculating the consumption of gas volume per month, the supplier can give the patient a predetermined delivery schedule. This will minimize patient apprehension as to whether his or her oxygen will be delivered on time. The patient now knows that at certain times each week oxygen will be delivered. The patient can also plan the week if he or she knows in advance what days deliveries will occur. By predetermining gas use per month, the supplier will also be gaining an awareness of the patient's general compliance with the prescribed oxygen. The supplier also benefits by knowing that someone will be home for the delivery. In summary, patient education regarding the usage factors of the gas system coupled with well-planned routing by the oxygen delivery personnel will usually result in a prudent patient, free of apprehension.

A relatively low cost of CGCs for the payor of services does not always mean this service is the most economical for the supplier of such service. Many overhead factors enter into the cost of delivering an oxygen cylinder, such as the cost of delivery vehicle, its operating cost, including insurance, gas and oil, and maintenance, the wages and benefits of the home care technician, maintenance of regulators and flow-metering devices, wages and benefits of office personnel for processing and billing, and storage costs of cylinders on site, including demurrage, a fee paid per tank per month to the wholesaler for use of the cylinder. There are also the costs of miscellaneous items supplied with CGCs that are needed but not always charged for, e.g., cannulas, humidifiers, extension tubing, etc. Table 3–3 shows a sample cost calculation.

An advantage to CGCs is for long-term storage and intermittent use. An example of long-term storage would be as the emergency backup cylinder used in conjunction with the electrically operated oxygen concentrator. CGCs may also be required as an emergency power source for a pneumatically powered standby mechanical ventilator in the home.

The smaller E-size CGC used as a portable source of oxygen outside the home is an example of intermittent use and storage. It is favored for the patient leaving the home for only brief periods.

A CGC can also be used in the home as 50-psi pressure source for the application of certain mechanical ventilators. Today those usages would probably be limited to the standby ventilator or as a backup bank of reserve oxygen for the extremely high-volume user on a ventilator (*see* Chapter 8).

The other major advantage to using CGCs is that they are not electrically operated. The patient is almost always financially responsible for the increases in electrical consumption produced by the in-home medical equipment (exceptions are very rare). The fact that CGCs are not electrically operated allows them to be used in regions experiencing frequent power outages or that are without electric power completely.

Disadvantages. The disadvantages of CGC in the home are listed in Table 3–1. An obvious disadvantage to having large oxygen cylinders in the home is that they must be secured from falling. The methods used to ensure safety of persons and possessions in the home from the damage that may occur if they fall adds to the unpleasant appearance of the cylinder itself in the individual's home.

TABLE 3–3. COST ASSOCIATED WITH DELIVERING ONE H-CYLINDER*

Administrative Costs (Costs involved in processing the order):

Wages: for 2 min at $6.00/h	$0.20
Miscellaneous: paper, rent, electricity, etc.	0.05
	Total $0.25

Cylinder Costs (Costs involved with filling, delivery, and demurrage):

Delivery to vendor for one H-cylinder	$0.50
Cost of oxygen per 282 cu ft	3.50
Rental (demurrage) of H-cylinder per week	0.63
	Total $4.63

Delivery Costs (Labor, gasoline, and vehicular maintenance):

Labor for half an hour	$ 4.35
Gasoline for 10 miles	0.91
Vehicular costs	
Monthly payments	254.35/mo
Oil change and lubrication	26.00/mo
Depreciation	170.00/mo
Misc (wash, repairs, fluids)	25.00/mo
	Subtotal $475.35/mo
10 miles = 0.004% of monthly travel; 0.004% × $475.35	$ 1.90

Thus

Administrative costs	$ 0.25
Cylinder costs	4.63
Delivery costs	5.26
Vehicular costs	1.90
Total	**$12.04**
Final cost:	**$12.04**

*These figures are estimates of what it costs Northcoast Oxygen Company, Inc., in Cleveland, Ohio, to deliver one H-cylinder to one patient, including return trip to service center. Obviously these costs will vary from company to company, but the major factors involved in getting the cylinder to the patient's home have been included.

Basic assumptions made to arrive at the costs listed are:

1. Each stop will take $\frac{1}{2}$ hour
2. Allowance of 10 mi round trip travel for one delivery
3. Assume the delivery vehicle attains 12 miles per gallon fully loaded
4. Gas prices reflect $1.10 per gallon
5. The full tanks are delivered to the service center from the manufacturer at $10.00 per delivery and 20 tanks per delivery
6. The truck travels approximately 2500 miles per month

A cylinder stand is most commonly employed to secure the cylinders; these come in many sizes and shapes. One consideration when choosing a cylinder stand is a protective bottom. A bottom will protect the patient's floor from the dirt, rust, or melting snow that will inevitably be found on the cylinder bottom (Fig 3–2).

Many patients prefer to fabricate their own securing devices. If this is the case, we generally require the individual to place chain holders or eyebolts into the wall studs to ensure maximum strength. This way the chain or securing strap can be pulled tight without damaging the wall.

A second disadvantage to the use of CGC is that of waste and resultant

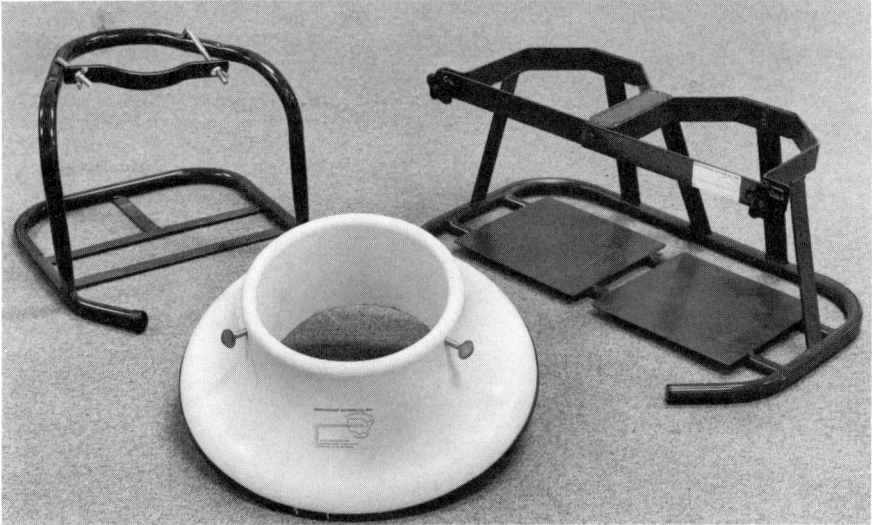

Figure 3–2. Various types of large cylinder stands that are used in the home.

additional expense if the cylinders are not operated properly. Because of their silent operation, patients may forget to turn the cylinder off when it is not in use, only to find it empty when they are ready to use it again. Children must be instructed not to play with the cylinder valves and flowmeters for the same reason.

A relatively serious disadvantage of placing CGCs in the home is the obvious need to have them replaced on a regular basis. Many patients confined to the home worry about running out of oxygen. Much of their time is spent watching the pressure gauge and "metering out" oxygen sparingly, so they do not run out. This adds to the stress and anxiety of the entire disease state.

The anxiety and apprehension relating to the delivery of oxygen should be minimized or alleviated by the supplier if at all possible. The additional emotional stress can be so significant with some patients who "watch their oxygen" that changing to another system may be justified.

The disadvantage of the H-cylinder's size truly relegates it to a stationary role in the home. A height of 55 in, a width of 9 in, a weight of 165 lb when full, and the fact that it is chained to the wall mean the H-cylinder is not portable from room to room. This means the cylinder must be placed in a centralized area of the home, which may not be desirable for the patient or family, or may mean that unwieldy oxygen connecting tubing must be used.

The other major disadvantage to CGCs in the home are the difficulties of operation imposed on the blind or physically handicapped patient. It

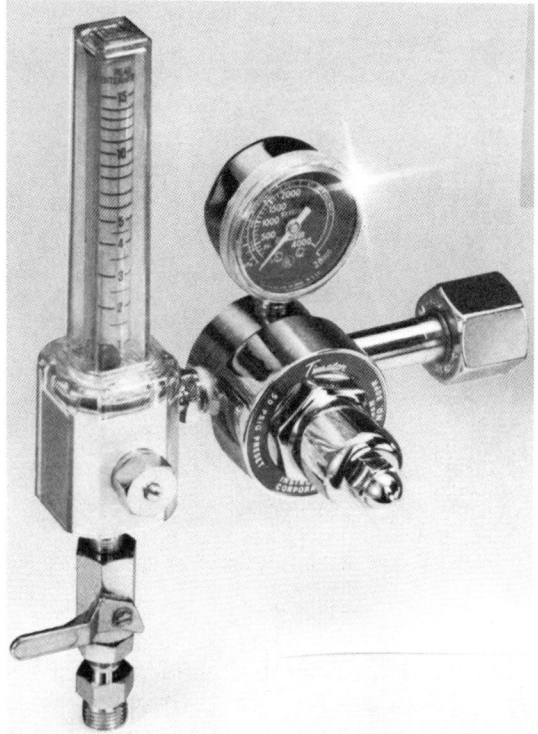

Figure 3–3. Example of a locking flowmeter with lever activation for use with the blind or physically handicapped oxygen-dependent patient.

is much easier to push the on-off switch on the oxygen concentrator than to manipulate a cylinder valve and flow control. If a cylinder must be used for the blind or manually handicapped patient, a locking flowmeter and lever-operating regulator should be employed (Fig 3–3).

Oxygen Concentrators

A second, and probably the most popular, oxygen delivery system for home use is the OC. The OC has many advantages and disadvantages for the patient, but there are advantages for the supplier, also, that contribute to its immense popularity.

The points that make the concentrator attractive for the equipment supplier include:

1. The rate of reimbursement relative to degree of service required is higher than with CGC or LOX.
2. Specially equipped delivery vehicles are not necessary for delivery of the unit.
3. Practically every portion of the oxygen concentrator is replaceable, therefore allowing many years of service in return for a comparatively small purchase price.

When the costs of service and delivery of the oxygen cylinder and liquid oxygen vessel are compared to those of the oxygen concentrator, the oxygen concentrator is by far the greatest profit generator.

The modern OC can be delivered by one person, in a car if necessary. The improved assembling techniques, volume of production by the manufacturers, and level of technology have just about halved the cost of the concentrator for the supplier in past years. During those same years, however, the rental rates and rates of reimbursement for this device have steadily increased, which can only translate to greater profit margins for this inexpensive modality for administering oxygen.

The popularity of this unit has increased in this country year after year. The OC affords the patients in their home and those traveling about the country many benefits (*see* Table 3–4). These are detailed below.

TABLE 3–4. ADVANTAGES AND DISADVANTAGES ASSOCIATED WITH THE USE OF THE OXYGEN CONCENTRATOR

Advantages	Disadvantages
1. Uninterrupted continuous use	1. Higher cost per month for intermittent oxygen user*
2. Easily manipulated by the blind and/or handicapped user	2. Not designed for greater than ambient pressure applications (e.g., driving a pneumatically powered ventilator, oxygen source for Venturi masks)
3. No regular deliveries required	3. Not designed for high-flow applications (i.e., greater than 4 lpm, depending upon model and manufacturer)
4. Relatively pleasing appearance	4. Condensation and accumulation of water in long delivery tubing
5. Low-pressure system	5. Loss of oxygen supply associated with electrical power failure
6. Relatively mobile within the home	6. Noisy
7. Easily placed in the car, making travel much easier	7. Generation and expulsion of heat
	8. Increased operational costs resulting from increased electrical power consumption for the user
	9. Occurrence of subtle internal malfunctions that can dramatically reduce oxygen concentration without patient's awareness

*Recent changes in the reimbursement guidelines from Medicare have broken down the usage of the concentrator to cubic feet used per month as stated on the physician prescription. Concentrators are now reimbursed according to their relative rates of use, not on a single rental price per month as in the past.

Advantages. The OC offers the patient almost uninterrupted continuous use of oxygen without the fear of running empty and without the disadvantages associated with regular deliveries. The blind and/or handicapped patient can easily manipulate the OC. By presetting the flow rate and combining the use of prefilled humidifiers, which need not be disassembled, cleaned, and reused, the delivery of oxygen to this patient group is almost trouble-free.

Important to mention at this time is the delivery of low-flow oxygen without humidification altogether, for the ease and convenience of the blind or handicapped patient. This method of delivering oxygen without supplemental humidity has been supported by The American College of Chest Physicians (ACCP) and others (American College of Chest Physicians, 1984; Lasky, 1982). Receiving low-flow oxygen in this manner, the patient has no humidifier to care for, which dramatically simplifies oxygen delivery in the home. Not only does the patient save money on cleaning solutions, but a major problem-producing area in the treatment has been eliminated. The humidifier is no longer a source of oxygen leaks or pressure-relief valves that stick open and allow gas to escape to the atmosphere without indication. One drawback to delivering oxygen without the humidifier is that the audible pressure-relief valve has been eliminated: When present this provides a useful indication to the patient if the connecting tubing is blocked or crimped. The water-filled humidifier can also be used as a crude visual indicator of oxygen flow through the system. Therefore deletion of the humidifier also removes the pressure relief valve and visual indication of flow. A unique device called the Flow Alert that has recently appeared on the market allows a pressure-relief indicator and a visual flow indicator on an oxygen delivery system to be used without a humidifier (Fig 3–4).

The OC obviously requires no regular deliveries. The anxiety associated with running out of oxygen is minimized for the patient. The OC should be set up in the patient's home with an emergency backup cylinder for use in the event of electrical power failure or mechanical breakdown of the unit. Ideally, the OC in the home should be associated with oxygen use throughout the major portion of the day (14 to 24 hours). The insurance dollar is most effectively spent when the OC is used in this manner. If the patient requires oxygen through the major portion of the day, the backup oxygen cylinder should be supplied with the OC. The oxygen cylinder supplied should offer the patient a minimum of 24 hours use at the prescribed liter flow.

Example:
The patient is going to bed at 10 PM and the OC has malfunctioned; now the patient is without oxygen during the most important period of the day (Nocturnal Oxygen Therapy Trial Group, 1980). The patient now calls the oxygen supplier and must wait until either a replacement OC or backup cylinder is

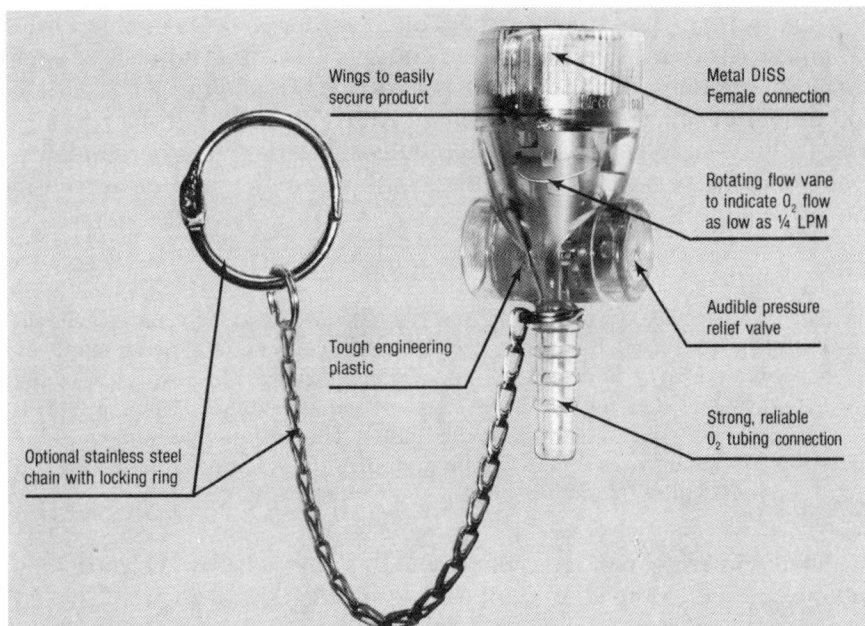

Figure 3–4. The Flow Alert pressure relief valve and visual flow indicator for use on oxygen delivery systems without humidifiers. *(Courtesy of Precision Medical, Bath, Pa.)*

delivered. This action has again produced anxiety and frustration for the patient as well as the supplier. The cost of delivering that backup cylinder probably would be more than if the supplier had left one on the initial setup for use in an emergency such as this (*see* Table 3–3).

Since the patient was not at fault in this situation associated with a mechanical breakdown, no service charge should have been involved. Thus the supplier suffers a financial loss and the patient an avoidable emotional upset. These problems can be avoided by placing the backup cylinder at the time of setup.

The distance the patient lives from the supplier, coupled with the prescribed rate of use, will determine the size of the backup cylinder supplied.

Another advantage associated with the OC is its pleasing appearance in the home. Many patients have refused to use oxygen because the oxygen cylinders are "ugly," disrupt the decor of the home, and provide obvious signs of oxygen being in the home, which is a constant reminder of disability to patient and visitor. Many people express greater fear of explosion with the presence of cylinders than with any other oxygen supply system in the home.

It is our policy to briefly discuss all oxygen systems available to the patient briefly and to present the advantages and disadvantages of each during the initial setup and instruction period. This informs the patient and family of other modes of oxygen delivery in the event the patient's needs or physical condition change, requiring the use of another modality. This policy may at times hinder the most economical use of oxygen in the home.

> ***Example:***
> The supplier and referral sources may have already decided the patient should use cylinders for nocturnal use only. This particular patient, being relatively affluent and living in one of the "nicer" neighborhoods in town, refuses the cylinders and opts for the OC because of the appearance. The supplier in this case really has no choice in the matter. This is a private home and the supplier cannot force a situation on an individual who does not want it and ultimately will not comply with it.

Many times the aesthetics of the OC are of great benefit because they enhance patient compliance with the prescription. Knowing that the oxygen source will not run out and because the OC appears more like a piece of furniture than a torpedo, the patient is more likely to use it.

The fact that the OC is a low-pressure delivery system (*see* Chapter 2) can be viewed as an advantage. If the concentrator is accidentally mishandled, abused, or frequently placed in the car for travel, the worst that can happen is that its casing will break or dent or the unit will become nonfunctional. The oxygen cylinders must be handled and transported with much more care and consciousness of what one is doing. We are all familiar with the "missile" hazard caused by high pressure, if the cylinder valve is damaged or broken off.

The OC is very light in comparision with the stationary oxygen cylinder (*see* Chapter 2) and the OC usually incorporates wheels or casters, which allow ease of mobility within the home. This is an advantage for many people who cannot tolerate sleeping with the continuous noise and heat generated by the OC at the bedside. Patients can easily place the OC in the hallway or spare room close to the bedroom, or whatever room they please.

The size, weight, and compactness of the OC make relatively short driving trips much easier for the patient. The OC can be safely packed in the trunk or backseat and used in a motel or relatives' home upon arrival. An E-size portable cylinder, if needed during the drive, can allow up to five hours' oxygen supply at 2 lpm. The E-size cylinder can be refilled by a supplier at the destination for the trip home.

Disadvantages. As widely used as the OC is today, it is not suitable for every patient and, like each oxygen delivery system, it has inherent disadvantages (*see* Table 3–4).

The first disadvantage here is the cost for the intermittent user and his or her insurance carrier. The issue of cost is a difficult subject to approach at this time. The Health Care Finance Administration (HCFA) and Medicare are changing reimbursement guidelines for all home care equipment very rapidly. It is not within the scope of this book to give adequate guidelines on this volatile issue. At present HCFA and Medicare are providing more equitable reimbursement schedules for all types of oxygen systems and respiratory care equipment than ever before. Until October 1985, the standard monthly rental rate for a concentrator was reimbursed no matter what the patient's use was. Since then, HFCA, along with Medicare, has tightened these guidelines and broken down the reimbursement rate to coincide with the cubic feet used per month as prescribed by the physician. The reader should keep abreast of Medicare changes in his or her area.

The OC is not designed for use in pressure applications in excess of ambient pressure. Most OCs today do incorporate pressure-compensated flowmeters, although that pressure compensation is calibrated to the unit's driving pressure, which is usually in the range of 4 to 10 psi. Any significant downstream resistance will severely affect the flow rate capabilities of the unit. The OC is not suitable for use with Venturi masks and oxygen supply sources for pneumatically powered ventilators, etc. The OC can be applied as an oxygen source for ventilators if used as a downstream bleed-in source for oxygen.

The OC also cannot deliver oxygen in the 90% range in excess of 4 lpm. (Depending upon manufacturer and model, some cannot supply 90% oxygen in excess of 2 lpm.)

The addition of long oxygen extension tubing, usually in the range of 14 ft to 50 ft, will result in humidity condensation and annoying accumulation of water in the tubing. This is due to the ambient air being drawn in and compressed by an air compressor within the unit. When the air is compressed, its temperature increases above ambient. As this warmer-than-room-temperature gas passes through the humidifier it holds more water vapor than the surrounding room temperature air. As this warmer saturated gas passes through the oxygen extension tubing (usually lying on the floor) it cools to room temperature and the dew point temperature is reached. This allows the excess water vapor to condense and accumulate in the tubing. The patient should always be made aware of this consequence so he or she may take action to correct it and not feel the OC is malfunctioning. This author generally instructs the patient to empty the humidifier and continue to use the OC as always and the dry gas will eventually evaporate the water in the tubing; then the humidifier should be refilled and used as directed. Other solutions to this problem include shortening the extension tubing—but this hampers mobility within the home—and placing the long extension tubing between the outlet of the concentrator and the humidifier, then attaching only the nasal cannula to the humidifier (Fig 3–5).

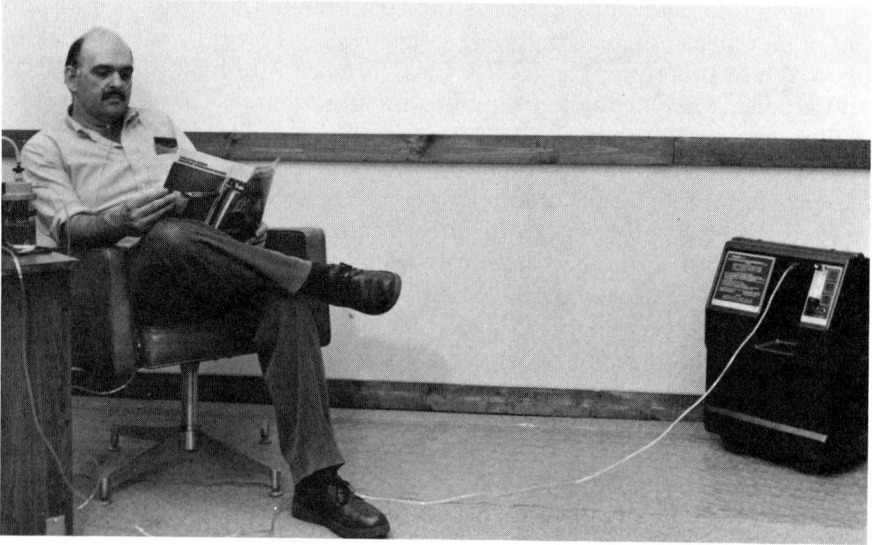

Figure 3–5. Keeping the humidifier close to patient may prevent annoying water accumulation in the connecting tubing when an oxygen concentrator is used.

The OC will obviously not function in the event of electrical power failure. In households where this occurs frequently the OC may not be the system of choice.

The increased cost to the patient as a result of electrical consumption should also be considered when choosing the appropriate oxygen delivery system. As a rule the insurance carrier will not pay for the increase in the patient's electric bill. The electric supply company usually does not offer financial aid here either. The patient is almost always responsible for the increased electrical cost of operating the OC and should be made aware of this at the time of setup.

In the greater Cleveland area, the patient using his or her OC on a continuous basis (20 h/day) can expect an approximate 20-dollar-per-month increase in his or her electric bill (Table 3–5).

Oxygen Enricher

The close cousin to the OC is the oxygen enricher, which has not enjoyed the same popularity as the OC (OECO, 1984).

The oxygen enricher (OE) employs a permeable membrane to separate and also concentrate the oxygen molecules, thus increasing the oxygen concentration in the gas exiting the unit (*see* Chapter 2). The OC provides oxygen concentration in excess of 90% to 96% throughout its range of applicable flow rates, unlike the OE. The OE provides a constant oxygen concentration of 40% throughout its range of flow rate capabilities.

TABLE 3–5. FORMULA FOR ELECTRICAL CONSUMPTION COST WITH USE OF AN OXYGEN CONCENTRATOR

Hours per month unit is used	×	Kilowatts per hour unit consumes	×	Cost per kilowatt hour	=	Total operational cost per month

Example: Mr Smith uses his oxygen concentrator continuously (20 h/day/30 days/mo). He is using the Devilbiss DeVo/44 concentrator that consumes 375 watts per hour (0.375 kW per hour), and his cost per kilowatt hour is 9 cents.*

(20 h/day × 30 days/mo) = 600 h/mo

600 h/mo × 0.375 kW/h × $0.09/kW hour = $20.25

*The simplest method in determining cost per kilowatt hour is to take the electric bill and divide the total cost by the total number of kilowatt hours consumed for that month.

The OE is based on the theory that if 1 lpm of 100% oxygen produces an expected rise in arterial oxygen tension, then 3 lpm of 40% oxygen should produce similar results. In other words, the patient receiving three to four times the liter flow of 40% oxygen should receive the equivalent inspired oxygen concentration that would normally be expected with 1 to 2 lpm of 100% oxygen. This is true to a degree.

Consider the following patient parameters:

Tidal volume (V_T)	500 ml
Respiratory rate (RR)	20 per minute
Inspiratory time (T_I)	1 second
Expiratory time (T_E)	2 seconds
Anatomic reservoir volume	50 ml

Assume a nasal cannula with an oxygen flow rate of 2 lpm or 33 ml/s and 100% oxygen. Specifically, how will this oxygen be utilized during ventilation to produce a given inspired oxygen percentage?

During the "static flow" period of exhalation (the final 0.5 seconds of exhalation) the anatomic reservoir, consisting of nose, nasopharynx, and oropharynx, will fill with 16.5 ml of 100% oxygen. The inspiratory time is 1 second; therefore the flow rate from the cannula will provide 33 ml of 100% oxygen. The remainder of the inspired gas volume is 450.5 ml of room air, which contains 21% oxygen. This will result in the inspiration of 94.5 ml of 100% oxygen from the room air (0.21 × 450.5).

Taking these figures we can calculate the following:

16.5 ml of 100% oxygen in the anatomic reservoir

33 ml of 100% oxygen from the cannula flow rate

94.5 ml of 100% oxygen from the room air

EQUALS

$$\frac{144 \text{ ml of } 100\% \text{ oxygen}}{500 \text{ ml of total inspired gas volume}} = 28.8\% \text{ or } 29\% \text{ oxygen}$$

If we assume the same patient parameters but double the flow rate to 4 lpm or 66 ml/s of 40% oxygen from the OE we will calculate the following inspired oxygen concentration.

During the static flow period of expiration, the anatomic reservoir will accumulate 33 ml of 40% oxygen. (This volume is 33 ml because the static flow period is 0.5 seconds.) The inspiratory time is 1 second; therefore 66 ml of 40% oxygen will be inspired. The remainder of the inspired gas volume is 401 ml of room air containing 21% oxygen. This calculation now changes slightly because we must convert the following 40% oxygen volumes to 100% oxygen volumes.

$$\begin{array}{ccc} \text{33 ml of 40\% oxygen} \\ \text{in anatomic reservoir} \end{array} \text{ becomes } \begin{array}{c} \text{13 ml of} \\ \text{100\% oxygen} \end{array} = 0.40 \times 33 \text{ ml} \\ = 13 \text{ ml}$$

$$\begin{array}{ccc} \text{66 ml of 40\% oxygen} \\ \text{from cannula flow rate} \end{array} \text{ becomes } \begin{array}{c} \text{26 ml of} \\ \text{100\% oxygen} \end{array} = 0.40 \times 66 \text{ ml} \\ = 26 \text{ ml}$$

THUS

13 ml of 100% oxygen in anatomic reservoir
26 ml of 100% oxygen from cannula flow rate
84 ml of 100% oxygen from inspired room air

EQUALS

$$\frac{123 \text{ ml of 100\% oxygen}}{500 \text{ ml of total gas volume}} = 24–24.5\% \text{ oxygen}$$

The operating concept of the OE demonstrates that to some degree higher flow rates of 40% oxygen can produce similar results to those of the OC. That degree ends at 8 lpm of 40% oxygen, which will attain approximately 29% to 30% inspired oxygen concentrations.

Many patients with COPD experience air hunger, dyspnea, and shortness of breath. Some patients at home have been observed to use fans to blow air into their faces. This air flow somewhat relieves the feelings of air hunger and shortness of breath. This is also a reason why many patients request or attempt to turn up their oxygen flow rates in the hospital. The Venturi mask also relieves the described sensations because of its high-flow functions.

This is one benefit derived from the OE, the higher flow rates without the corresponding high oxygen concentrations.

The membrane separation principle of the OE also allows water vapor to pass through, thereby eliminating the need for the typical bubble-type humidifier. Carbon dioxide also crosses the membrane and is concentrated from the 0.03% found in the atmosphere to approximately 0.12%.

This concentration is not significant enough to cause concern or to contribute to further hypercapnia.

The OC and, to a much lesser extent, the OE have revolutionized oxygen delivery in the private home. Continued technological advancements will probably enhance their popularity, and they will continue to be the mainstay of long-term home oxygen delivery systems. Although they do have a number of disadvantages, it must be repeated that no one delivery system is adequate for all patient applications.

Liquid Oxygen

This brings us to the third home oxygen delivery system, liquid oxygen. As with the cylinder and regulator, oxygen concentrator and oxygen enricher, the construction and function of the liquid vessels is detailed in Chapter 2.

LOX has only recently been applied widely in the home marketplace. It is our belief that a number of new trends in medicine have been responsible for the greater use of LOX in the home. These major trends include:

1. Rapidly growing emphasis on cardiac and pulmonary rehabilitation.
2. A new emphasis on patient mobility, travel, and the maintenance of the individual's postdischarge social life.
3. The introduction of federal legislation responsible for the hospital-based diagnosis-related group (DRG) system. This system is ultimately sending patients home earlier, sicker, requiring the use of relatively high oxygen flow rates during treatment at home.

As with the other home oxygen-delivery systems, LOX also has advantages and disadvantages (Table 3–6).

TABLE 3–6. ADVANTAGES AND DISADVANTAGES ASSOCIATED WITH LIQUID OXYGEN (LOX) SYSTEMS IN THE HOME

Advantages	Disadvantages
1. The system of choice for the continuous *high-volume* user	1. Oxygen waste and additional expense incurred as a result of evaporative losses if not used on a nearly continuous basis
2. Ability of active patient outside the home to fill his or her own portable system	2. Regular deliveries are required
3. No electrical operation	3. Personal injury may occur from handling of extremely cold transfilling fittings by patients or home care personnel
4. Large-volume capacity in small space	
5. Capable of being used in a wide range of pressure applications	

Advantages. The variety of volume measurements of liquid oxygen can be confusing. Liquid oxygen volume can be expressed as pounds, gallons, liquid liters, gaseous liters, liquid cubic feet, gaseous cubic feet, etc. For purposes of our discussion, pounds, liquid liters, and gaseous cubic feet will be used. Table 3–7 on pages 78 and 79 is an oxygen conversion chart.

The concept of high-volume oxygen use has been discussed earlier in this chapter.

LOX is best suited for the high-volume oxygen user for a number of reasons:

1. The oxygen concentrator cannot provide high flow rates (in excess of 4 to 5 lpm); the newest liquid vessels can, if necessary, provide flow rates up to 10 lpm.
2. Less-frequent deliveries are made to the patient using LOX than for CGCs because of the LOX reservoir's large-volume capacity. For example, the Cryo$_2$ Corporation's Grandeair II Model is a stationary liquid vessel for the home with a cylinder. The total full weight of this reservoir is 140 lb; 93 lb is LOX. The height of the vessel is 33 in and its diameter is 16 in (Cryo$_2$ Corporation). If the LOX were converted to gaseous liters, it would provide 31,908 L. This is comparable to the volume of four H-size cylinders, which, with manifolds, would occupy approximately 62 in or slightly more than 5 ft of wall space in the patient's home. The four H-cylinders would weigh approximately 660 lb.
3. LOX should be used on a continuous basis for optimal economical operation because of the evaporative losses experienced during nonuse.

The second advantage to using LOX is that it permits the active patient to remain active outside the home. When this patient wishes to leave home to socialize or simply to mow the lawn, the patient can fill his or her own portable from the stationary unit. If this patient were using a concentrator or oxygen cylinders, the supplier would need to deliver a portable CGC (or a number of portables) to last the patient for the week. If more than one portable CGC is delivered, the patient must change the regulator from cylinder to cylinder as each one empties; whereas the patient using LOX can fill the portable at will and go. The patient does not have to wait for delivery, store a number of portable cylinders in the home, or change regulators from tank to tank. (Liquid portable units do not incorporate insulating material as do the stationary units. Therefore, this author generally instructs the patient to use the portable until it is empty before switching back to the stationary reservoir. An average figure to consider when speaking of normal evaporative losses can be approximately 0.055 lb/hr. This means that a portable unit containing 2.5 lb of LOX will lose approximately one half pound of liquid oxygen for each nine-hour period of nonuse.)

The ease of using the LOX portable may also improve the patients' compliance in using oxygen. The LOX portable is smaller, lighter, less conspicuous, and offers greater longevity than any other compressed gas portable. These characteristics, along with its ease of use, may be responsible for patients using their oxygen for longer periods and maintaining a level of activity outside the home that they might not otherwise achieve.

The person who wishes to maintain his or her social travel and personal activities outside the home while using oxygen is one of the prime candidates for LOX whether the patient is a high-volume user or not. Even the low-volume user, 1 lpm or less continuously, who wishes to maintain outside activities should be placed on LOX. Another advantage of LOX, as with the CGC, is that it does not require electrical operation, which can further add to the patient's out-of-pocket expense for this medical treatment at home.

LOX can be adapted and used as the primary oxygen source for high-volume oxygen users on mechanical ventilators. The advantage here again is the large-volume capacity in a relatively small space, along with the possibility of attaining 50 psi (or greater) driving pressures either for powering the ventilator itself or, more commonly, supplying the air-oxygen blender within the ventilator at a 50-psi source pressure (e.g., the MA–1 ventilator by Puritan-Bennett or the PLV–102 home ventilator by LIFECARE, both requiring 50-psi oxygen inlet pressures).

A typical large Dewar (pronounced doer) used by the home care company to fill the patient's stationary liquid vessels in the home can be adapted as the primary oxygen source for this high-volume user on the ventilator. This Dewar, assuming it contains 180 L of liquid oxygen, will supply 154,800 L of gaseous oxygen for this patient's application (the equivalent of 19 H-cylinders) (Fig 3–6).

This method of oxygen supply can also be used by other patients requiring extremely high-volume oxygen use. These patients require flow rates in the range of 6 to 8 lpm or higher for long periods of time (e.g., Venturi masks, simple oxygen masks, pediatric or adult mist tents requiring relatively high oxygen concentrations, etc.).

Disadvantages. The primary disadvantage to LOX use in the home is costly waste (*see* Table 3–6). The liquid oxygen vessels are designed to be used. If they are not used on a nearly continuous basis (greater than 14 to 16 hours per day) the wasteful evaporative losses will add to the overall cost of providing oxygen in the home. No one benefits from the evaporative losses, but someone pays for it. Let us assume the patient has been placed on LOX at 2 lpm and only uses it 12 hours per day. The manufacturer states that the normal evaporative loss from the patient's vessel is 0.062 lb per hour at 70°F during nonuse. This is equivalent to losing 254 gaseous liters during the 12 hours that the patient is not using

TABLE 3–7. OXYGEN CONVERSION FACTORS

	Liters Gas NTP	Cubic Feet Gas NTP	Pounds	Grams	Liters Liquid NBP	Cubic Feet Liquid NBP	Gallons Liquid NBP
				Quantities*			
Liters gas NTP	1	0.0353	0.002924	1.327	0.00116	0.000041	0.000307
Cubic feet gas NTP	28.317	1	0.0828	37.558	0.0329	0.00116	0.00869
Pounds	342.07	12.08	1	454	0.397	0.01403	0.105
Grams	0.753	0.0266	0.002205	1	0.000874	0.0000309	0.000231
Liters liquid NBP	860.94	30.40	2.517	1143	1	0.0353	0.264
Cubic feet liquid NBP	24379	860.94	71.27	32357	28.317	1	7.48
Gallons liquid NBP	3258	115.1	9.527	0.02098	3.788	0.1337	1

Gaseous Flow Rates (NTP)	Pounds/Hour	Liters/Minute	Cubic Feet/Minute
Pounds/hour	1	5.7	14.35
Liters/minute	0.175	1	0.0353
Cubic feet/minute	4.968	28.317	1

Equivalent Liter/Minute Gas Use Rate and Pounds Oxygen/Hour

Liter/Minute Flow Rate	Pounds of Oxygen/Hour
1	0.175
1½	0.263
2	0.351
2½	0.439
3	0.526
4	0.702
5	0.877
6	1.05
7	1.23
8	1.40

*NBP = Normal boiling point (−297.3°F); NTP = Normal temperature and pressure (70°F & 14.7 psia).

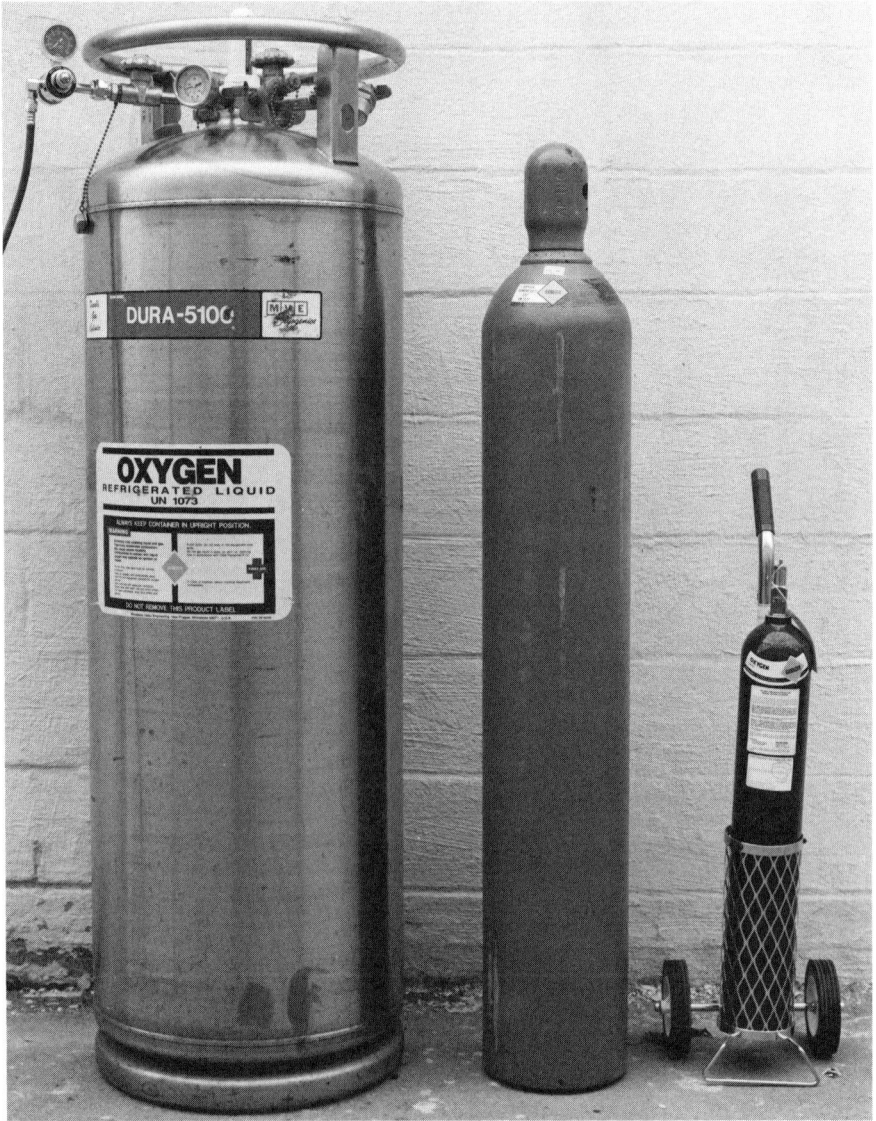

Figure 3–6. A comparison view from left to right of a 180-L liquid vessel and an H-cylinder and E-cylinder. This liquid vessel can, at times, be used at the patient's home for oxygen delivery for high-volume uses.

it. In one month the evaporative loss will equal at least 7,633 gaseous liters, or the approximate equivalent of 1 H-cylinder per month, 12 per year. This may not seem like too much but consider these figures:

$$7{,}633 \text{ gaseous liters} = 22.3 \text{ lb of LOX}$$

$$22.3 \text{ lb of LOX at } \$1.25 \text{ per pound} = \$28/\text{mo}$$

$28 per month $\times$ 12 months = $336/patient/yr

$336 $\times$ 50,000 hypothetical patients in the USA = $16,800,000/yr

That is almost 17 million dollars per year!

The evaporative losses associated with nonuse are compounded by the gaseous waste that occurs during filling of the stationary vessel by the home care supplier and those wastes produced by filling of the portable by the patient. (These losses or wastes are unavoidable, however.)

The second major disadvantage to LOX is that regular deliveries must be made. The hazards associated with delivery schedules and the patient's fear of running out of oxygen are the same as those mentioned in the discussion of CGC.

The last major disadvantage to using LOX in the home is one of personal injury that may occur through accidental handling of the extremely cold filling connections by the patient during transfilling of the portable. This thermal "burn" produces tissue damage similar to that experienced with frostbite. The difference is that it occurs much faster. This can be avoided with proper patient instruction. This author has never had a patient experience this hazard during six years of experience.

After determining which oxygen storage and delivery system is best suited for the patient's environment, physical condition, and prescription, we must now consider how to optimize the patient's use of the oxygen.

MANAGEMENT OF PATIENT AND OXYGEN SYSTEM TO PROVIDE FOR OPTIMAL BENEFIT

The best place to start is at the beginning, during the predischarge period. It is at this time, in the hospital, when the patient has been determined to need long-term oxygen use at home, that training begins. This educational process must also include the family. Teaching the patient and family early will make their home experience with oxygen more beneficial. During the predischarge period coverage of certain important topics can make this hospital-to-home transition easier. These topics should include:

- Description of disease process: how the disease was acquired and basic pathophysiology.
- Instructions on self-care and environmental hazards to avoid.
- How oxygen use will improve personal performance, and what basic physiologic changes occur with oxygen use as prescribed.
- Providing actual home equipment in the hospital for patient and family instruction and use before discharge.
- Encouragement of outside activities and continuation of social life.
- Maintenance of patient's self-image.
- Psychologic evaluation of patient and interfamily relationships.

- Predischarge insurance verification for the home-going equipment and services. Patient and family informed of out-of-pocket expenses before discharge.

Coverage of this basic information in the hospital can alleviate much of the stress, anxiety, and frustration of the discharge period. The patient and family have time to plan for the changes about to occur in their life styles. Many of the surprises are taken out of that initial discharge period. Consider how the patient sees oxygen therapy in the hospital. Oxygen therapy in the patient's eyes consists of a flowmeter in the wall and a length of oxygen tubing. Oxygen therapy at home is obviously much different and can be distressing, if not overwhelming, initially. The groundwork for noncompliance with ordered therapy should not be laid on the day of discharge! If the patient and family are prepared before discharge, compliance with oxygen therapy at home will probably improve. This subject will be covered in greater detail in Chapter 7.

There has been a technological explosion related to the home health care market. Every piece of home health care equipment has either been improved or "reinvented" in the past 5 years. New equipment types and procedures are being introduced each month. Many of these advances have directly improved the quality and function of home oxygen therapy systems.

The technological advances responsible for improving home oxygen therapy equipment and procedures can also be viewed as improving patient home care in many respects. The most outstanding improvements related to home oxygen therapy include:

- Oxygen-conserving devices and techniques.
- Compact, lightweight, aesthetically pleasing equipment.
- Equipment designed for travel or use away from 115-volt current availability.
- Equipment designed for patient use and patient understanding.

There is a myriad of equipment and procedures types that could be discussed in association with the above-mentioned improvements. To list and describe them all is well beyond the scope of this chapter. We believe the single most important determinant of quality home oxygen therapy and its availability to the huge patient population requiring it will be cost. The previously mentioned oxygen-conserving devices (OCD) and techniques deserve special attention.

Oxygen Conserving Devices and Related Techniques

The most notable OCDs and techniques on the market at present are:

1. The "pulsed dosing" method of delivering oxygen only during inspiration.
2. The reservoir nasal cannula.
3. Transtracheal oxygen therapy (TTOT).

Pulse Dosing. The principle of pulse-dosed oxygen is that of delivering oxygen during inspiration, thus reducing the waste of oxygen delivery during expiration.

One device available is a demand valve (demand oxygen controller, $Cryo_2$ Corporation) incorporated within a portable liquid oxygen reservoir called the Pulsair (*see* Fig 3–7). A fluidic sensor detects the initiation of inspiration by the patient through the nasal cannula and delivers a preset volume of oxygen. Conventional flow rate settings are marked on the device but only equivalent inspiratory "doses" of oxygen are delivered when used in the pulse mode.

Example:
When the device is set to deliver 1 lpm, approximately 17 ml is delivered during inspiration in the pulse mode, 2 lpm = approximately 35 ml, 3 lpm = approximately 51 ml, etc.

If the pulse mode fails, the patient has the option of switching the unit to the conventional continuous-flow mode. The most important factor to be considered with this device is a potential oxygen saving of 60% or greater over the conventional liquid oxygen portable. This translates to much smaller inconspicuous liquid portables that allow longer duration for the active patient outside the home. The major disadvantages to this system include: (1) technical complexity resulting in operational failures;

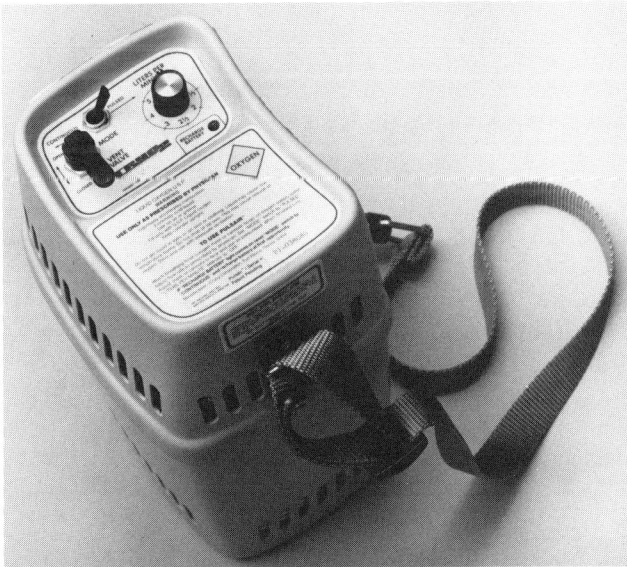

Figure 3–7. The Pulsair liquid portable, which provides "pulsed dose" oxygen administration during the inspiratory phase only. *(Courtesy of Cryo₂ Corporation, Fort Pierce, Fla.)*

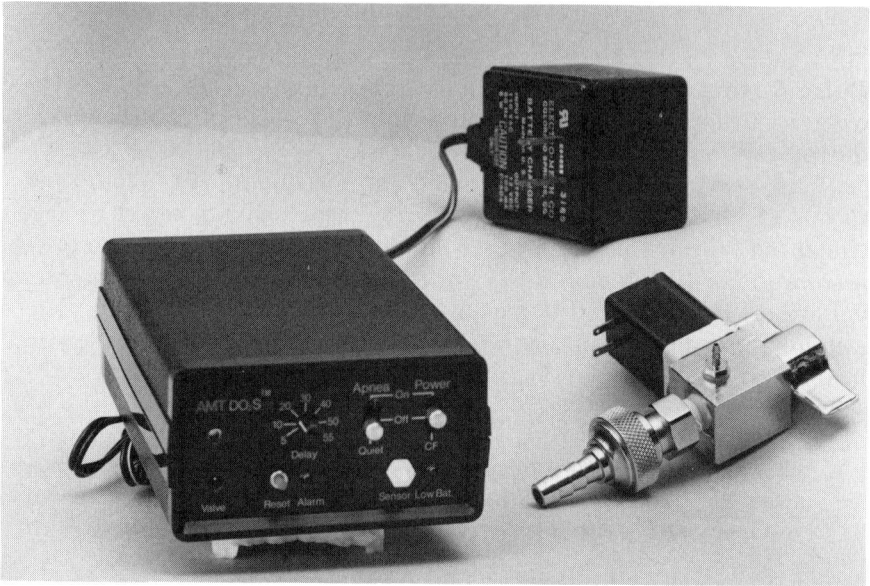

Figure 3–8. The DO$_2$S demand valve for use with any type oxygen portable system. *(Courtesy of Applied Membrane Technology, Inc, Minnetonka, Minn.)*

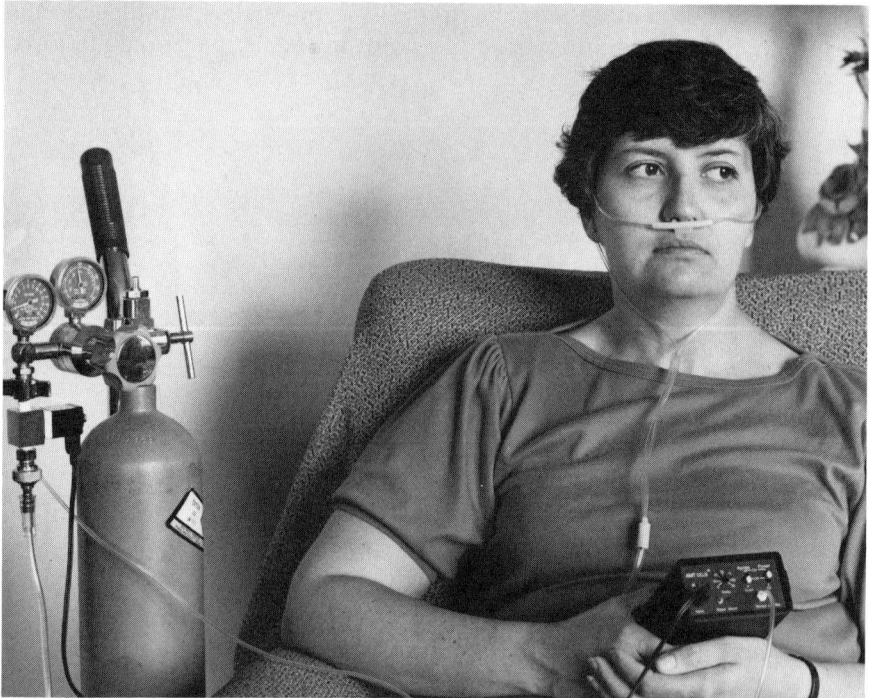

Figure 3–9. Patient using a self-contained demand valve which can be applied to any liquid oxygen or compressed gas portable unit.

(2) high initial costs, which would be offset in time with oxygen savings; and (3) the device is limited to use with the liquid portable unit only.

A second type of pulse dosing device is the self-contained demand oxygen saver system (DO_2S, Applied Membrane Technology, Inc.) (Fig 3–8).

The major difference associated with this device is that it can be attached to stationary oxygen-delivery vessels such as the CGC and the stationary LOX vessel as well as to their portable counterparts (Fig 3–9). This manufacturer claims a 50% to 75% oxygen savings. To date there is no pulse-dosing system that can be used with, or is incorporated within, an oxygen concentrator, but this is sure to change in the near future.

These devices are examples of the expanding technology that allows oxygen-dependent patients more freedom and ease of travel, all contributing to enhanced compliance with ordered therapy.

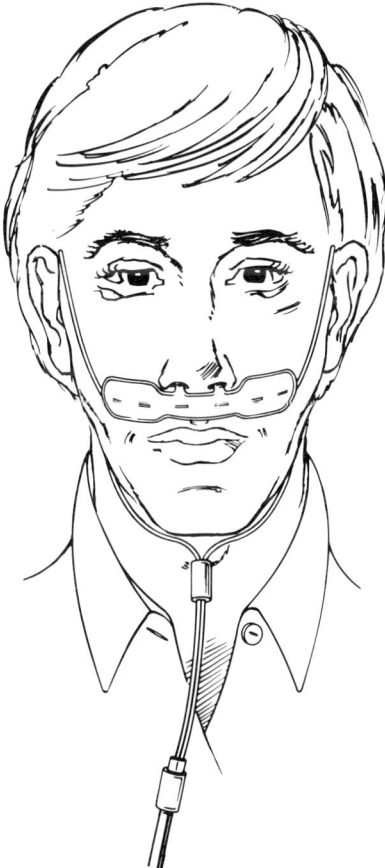

Figure 3–10. An oxygen-conserving device, the reservoir cannula.

Reservoir Nasal Cannula. A nasal cannula has been developed incorporating a reservoir space below the nose, which also minimizes oxygen waste during the expiratory phase (Oxymizer, Chad Therapeutics) (Fig 3–10).

The manufacturer claims a 50% oxygen savings with the use of this device. Its major disadvantage is the obvious presence of the reservoir on the face. Many patients object to its appearance; therefore the manufacturer also offers a pendant-style reservoir that hangs about the chest (Fig 3–11). The major advantage to this type of OCD is the minimal cost when compared with the pulse-dosing demand valves.

Transtracheal Oxygen Therapy. This relatively new method of oxygen delivery (initially introduced and reported by Dr H.J. Heimlich in 1982) has spawned an entirely new segment, from manufacturing to marketing, in the respiratory home care field (Heimlich, 1982; Heimlich & Carr, 1985). More importantly, TTOT has literally changed the lives of many patients using this exciting new practice of oxygen administration (Fig 3–12).

Heimlich's original technique consisted of administering oxygen di-

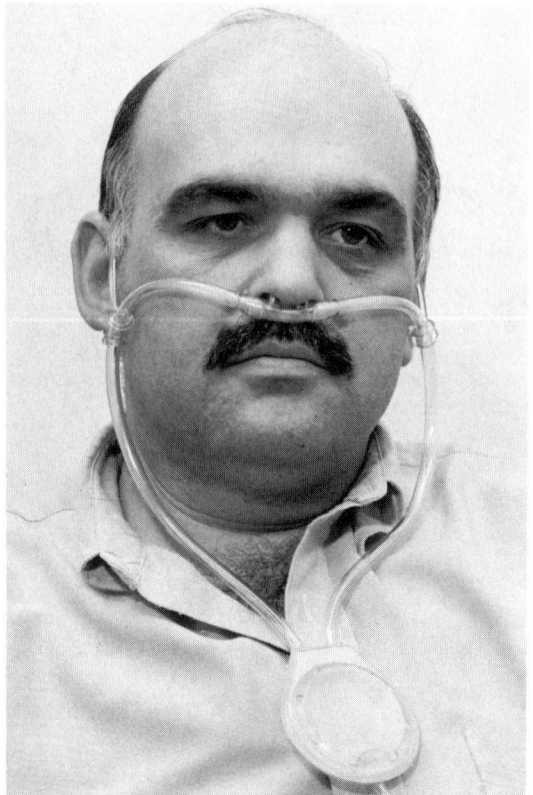

Figure 3–11. The Pendant-style reservoir nasal cannula.

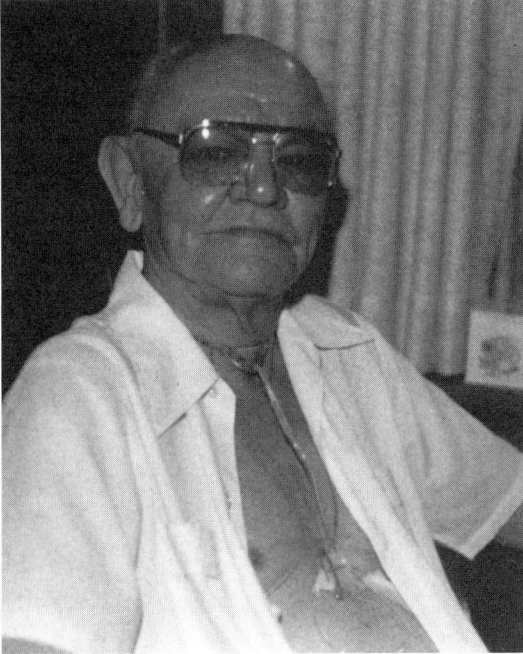

Figure 3–12. This patient had a transtracheal-oxygen-administering catheter placed by Heimlich. His oxygen use was reduced by almost half immediately after catheter placement.

rectly into the trachea via a 16-gauge intravenous catheter, which was inserted between the second and third tracheal rings and sutured to the skin.

Direct oxygen administration into the trachea resulted in a number of benefits (Table 3–8) not the least of which was a 50% to 60% oxygen savings. The most important benefits realized from TTOT are: (1) the ability to conceal the oxygen catheter under clothing; (2) the oxygen portable used by the patients can be half the size they normally required with nasal cannula use; and (3) the procedure has allowed many patients to return to work or increase their ambulation time outside the home. Transtracheal oxygen therapy, in this author's opinion, is probably the single most influential technique developed in home oxygen therapy. Transtracheal oxygen therapy has provided a productive, useful, self-image-restoring life style for the patient.

An interesting "extension" of Heimlich's original method of delivering transtracheal oxygen is the method devised by Dr B.T. Spofford and Dr K.L. Christopher at the Institute for Transtracheal Oxygen Therapy, Presbyterian Denver Hospital in Denver, Colo (Christopher, Spofford, McCarty, et al, in press). The basic concept of administering oxygen directly to the trachea via small-bore catheter is the same as Heimlich's in principle, but this is where the similarities end. Spofford and Christopher have developed what they call the SCOOP transtracheal procedure. (SCOOP is an acronym for *Spofford Christopher Oxygen Optimizing Prosthesis.*)

TABLE 3–8. BENEFITS AND COMPLICATIONS ASSOCIATED WITH TRANSTRACHEAL OXYGEN THERAPY

Benefits	Complications
1. Significant reductions in oxygen flow rate over that of the nasal cannula to maintain the same Pao_2 (50%–60% savings)	1. Inadvertent catheter dislodgement
	2. Mild transient increase in sputum production
2. Elimination of irritation and soreness at the nares, face, and ears caused by continued application of nasal cannula	3. Transient hoarseness
	4. Minor bleeding at site and time of insertion (10ml)
3. Elimination of drying effects on the nasal and oropharyngeal mucosa caused by nasal oxygen administration	5. Coughing catheter into cephalad position
	6. Tract tenderness
4. Improved patient appearance and self-image because of nearly total concealment of transtracheal catheter	7. Subcutaneous emphysema in head and neck region (usually resolve spontaneously)
5. Improved patient mobility resulting from use of smaller portable vessels	
6. Prolongation of patient activity outside the home as a result of increased longevity of portable with lower liter flow	
7. Improved patient compliance with prescribed *continuous* oxygen therapy resulting from enhanced overall comfort	
8. Subjective improvements reported include: Enhanced sense of smell, improved appetite and ability to sleep, reduction of dyspnea, and enhanced exercise tolerance	

The SCOOP technique differs from the Heimlich technique in a variety of ways (Figs 3–13 and 3–14).

The SCOOP approach is an entirely packaged system that includes a printed procedure, specifically designed products, and full instructions for both the patient and physician. Figure 3–15 is an example of their literature and procedure. The products and literature designed for use with SCOOP procedure are sold and marketed through Transtracheal Systems, 601 East 18th Avenue, Suite 200, Denver, CO 80203.

Yet another system administering oxygen transtracheally is undergoing a clinical trial at the Swedish Hospital Medical Center in Seattle, Washington (Johnson & Cary, 1987). Dr L.P. Johnson and Dr J.M. Cary have experimented with permanently implanted polymer oxygen tubing

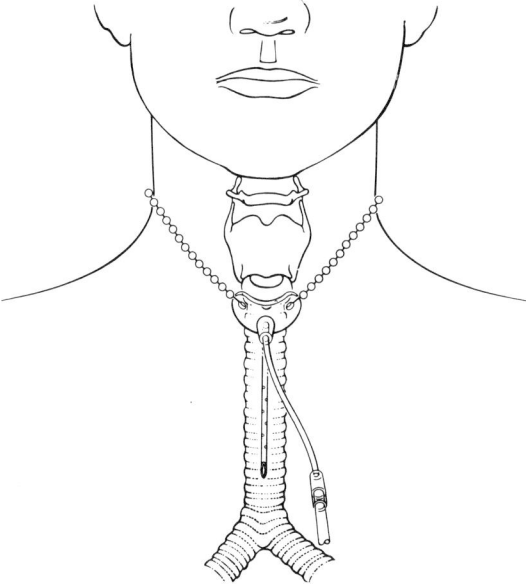

Figure 3–13. Frontal view of SCOOP transtracheal catheter after placement.

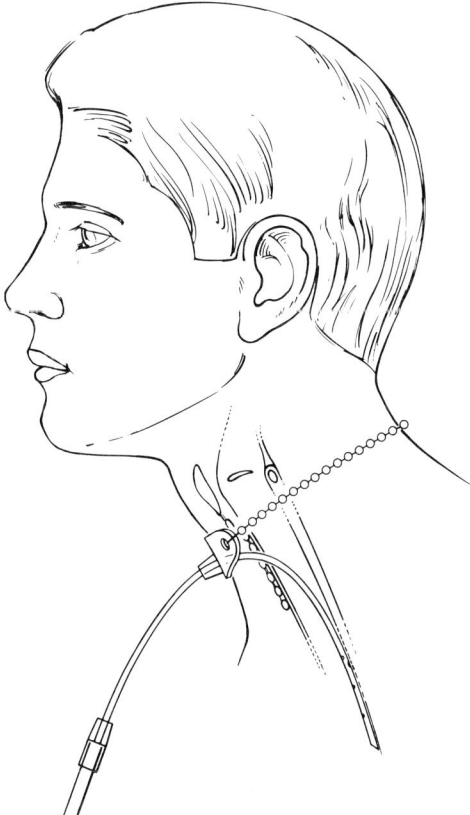

Figure 3–14. Anatomical side view of the SCOOP transtracheal oxygen catheter after placement.

CATHETER CLEANING

Regular cleaning of your SCOOP-2 catheter will ensure its proper function. Cleaning twice daily is recommended; however, your doctor may prescribe cleaning more often. The cleaning procedure requires an exchange with a second clean SCOOP-2 catheter.

Review all steps before you begin.

1. Gather the following materials:
   - A second clean SCOOP-2 catheter
   - Nasal cannula
   - Cotton-tipped applicator
   - Mild soap
   - Cleaning rod
   - Antibacterial soap (e.g., Hibiclens, PhisoHex)
   - Water-soluble jelly (e.g., Surgilube)
   - Clean, disposable latex or vinyl gloves

2. Wash your hands and position yourself in front of a mirror with good lighting.

3. Disconnect the SCOOP oxygen hose from the catheter.

4. Connect the nasal cannula to the oxygen source and use nasal oxygen at your nasal cannula flow rate throughout the exchange procedure.

5. With the SCOOP-2 catheter in place, use a cotton-tipped applicator and mild soap to clean mucus crusts from around your tract opening **(A)**. Blot the area dry with tissue.

6. Put on clean, disposable latex or vinyl gloves.

7. Apply a small smount of water-soluble jelly to the tip of the clean second catheter.

8. Disconnect the bead chain necklace and remove the first catheter from your tract **(B)**.

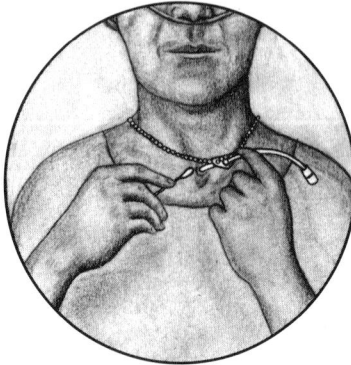

A. Clean mucus crusts from tract opening

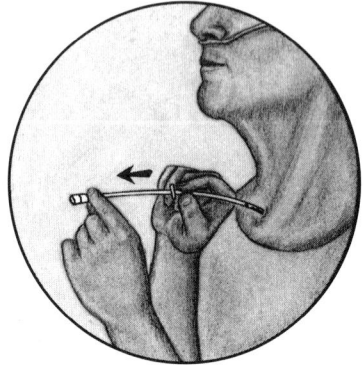

B. Remove catheter from tract

Figure 3–15. Example literature of the SCOOP transtracheal oxygen therapy system. (*Reproduced with permission from:* SCOOP-2 Transtracheal Catheter: Patient Instructions, *Transtracheal Systems, Denver.*)

9. Insert the clean catheter (C). The tip should be placed into your tract opening, and the catheter gently pushed straight back. Do not try to turn the catheter downward—it will turn itself. If resistance is met, twirl the catheter as it is inserted. It is normal to experience a tickle and cough as the catheter enters your trachea.

Caution: catheter should be out only briefly.

If you cannot reinsert the catheter, call your doctor immediately.

10. Reconnect the bead chain necklace. When properly reinserted, the SCOOP label will be upright and readable.

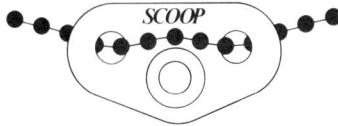

11. Reconnect the SCOOP oxygen hose to both the oxygen source and to the SCOOP catheter and return to the SCOOP-2 flow rate. Remove the nasal cannula. The exchange step is complete.

Cleaning the Soiled Catheter:

1. Rinse mucus off the catheter using running water. Pay special attention to clearing the oxygen ports at the tip. Run the cleaning rod through the inside of the catheter until it is clean (D).

2. Use a few drops of antibacterial soap and wash the catheter under warm, running water.

3. Rinse the outside and the inside of the catheter thoroughly to remove all soap residue.

4. Dry the catheter with a clean paper towel, then let air dry.

5. Store the SCOOP-2 catheter and cleaning rod in its original package in a clean, dry place out of direct sunlight.

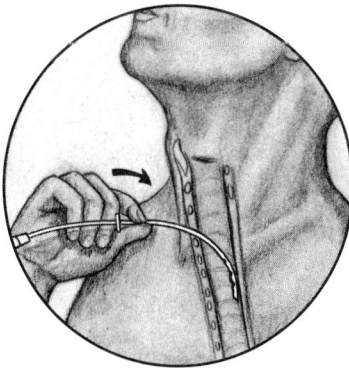

C. Insert clean catheter   D. Clean soiled catheter

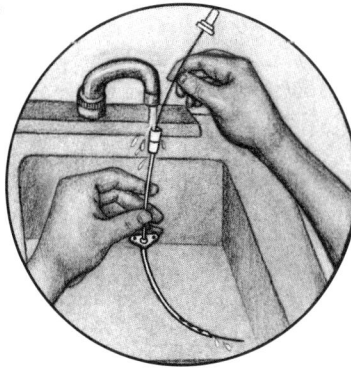

Figure 3–15. (cont.)

PATIENT PRECAUTIONS

1. SCOOP transtracheal catheters should only be used with tracts created by the SCOOP transtracheal procedure. Tracts created by other techniques may be the wrong size or positioned in an unacceptable location.

2. SCOOP-2 should always be removed for cleaning. It cannot be properly cleaned in place like SCOOP-1.

3. Follow the ten SCOOP rules on the back panel of these instructions.

4. Call your doctor immediately if you have any of the following:
   • SCOOP-2 cannot be reinserted
   • Increasing cough or sputum
   • Increasing shortness of breath
   • Blueness of lips or fingernails
   • Extreme nervousness
   • Irritation of tract opening
   • Fever

REPLACEMENT SCHEDULE

1. Replace this SCOOP product routinely at three months. Earlier replacement is required if it develops cracks, breaks, permanent kinks, or a foul odor.

2. Record the catheter model (e.g., SCOOP-2), date first used, and the scheduled replacement date in your *Patient Record* booklet.

Figure 3–15. (cont.)

that is placed subcutaneously from a tracheal insertion point to skin exit site that is usually in a convenient area beneath the breast (Fig 3–16).

This approach allows the user to completely hide all evidence of the oxygen-administering catheter and associated oxygen-delivery tubing. This oxygen catheter placement may be an interesting technique and option available in the near future.

As with all invasive procedures, TTOT is not without its inherent complications (*see* Table 3–8). Although the complications do exist, they are relatively minor in the degree of severity, percent of occurrence, and in comparison to the potential benefits.

FUTURE CONCEPTS REGARDING LONG-TERM HOME OXYGEN THERAPY

We are entering an exciting era of change in the respiratory home care field. An extraordinary future is about to unfold. Long-term home oxygen therapy is about to undergo dramatic change in the very near future. This change will be responsible for vast improvements in the patient's acceptance, use, and mobility with oxygen. The need to conserve oxygen to

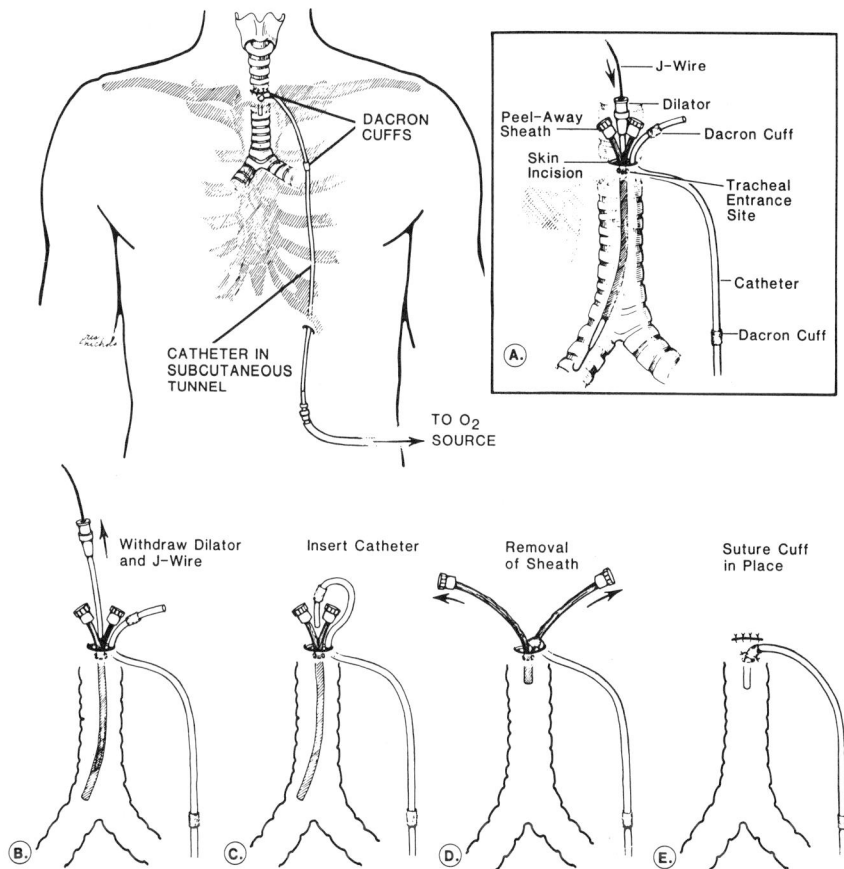

Figure 3–16. Procedure showing subcutaneous oxygen tubing and catheter placement, thereby hiding all evidence of oxygen-administering hardware.

reduce costs of LTDO$_2$ will result in many new lines of equipment and equipment changes. Compact, battery-operated oxygen concentrators will soon be available. Oxygen-conserving devices and related procedures will further streamline all oxygen delivery.

As the importance of LTDO$_2$ is further realized and no longer viewed as "tanks in the home" and "basic oxygen therapy," it is to be hoped that more hospital-based professionals will improve predischarge practices. As the field of respiratory home care continues to grow, more medical professionals will enter it; standards must be designed and accepted that will upgrade patient care at home to a much higher level. Home care dealers and suppliers must promote the new procedures and equipment responsible for conserving oxygen and ultimately reduce costs for home care.

Private and federal insurance carriers must employ qualified medical professionals to guide and advise them on new equipment developments and practices relating to the changing home care marketplace. This will ensure an intelligently spent insurance dollar and help foster further improvement in patient care techniques and equipment. Respiratory home care is and will continue to be a rapidly changing and volatile field as long as improvement in meeting patient-care needs continues and existing problems are solved. Present technology will improve and expand, new industries will be formed, and many people will be employed. We must not lose sight of the prime beneficiaries of this exciting change—the patients and their families.

REFERENCES

American College of Chest Physicians: National Conference on Oxygen Therapy. *Respir Care* 1984;*29*:922.

Ashutosh K, Mead G, Dunsky M: Early effects of oxygen administration and prognosis in chronic obstructive pulmonary disease and cor pulmonale. *Am Rev Respir Dis* 1983;*127*:399.

Christopher K, Spofford BT, McCarty DC, et al: Transtracheal oxygen therapy. *JAMA*, 1987.

Cryo₂ Corporation: *Grandair/Stationair Operations Manual.* Fort Pierce, Fla.

Flasterstein F, & Klocke RA: Outpatient oxygen therapy. *Primary Care* 1982;*9*:127.

Heimlich HJ: Respiratory rehabilitation with transtracheal oxygen system. *Ann Otol Rhinol Laryngol* 1982;*91*:643.

Heimlich HJ, Carr GC: Transtracheal catheter technique for pulmonary rehabilitation. *Ann Otol Rhinol Laryngol* 1985;*94*:502.

Johnson LP, Cary JM: The intratracheal oxygen catheter: A novel and efficient approach for long-term oxygen therapy. Read before the World Congress on Oxygen Therapy and Home Care, Denver, Colo, February 21, 1987.

Krop HD, Block AJ, Cohen E: Neuropsychological effects of continuous oxygen therapy in chronic obstructive pulmonary disease. *Chest* 1973;*64*:317.

Lasky MS: Bubble humidifiers are useful: Fact or myth. *Respir Care* 1982;*27*:735.

Levine BE, Bigelow DB, Hamstra RD, et al: The role of long-term continuous oxygen administration in patients with chronic airway obstruction with hypoxemia. *Ann Intern Med* 1967;*66*:39.

Nocturnal Oxygen Therapy Trial Group: Continuous or nocturnal oxygen therapy in hypoxemia chronic obstructive lung disease. *Ann Intern Med* 1980;*93*:391.

OECO: *Oxygen Enrichment Company, Ltd., Operations Manual.* Schenectady, NY, OECO, 1984.

4

Traveling with Oxygen

G. SLEEPER, RRT

AMBULATION AT HOME

An essential aspect of oxygen therapy in the home environment is mobility; it must become integrated into the patient's day-to-day activities in as natural a manner as possible. All too often, the presence of an oxygen system is allowed to impose a sentence of imprisonment on the fearful patient. The patient becomes trapped in a vicious cycle: lack of activity promotes deconditioning of the cardiopulmonary system and general muscle wasting, which further increases dependence on oxygen, which in turn even further reduces level of activity.

The first step to avoid this inevitably fatal cycle is as simple as providing the patient with a 50-foot extension tube and encouragement to use the oxygen while working around the house. For the housebound patient, this arrangement will allow mobility and may eliminate the need for more costly and complex portable oxygen systems. At this point, it is worthwhile to consider exactly why we are encouraging the chronic obstructive lung disease (COPD) patient to walk with oxygen.

Researchers have been studying the effects and potential benefits of portable oxygen since 1956 (Cotes & Gilson, 1956). Since then, numerous investigators have reported on the use of portable oxygen as an aid to exercise. While not all of the literature is in agreement, there is a general consensus that select patients are better able to exercise while using portable oxygen (Barach & Petty, 1975; Longo et al, 1971). Since the exercises in many of these studies involved walking on a treadmill, we can reasonably assume that any benefit granted to a patient in the laboratory will extend to similar activities in and about the home. These benefits include increased exercise endurance and tolerance, and reduced heart and respiratory rates (Barach & Petty, 1975; Bradley et al, 1978; Pierce et al, 1965). Further, some of the patients reported that they felt better when exercising with oxygen even when there were no measurable physiologic improvements (Lilker et al, 1975). When investigators began to measure the patient's subjective evaluation of breathlessness separately from exercise capacity, they found significant improvement in breathlessness scores when the patient exercised with portable oxygen (Waterhouse & Howard, 1982). Therefore, we cannot discount the patient's increased sense of well-being as unimportant, even if we cannot document objective improvement. In addition, if a formal exercise program is prescribed for the patient, portable oxygen can be used to reduce the stress of exercise and training (Pierce et al, 1965).

An important issue in prescribing portable oxygen is whether carrying a portable system increases the metabolic demands on the patient, effectively canceling the benefits of exercise with oxygen. In the first study to investigate this, Leggett and Flenley (1977) found that carrying a portable system on the shoulder negated any gain in exercise tolerance; this gain was restored when the patient pulled the portable system in a cart. Two subsequent studies found that carrying a portable system did not reverse the benefits of supplemental oxygen (Brambilla et al, 1985; Woodcock et al, 1981). Considering these studies, we feel that most oxygen-dependent patients can carry their portable oxygen without additional burden. Patients who do find this to be a problem may be directed to buy a two-wheeled shopping cart to tow their oxygen. It should be noted that these carts are generally not reimbursable by third-party payers.

For the last 30 years, numerous studies have demonstrated the benefits of portable oxygen for the chronically hypoxic patient. Clearly, it is imperative that even the housebound patient be provided with both the appropriate equipment and necessary encouragement to remain as active as the disease process allows.

GENERAL CONSIDERATIONS OF TRAVEL WITH OXYGEN

Most nonhousebound patients receiving long-term oxygen therapy are going to require some form of portable oxygen system. Recent developments in portable oxygen cylinders, liquid oxygen systems, and oxygen concentrators have helped to provide mobility to these patients.

Oxygen Cylinders
Conventional steel oxygen cylinders are commonly used for travel. Cylinder sizes B (M9), D, and E are small enough to be considered "portable" and may be used depending on the patient's oxygen rate of consumption and travel needs. The E-cylinder is the most commonly used tank for traveling to the doctor's office or taking a walk in the backyard or neighborhood. At approximately 16 lb, it must be placed in a wheeled cart to allow the patient to pull the cylinder behind him or her. Table 4–1 lists these cylinders and compares their weight, size, volume, tank factor, and duration while running at 2 lpm. More recently, aluminum cylinders have been manufactured for portable use. These cylinders are up to 40% lighter

TABLE 4–1. PORTABLE STEEL MEDICAL OXYGEN CYLINDERS*

Cylinder Size (Code Letter)	Weight (Lb Full)	Dimensions (D × Length)	Volume (Cu Ft/L)	Tank Factor (L/psi)	Duration (Hr at 2 lpm)
B	5.6	3.1 × 16	7.4/210	0.1	1.8
D	12.2	4.1 × 20	15/425	0.19	3.5
E	16.0	4.1 × 30	24.9/705	0.32	5.8

*All specifications are approximate and will vary somewhat among manufacturers. Specifications are based on a service pressure of 2015 psig and overfilled by 10%. The M9 is not generally available as a steel cylinder.
Courtesy of Air Products.

than comparably sized steel tanks and are available with leather carrying cases to allow the patient to carry these cylinders over their shoulders. A comparison of currently available aluminum cylinders is shown in Table 4–2.

Refilling Oxygen Cylinders. An important concern of the patient using portable oxygen cylinders is refilling the cylinders during travel. For short trips away from home, the home care company may simply supply the patient with enough cylinders because they may be transfilled from a stationary H-cylinder in the home by the patient or patient's family. However, there is considerable disagreement concerning the advisability of transfilling cylinders at home. This process has been documented as safe and convenient (Heiny, 1974; Petty, 1974), with the recommendation that a respiratory therapist instruct the patient in accordance with the manufacturer's instructions and evaluate the patient's ability to perform the procedure correctly. However, most manufacturers do not recommend this, and the National Fire Protection Association's recommendations specifically prohibit transfilling cylinders in the home (National Fire Protection Association, 1981).

For longer trips, the patient must plan the itinerary and identify home care dealers along the proposed route who can fill the cylinders. This involves knowing the capacity of the cylinders, the rate of usage, the cost of refills, and how these charges will be billed. Because of the potential

TABLE 4–2. PORTABLE ALUMINUM MEDICAL OXYGEN CYLINDERS*

Cylinder Size (Code Letter)	Weight (Lb Full)	Dimensions (D × Length)	Volume (Cu Ft/L)	Tank Factor (L/psi)	Duration (H at 2 lpm)
M9	3.9	4.4 × 11	8.8/248	0.1	2.0
D	5.5	4.4 × 16.5	14.6/415	0.19	3.4
E	8.1	4.4 × 25.6	24.1/682	0.31	5.7

*All specifications are approximate and will vary somewhat among manufacturers. Specifications are based on a service pressure of 2015 psig and overfilled by 10%.
Courtesy of Luxfor USA Limited.

complexities of planning the trips, the patient's home care company should provide the necessary information and assist in making arrangements with other dealers for refills and supplies.

Hazards. Traveling with oxygen cylinders is considered to be very safe if the patient observes the same safety rules that govern home use. In a nutshell, the cylinders must be protected from excessive heat and mechanical damage that might cause the cylinder valve to break. An oxygen cylinder should not be left in a car, as a car parked in the sun may well exceed 200°F. If the temperature rises significantly, the safety valve will rupture, causing oxygen to be released and creating a fire hazard. A full or partially full cylinder dropped down a flight of stairs could become a dangerous projectile if the valve were broken. Further, if the patient or family members are changing regulators or transfilling aluminum cylinders, care must be taken to avoid contaminating the system with combustable materials such as oil and grease.

Liquid Oxygen Systems

Liquid oxygen systems are excellent for the high-volume user who requires portable oxygen. The portable container is lightweight, weighing between 5 to 14 lb when full, and may be carried by means of a shoulder strap or pulled in a wheeled cart. When operated at flow rates of 2 lpm, a liquid portable unit can supply up to 10 hours of oxygen.

Two recent developments in portable liquid oxygen have come to the aid of the mobile oxygen user. The first is a trend toward smaller, lighter portable units. Although they do not provide as much volume as the heavier units, they are excellent for shorter trips and are easier for the debilitated patient to carry over the shoulder.

The second development is systems developed to deliver oxygen during inspiration only. Manufactured by $Cryo_2$, the Pulsair is an example of a demand system which is able to provide the patient with a longer duration of flow than a conventional liquid portable unit of comparable weight. See Chapter 2 for further information about these systems.

Refilling Liquid Oxygen Systems. The portable unit is filled by the patient or family from a base or reservoir unit in the home. This transfilling process is simpler and less potentially hazardous than transfilling aluminum cylinders. Each particular liquid portable unit can be filled only from a base unit from the same manufacturer; therefore, it is essential that the patient and home care dealer ensure compatible systems along the route of an extended trip. Often, the patient will take the base unit along on the trip. This reservoir unit may be fastened with a seatbelt in the backseat of a passenger car. By using a side-fill reservoir, this patient may fill his or her own portable unit in the car as well as minimize refilling visits to home care dealers. The authors would like to stress the advisability of additional restraints for securing the unit in the car. Additionally, the patient should be advised of all possible hazards involved in transporting large volumes of liquid oxygen.

Hazards. As with oxygen cylinders, travel with liquid portable oxygen systems is safe if the patient observes the same safety rules that govern home use. Because the liquid systems may lose as much as a pound or more of oxygen a day as a result of venting, the units should not be left in a closed car to avoid a fire hazard.

Oxygen Concentrators

Although not generally thought of as portable, oxygen concentrators do have a useful role in travel for the oxygen-dependent patient. Patients requiring only nocturnal oxygen may take the newer, lighter units with them in their vehicles. These units are in the 30- to 50-lb range and generally require an able-bodied spouse or traveling companion to heft the equipment. This type of travel arrangement eliminates the need for frequent stops for oxygen refills and the hazards of traveling with oxygen tanks or liquid vessels.

Recently, a portable oxygen concentrator has been introduced. The Roman Labs Freedom O_2 is available as a DC unit, which may be run from a car battery, or run from conventional AC with the use of a transformer pack.

Hazards. The hazards of traveling with an oxygen concentrator are no different from those of concentrator use in the home.

ORGANIZING A TRIP

Whether for recreation or business, many oxygen-dependent patients will take trips that necessitate at least one night away from home. With proper planning, these trips are pleasurable and relatively hassle-free. The following are considerations for a trip by private vehicle.

Travel by Car

Geographical Considerations. The distance to be traveled and the time required are two primary concerns to the oxygen-dependent patient and the home care company. If the patient is traveling with cylinders or liquid systems, stops must be planned in advance with the assistance of the home care company. If the patient will be at the destination for more than a couple of days, a local home care dealer should supply the patient with a system similar to what he or she has been used to. To avoid unnecessary stress, the patient should be well aware of the duration of the system being used, and the itinerary should not be so rigid that an unexpected delay would cause missing a refill stop! This need for forethought is where the home care company can be of immeasurable service to the patient.

Oxygen Requirements. The total volume of oxygen used per day is obtained by multiplying the ordered liter flow per minute by the ordered duration in hours and then multiplying by 60 minutes per hour. This formula will aid in choosing the appropriate portable system.

Traveling Prescriptions. It is essential that the patient traveling with oxygen obtain a written prescription for oxygen from the physician. A home care supplier is unlikely to fill an oxygen vessel without a prescription. As with any other such prescription, it must state flow rate, duration, and frequency.

Conserving Oxygen. An oxygen-conserving cannula may be used to extend the duration of a portable cylinder or liquid unit, lengthening the range of the oxygen-dependent patient. Conventional steady-flow cannulas are highly inefficient because they deliver oxygen continously during the respiratory cycle, although only about 15% to 20% of the total respiratory cycle actually results in inspired gas entering the alveoli (Tiep et al, 1985). Researchers have investigated various means of delivering oxygen during the inspiratory phase only. The Oxymizer and Oxymizer Pendent oxygen-conserving devices are two commercially available nasal cannulas that allow reduced oxygen flow rates while supplying oxygen concentrations comparable to conventional cannulas at higher flow rates. In one clinical evaluation, a liter flow of 0.5 lpm resulted in an oxygen saturation equivalent to a conventional cannula running at close to 2 lpm, a nearly fourfold savings in oxygen (Tiep et al, 1983). This savings is accomplished by a 20-ml reservoir and collapsible membrane arrangement. This design allows delivery of oxygen-enriched air on inspiration only; oxygen collects in the reservoir during the expiratory phase. Potential drawbacks to these devices include increased cost and the manufacturer's recommendation that the device be replaced at least once per week. The device also requires minimal nasal breathing to function correctly.

Altitude. Of special concern to the oxygen-dependent patient is traveling from locations of low altitude to those of higher altitudes. As altitude increases, there is a nearly linear decrease in the pressure of the atmosphere and, proportionally, the partial pressure of oxygen. For example, if a patient were to drive from Cape Cod (sea level) to Denver (about 5000 ft above sea level), he or she would encounter a drop in Po_2 of almost 30 torr. Therefore, it is essential that patient and physician carefully

TABLE 4–3. EFFECTS OF ALTITUDE ON ATMOSPHERIC AND ARTERIAL
OXYGEN PRESSURES

Altitude (feet)	Barometric Pressure (torr)	Atmospheric P_{O_2} (torr)	Arterial Blood P_{O_1} (torr)
Sea level	760	159	96
2000	611	148	87
4000	653	137	79
6000	604	126	71
8000	558	116	63

consider the advisability of trips involving significant increases in altitude. Table 4–3 displays the effects of altitude on atmospheric and oxygen pressures and Table 4–4 lists the altitudes of major US cities.

Travel by Air
For most passengers, commercial aviation offers a safe and convenient means of travel. However, for the oxygen-dependent patient, flying presents hazards that must be considered to determine whether the patient is fit to travel aboard an aircraft (Mills & Harding, 1983).

TABLE 4–4. TWENTY MAJOR CITIES AND THEIR ALTITUDES

Cities	Altitudes (ft)
Atlanta	1050
Boston	21
Chicago	595
Denver	5280
Detroit	585
Washington, DC	25
Houston	40
Indianapolis	710
Kansas City, MO	750
Las Vegas	2030
Los Angeles	340
Louisville	450
Memphis	275
Milwaukee	635
Minneapolis	815
New York City	55
Orlando, Fla	70
Philadelphia	100
Phoenix	1090
Seattle	10

ALTITUDE CONSIDERATIONS

As discussed in the previous section, an increase in altitude is associated with a fall in atmospheric pressure. For instance, as a plane ascends from sea level to a cruising altitude of 35,000 ft, the air pressure drops from 760 mmHg (14.7 psi) to 176 mmHg (3.40 psi) (AMA Commission on Emergency Medical Services, 1982). In addition, there is a parallel drop in atmospheric temperature and density (Harding & Mills, 1983).

The sigmoidal shape of the oxygen dissociation curve provides protection against hypoxia to the normal passenger up to 10,000 ft. At this altitude, the alveolar Po_2 will have dropped to about 60 mmHg from a sea level measurement of about 103 mmHg. However, the oxygen saturation will have only dropped from about 97% to just below 90%, because of the plateau on the dissociation curve (Harding & Mills, 1983). Much beyond this altitude, the lowered alveolar pressures will reach the steep portion of the oxygen dissociation curve, resulting in a precipitous drop in oxygen saturation and causing severe hypoxia (*see* Fig 4–1).

Aircraft Operational Considerations. To protect against the dangers of altitude-induced hypoxia, the cabins of commercial aircraft are pressurized by drawing in external air and controlling the outflow. However, it is neither practical nor necessary to pressurize the cabins to sea level. Instead, the cabin is pressurized to pressures equivalent to flying at lower altitudes, usually not to exceed 8000 ft. This is termed "cabin altitude." The difference between the aircraft altitude and the cabin altitude, expressed in psi, is known as the pressure differential, which is close to 9 psi. For example, if an aircraft is flying at 35,000 ft, the atmospheric pressure is about 3.4 psi. If the pressure differential in this particular aircraft at this altitude is 8.6 psi, the resulting cabin pressure will be 12 psi, which is equivalent to a cabin altitude of 5500 ft (AMA Commission, 1982).

Recommendations. Because a normal passenger's alveolar Po_2 will decrease by about 40% at a cabin altitude of 8000 ft (Harding & Mills, 1983), the AMA Commission on Emergency Medical Services has issued several recommendations for oxygen-dependent patients considering air travel (AMA Commission, 1982). Among them are:

1. All patients with chronic cardiovascular or pulmonary problems should have supplemental oxygen during flights with cruising altitudes above 22,500 ft. Examples of these pathologic conditions are: cystic fibrosis; chronic emphysema; cyanotic congenital heart disease; chronic asthma; coronary insufficiency; fibrotic pulmonary conditions.
2. A recent arterial blood gas should be obtained; the Po_2 should be above 50 mmHg. If the patient with a low Po_2 must fly, the medical

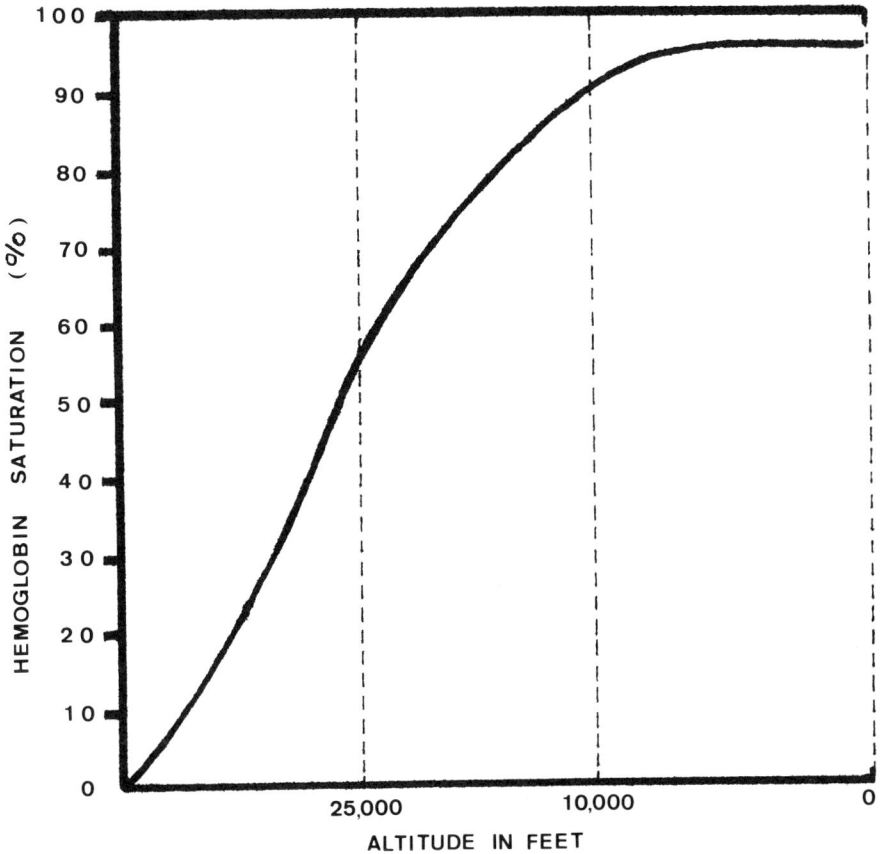

Figure 4–1. Relationship between hemoglobin saturation and altitude.

department of the airline should be consulted and supplemental oxygen should be provided.

Most airlines will supply supplemental oxygen if given advanced notice. In general, most commercial airlines require the following:

1. Advance notice of 48 to 72 hours.
2. Fee for oxygen of $50 per flight.
3. Prescription or medical certificate from the patient's physician stating liter flow and duration of oxygen, assuming a cabin altitude of 8000 ft. Also included should be a statement of fitness to fly and the physician's name and phone number.

In addition, some airlines require a patient to be accompanied by an able-bodied person. No airline will accept the patient's own full tanks or liquid vessels, but most will accommodate empty tanks or vessels that comply with the baggage weight restrictions. Table 4–5 lists a summary of airline specifications for patients traveling with oxygen.

TABLE 4–5. COMMERCIAL AIRLINE SPECIFICATIONS

Airline	Equivalency at 35,000 Ft	Equivalency at 40,000 Ft	Oxygen Charge	Advance Notice	Comments
American	5200–5500 ft	—	$40 per nonstop flight	24 h	American uses solid state oxygen only
Continental	O_2 not supplied	—	—	—	Continental does not transport persons requiring oxygen
Delta	7000–8000 ft	—	$40 per nonstop flight	24 h	Signed statement from physician giving O_2 requirements needed
Eastern	8000 ft	—	—	24–48 h	Physician or therapist required to adjust system at departure; letter giving O_2 requirements needed
Northwest	7200 ft	8300 ft	$40	24 h	If adjoining seat needed for equipment, it must be purchased

Airline					
Pan Am	5000 ft	7000 ft		48 h	Stretcher service available at 9 times regular economy fare; physicians letter for O_2 required
TWA	5400 ft	—	$25 instal-fee $15 per canister used	48 h	Passenger must pay for extra seat for equipment if needed
United	6500 ft	7500 ft	—	—	United's physician will contact patient's physician to determine equipment needs
Western	—	—	$50	—	Consultant firm AIR MEDIC contacts patient's physician to determine equipment needs

Courtesy of Erie Manufacturing Company.

Travel by Bus and Railway

Buses and trains are excellent means of travel for the hypoxic patient unable or unwilling to tolerate the lowered pressures experienced in commercial flight. In addition, they are ideally suited for inexpensive local travel. The major bus lines, including Greyhound, Trailways, and Bluebird Coach Lines, as well as the major passenger railways, such as Amtrak, have few restrictions on portable oxygen use. Greyhound requests that

---

TRAVEL ARRANGEMENTS

When a patient contacts the office in need of oxygen and related equipment for travel purposes, obtain the following information from the patient:

1. Patient's home address and telephone number including area code.
2. Destination address (as complete as possible).
3. Length of stay at destination (dates of arrival & departures).
4. Type of equipment needed.
5. Mode of travel.
6. Planned stops along the way, and length of stay at each stop.

Once this information has been obtained:

1. Locate area code of city of destination.
2. Phone 1 (area code) 555–1212.
3. Ask for phone number of any hospital in that town.
4. Phone that hospital and ask for Respiratory Therapy Department or discharge planner.
5. Inform Respiratory Therapist or discharge planner that a patient is coming to that area and would like a referral to an independent home care company.
6. Phone home care company and relay information on patient (date of arrival, place; etc).
7. Question if they will:
    a. pro-rate their charges.
    b. bill your company.
   If patient uses a cylinder ask:
    a. do they transfill
       1) steel portable.
       2) aluminum portable.
       3) M–60 with American/Canadian standard safety system.
   If patient uses a liquid system ask if they:
    a. supply same type of system as patient has.
    b. provide portable.
8. Obtain complete name, address, phone, and contact person of company.
9. Inform patient of completed details:
    a. company name.
    b. contact person's name.
    c. company's complete address and phone number including area code.
    d. our phone number, including area code.

Figure 4–2. Sample form for travel arrangements.

the oxygen user sit in one of the first three rows, and Amtrak requests a letter from the physician approving the patient's fitness for travel.

THE RESPONSIBILITIES OF THE HOME CARE DEALER

Twenty years ago, much home medical oxygen was purchased from welding companies. Today, the range of services provided by the professional home care company extends well beyond simple delivery and billing. It is the authors' opinion that the home care company should help the oxygen-dependent patient who wishes to travel in any way possible. When this patient wishes to travel out of town, the home care company should make arrangements to provide the necessary services. For the national companies, this is often simply a matter of calling another branch. For the small independent dealer, this necessitates contacting other dealers or hospitals to arrange services. Independent dealers will often accumulate a list of dealers whom they trust to provide good out-of-town service. In addition, most manufacturers of liquid oxygen systems will make available to the home care dealer and patient a listing of dealers across the country who use their systems. These lists enable the home care dealer to arrange a patient's itinerary with compatible systems coast to coast. Figure 4–2 shows the procedure a home care company uses to arrange for a patient travel with oxygen.

The home care company can also be of service in providing the patient's physician with guidelines for traveling prescriptions, medical certificates, and the various airline requirements.

Perhaps the greatest service that the home care company can provide is to help encourage the patient to live as normal a life as the disease process allows and to provide the means, through equipment and expert service, to make this possible.

REFERENCES

AMA Commission on Emergency Medical Services: Medical aspects of transportation aboard commercial aircraft. *JAMA* 1982;*247*:1007.

Barach AL, Petty TL: Is chronic obstructive lung disease improved by physical exercise? *JAMA* 1975;*234*:854.

Bradley BL, Garner AE, Billiu D, et al: The effect on exercise capacity; and arterial blood gas tensions. *Am Rev Respir Dis* 1978;*118*:239.

Brambilla I, Arlati S, Micallef E, et al: A portable oxygen system corrects hypoxemia without significantly increasing metabolic demands. *Am Rev Respir Dis* 1985;*131*:51.

Cotes JE, Gilson JC: Effect of oxygen on exercise ability in chronic respiratory insufficiency: Use of portable apparatus. *Lancet* 1956;*1*:872.

Harding RM, Mills JF: Problems of altitude. *Br Med J* 1983;*286*:1408.

Heiny LW: High-pressure medical oxygen equipment in the home. *Resp Care* 1974;*19*:521.

Leggett RJE, Flenley DC: Portable oxygen and exercise tolerance in patients with chronic hypoxic cor pulmonale. *Br Med J* 1977;284.

Lilker ES, Karnick A, Lerner L: Portable oxygen in chronic obstructive lung disease with hypoxemia and cor pulmonale. *Chest* 1975;*68*:236.

Longo AM, Moser KM, Luchsinger PC: The role of oxygen therapy in the rehabilitation of patients with chronic obstructive pulmonary disease. *Am Rev Respir Dis* 1971;*103*:690.

Mills JF, Harding RM: Fitness to travel by air. *Br Med J* 1983;*286*:1269.

National Fire Protection Association: National fire codes. Boston, National Fire Protection Association, 1981, vol 14.

Petty TL: The success and safety of home oxygen, editorial. *Resp Care* 1974;*19*:496.

Pierce AK, Paez PN, Miller WF: Exercise training with the aid of a portable oxygen supply in patients with emphysema. *Am Rev Respir Dis* 1965;*91*:653.

Tiep BL, Belman MJ, Mittman C, et al: A new oxygen saving nasal cannula (abstract). *Am Rev Respir Dis* 1983;*127*:4, (pt 2:86).

Tiep BL, Nicotra B, Carter C, et al: Evaluation of an oxygen-conserving nasal cannula. *Resp Care* 1985;*30*:19.

Waterhouse JC, Howard P: Breathlessness and portable oxygen in chronic obstructive airways disease. *Thorax* 1982;*38*:302.

Woodcock AA, Gross ER, Geddes DM: Oxygen relieves breathlessness in "pink puffers." *Lancet* 1981; 907.

5

Infant Apnea Monitoring

JAMES P. ORLOWSKI, MD, FAAP, FCCP

WHAT IS SIDS

In 1969 the Second International Conference on Sudden Infant Death Syndrome defined the sudden infant death syndrome (SIDS) as the sudden death of any infant or young child that is unexpected by history and in which a thorough postmortem examination fails to determine an adequate cause of death (Summary of Proceedings, 1971). As such, the diagnosis of SIDS cannot be made until after the death of the infant, and the pathologic diagnosis of the syndrome is one of exclusion in which no specific cause of death is found at autopsy (Naeye, 1977). Despite the uncertainties of the postmortem diagnosis, SIDS is a definite medical entity. It is the major cause of death in infants between 1 and 12 months of life and as many as 7000 infants die of SIDS annually in the United States for an incidence of about 2 to 3 per 1000 live births (Valdes-Dapena, 1980). Death seems to occur quickly, without apparent suffering, and almost always during sleep. Frequently, the infant may have a minor illness, such as a respiratory infection, but many victims are healthy prior to death (Table 5–1).

SIDS is at least as old as the Old Testament (I Kings 3:19–20) and occurred at least as frequently in the 18th and 19th centuries as it does now (Beckwith, 1976). Its incidence peaks in infants 2 to 3 months of age, decreases rapidly after 7 months of age, and becomes exceedingly rare after 12 months of age (Table 5–2) (Valdes-Dapena, 1977). The incidence of SIDS increases in the winter months (Merritt & Valdes-Dapena, 1984) (November to April in the northern hemisphere and May to September in the southern hemisphere) and is higher in blacks and lower socioeconomic classes. (Kleinberg, 1984; Naeye, 1980). SIDS is particularly frequent in infants of drug-addicted mothers (Brooks, 1982). There seems to be a familial predilection for SIDS, with various studies having found a three- to sevenfold increase of the syndrome in siblings of SIDS victims (Table 5–3) (Beal, 1983; Froggatt et al, 1971; Irgens et al, 1984;

110

TABLE 5–1. SOME BASIC FACTS ABOUT SIDS*

SIDS is a definite medical entity and is the major cause of death in infants of 1 month to 12 months of life.

SIDS is at least as old as the Old Testament (I Kings 3:19–20) and was as common in the 18th and 19th centuries as now.

SIDS victims appear to be healthy prior to death.

At this time SIDS cannot be predicted or prevented, even by a physician.

There appears to be no suffering; death occurs very rapidly, usually during periods of sleep.

SIDS is not caused by external suffocation, vomiting, or choking.

*SIDS = Sudden infant death syndrome.

TABLE 5–2. AGE DISTRIBUTION OF SIDS*

Age (Months)	Percent of Cases
0–1	4
1–2	25
2–3	27
3–4	17
4–5	11
5–6	7
6–7	3
7–8	2
8–9	2
9–10	1
10–11	1
1–12	0.2
over 12	≤0.1

*SIDS = Sudden infant death syndrome.

TABLE 5–3. RISK OF SIDS* IN SIBLINGS OF SIDS VICTIMS*

Author	SIDS/Sibs*	SIDS/1000 Sibs	Sib Risk†
Froggatt	4/360	11.1	3.7
	6/360	16.7	7.4
Peterson	11/567	19.0	9.5
Beal	6/302	20.0	10.0
Irgens	5/1043	4.8	3.7

*SIDS = Sudden infant death syndrome; Sibs = Siblings.
†Increased risk over normal population risk of 2–3/1000 live births.

TABLE 5–4. CHARACTERISTICS OF SIDS*

Incidence	2–3/1000 live births
Peak age	3–4 months of age
Time of death	Invariably during sleep
Seasonal variation	Higher in winter
Racial factors	Higher in nonwhites
Socioeconomic factors	Significant increase in lower socioeconomic class
Sex predominance	Higher in males
Birth weight	Higher in prematures and small-for-gestational-age babies
Multiple births	Higher in twins, highest in triplets
SIDS siblings	Very high incidence (3–7 times)

*SIDS = Sudden infant death syndrome.

Peterson et al, 1980). There is an increased incidence in multiple birth infants, including a number of simultaneous SIDS events affecting twins. There is a male preponderance of the syndrome and an increased risk among infants with low birth weights. Maternal smoking and young maternal age also appear to increase the risk of the syndrome (Table 5–4). The incidence of SIDS has decreased over the past few decades, paralleling the decline in infant mortality rates, but SIDS remains the major cause of postneonatal infant death (Table 5–5) (Schulte et al, 1982).

TABLE 5–5. SIDS* RISK FACTORS

Male (50%–75%)
Sibling of SIDS victim
Maternal drug addiction–especially opiates or methadone (10 times)
Low birth weight (3 times)–small for gestational age
Maternal smoking
Frequent or severe apneas
Bronchopulmonary dysplasia
Infant muscle tone abnormalities or neuromuscular disease
Young maternal age and low socioeconomic status
Abnormal pregnancy and perinatal complications—low Apgar scores
Upper respiratory tract infections
Failure to thrive or gain weight appropriately
Prematurity
Family history of SIDS

*SIDS = Sudden infant death syndrome.

Although many SIDS victims were perfectly healthy prior to death and the death appears to have occurred suddenly and unexpectedly, various pathologic studies have suggested that SIDS victims may have had many episodes of apnea and hypoxic stress that spontaneously aborted before the final fatal episode. These pathologic findings have included pulmonary artery hyperplasia similar to that seen in other chronic hypoxic states, increased right ventricular muscle mass, retention of periadrenal brown fat, increased extramedullary erythropoiesis, and astroglial proliferation in the brainstem (Ambler et al, 1981; Naeye, 1977). All of these pathologic findings have been interpreted to suggest recurrent undetected episodes of apnea and hypoxic stress prior to death. A finding suggestive of immaturity or maturational lag in the development of the brainstem was the finding of reticular dendritic spines in the brainstems of SIDS victims (Quattrochi et al, 1980). These dendritic spines are normally lost with perinatal maturation of the central respiratory neurons. These pathologic findings suggested to many physicians and researchers that not only was SIDS not a sudden and unexpected catastrophic event without premonitory warnings, but also that infants with recurrent episodes of apnea and infants who had sustained a cardiopulmonary arrest unexpectedly and had been resuscitated might provide important clues to the pathophysiology of SIDS. These infants began, therefore, to be referred to as near-miss or aborted SIDS victims.

WHAT IS THE INFANT APNEA SYNDROME

During the last decade a substantial amount of evidence has been accumulated that suggests that there may be a continuum from normally occurring periodic breathing and short respiratory pauses during sleep to life-threatening, long-lasting apneas with marked bradycardia or even cardiac arrest from which, however, the infant can be resuscitated (the near-miss for sudden infant death event) and finally, to SIDS. There are, however, still many missing links among these three phenomena, and it seems likely that the connection among all three is not a simple matter of degree of immaturity or dysfunction of the brainstem and cardiorespiratory control mechanisms. In fact, not all researchers or clinicians even agree that there is a continuum between the infant with apneas, the infant with a cardiopulmonary arrest who has been successfully resuscitated (the aborted or near-miss SIDS), and the SIDS victim (Fig 5–1).

Because of the uncertainty about the relationship among infants with apneas, infants who arrested during sleep but were fortuitously resuscitated, and the SIDS victim, and because many syndromes and diseases can present with apneas in infancy (Table 5–6), researchers and clinicians involved in SIDS agreed in 1980 to use the terminology infant apnea syndrome (IAS) for infants who present with apneas and to not use the

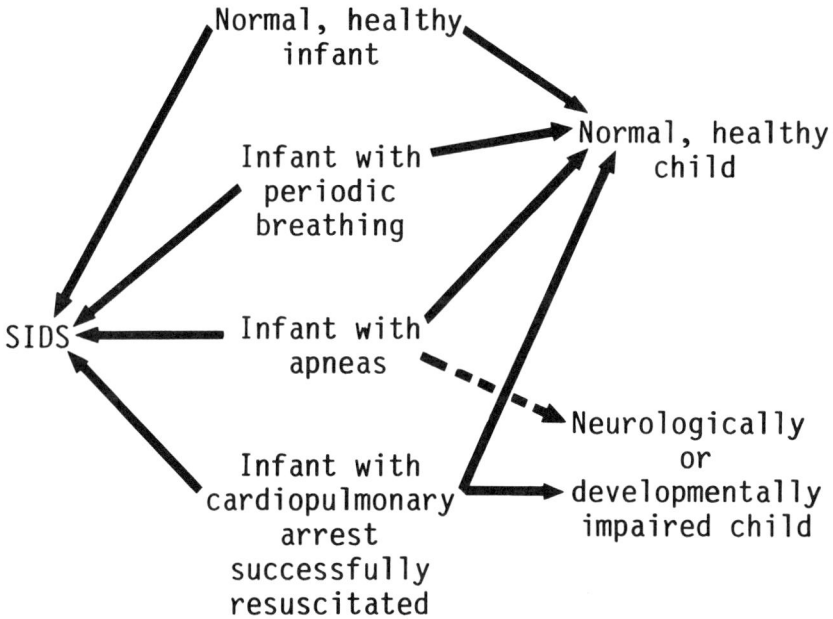

Figure 5–1. The ill-defined continuum between a healthy child and a diagnosis of sudden infant death syndrome (SIDS).

term near-miss SIDS until the relationship between these two entities could be better defined (Fig 5–2) (Nickerson, 1982). This differentiation is especially important because there are so many syndromes in infancy that can present with apneas that are clearly not related to SIDS, and likewise, some periodic breathing is normal in prematures and neonates.

TABLE 5–6. MEDICAL ENTITIES PRESENTING WITH APNEA IN INFANCY

Botulism	Neuromuscular disease
CNS* depression secondary to drugs	Patent ductus arteriosus
CNS* hemorrhage	Pneumonia
Congestive heart failure	Prolonged QT interval syndrome, and
Dehydration	other cardiac conduction abnormalities
Gastroesophageal reflux with aspiration	including Wolff-Parkinson-White
Hyaline membrane disease	syndrome and paroxysmal atrial
Hypocalcemia or hypomagnesemia	tachycardia
Hypoglycemia	Reye's syndrome
Hypophosphatemia	Seizures
Hypothermia or hyperthermia	Sepsis
Hypoxia	Shock, blood loss, or anemia
Kernicterus	Upper airway obstruction
Meningitis or encephalitis	Wilson-Mikity syndrome and
Metabolic acidosis	bronchopulmonary dysplasia

*CNS = Central nervous system.

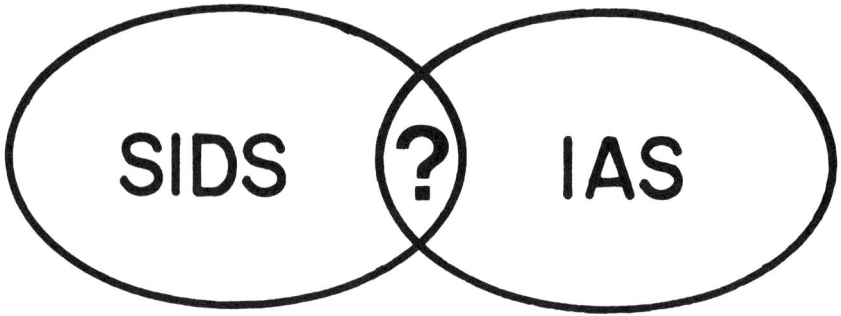

Figure 5–2. There exists an uncertain relationship between sudden infant death syndrome (SIDS) and the infant apnea syndrome (IAS).

Since SIDS is a diagnosis that can only be made after a thorough postmortem examination, it is difficult to define a near-miss SIDS or an aborted SIDS except retrospectively in the small number of infants who do die later and in whom a postmortem examination is consistent with SIDS.

An infant may be at risk for SIDS if it is a sibling of a previous victim or is experiencing apneas. Siblings of SIDS victims have been shown to be at a three-to sevenfold increased risk of SIDS over the general population. Apneas are not uncommon, especially in premature infants and neonates. Proposed causes for the idiopathic neonatal apneas of the premature infant include hypoxia from hypoventilation secondary to pulmonary airway instability, neurologic immaturity, altered sensitivity of either central or peripheral chemoreceptors, or possibly immaturity of the catecholamine-producing pathways (Table 5–7). During and after the neonatal period, apneas can occur for various pathologic reasons, and these disease states should be pursued as potential causes of the symptoms of apnea. Most of these medical entities can be excluded by a thorough history and physical examination and a minimum of laboratory studies (Table 5–8).

It is important to realize that only the occasional infant will be brought to medical attention because of the symptom of apnea. Rather than actually detecting apneas, parents may simply describe to the physician a

TABLE 5–7. PROPOSED ETIOLOGIES OF IDIOPATHIC NEONATAL APNEA

Hypoxia from hypoventilation or pulmonary instability
Neurologic immaturity
Altered sensitivity of central or peripheral chemoreceptors to CO_2 or O_2
Vagal overactivity
Immaturity of catecholamine-producing pathways

TABLE 5–8. MEDICAL EVALUATION FOR INFANT APNEA SYNDROME (NEAR-MISS SIDS*)

Complete physical examination
Complete neurologic examination including developmental assessment
Chest x-ray
ECG*
EEG*
Complete blood count
Blood glucose, electrolytes, calcium, magnesium, phosphate
Apnea and bradycardia monitoring
Polygraphic monitoring during sleep including
    EEG
    ECG
    EMG*
    EOG*
    Respirations
    Oxygen saturation
Additional evaluations to be considered if indicated by history or examination
    Sepsis workup including lumbar puncture
    Barium swallow or esophageal pH monitoring
    Arterial blood gases soon after apnea and during sleep
    CT* scan of brain
    Further cardiologic evaluation (e.g., echocardiogram)
    Otolaryngological evaluation including laryngoscopy and bronchoscopy

*CT = Computed tomography; EEG = Electroencephalogram; ECG = Electrocardiogram; EMG = Electromyogram; EOG = electro-oculogram; SIDS = Sudden infant death syndrome.

frightening episode in which the child did not look well. At other times parents may accurately describe cessations of breathing or apneas that require gentle or vigorous stimulation or in unusual circumstances, even cardiopulmonary resuscitation to abort the episode.

The physical examination should include a complete neurologic examination and assessment of any developmental delay or central nervous system (CNS) disease. The Amiel-Tison or Bailey Developmental Assessment Scales are useful. A chest x-ray film should be obtained to exclude pulmonary pathologic conditions, an electrocardiogram to exclude cardiac problems, and an electroencephalogram to detect subtle or subclinical seizures that may appear as apneas. Laboratory studies should include a complete blood count as well as measurement of blood glucose, electrolytes, calcium, magnesium, and phosphorous levels. If sepsis is considered a possible cause of the apneas, a complete sepsis workup including a lumbar puncture is mandatory. Additional evaluations that may be considered include a barium swallow or esophageal pH monitoring to rule out gastroesophageal reflux, arterial blood gases, especially if the infant was examined shortly after one of the apneic episodes, and transcutaneous monitoring of oxygen and carbon dioxide during sleep to look for signs of hypoventilation. A computed tomographic scan of the brain can confirm suspected CNS disease; an echocardiogram may be indicated if primary cardiac disease is suspected. Laryngoscopy or bronchoscopy may be used to search for a foreign body or anatomic abnormality that is compromising tracheal integrity. All infants hospitalized for suspected apneas should have continuous apnea and bradycardia monitoring while hospitalized. In selected cases a polysomnogram or polygraphic sleep monitoring may be employed to evaluate the occurrence of apneas during sleep. Polygraphic sleep monitoring employs simultaneous recording of electroencephalogram, electrocardiogram, electromyogram including chin and intercostal muscles, and an electro-oculogram, to continuously monitor the infant for an extended period during sleep (Fig 5–3); respiratory function and oxygenation are also monitored by means of a nasal air-flow monitor and transcutaneous oxygen tension or oxygen saturation monitors. Various studies have defined the number and duration of apneas (defined as respiratory cessations greater than 10 seconds in duration) and respiratory pauses (defined as respiratory cessations between 3 and 9 seconds duration) that are normal and abnormal at different ages and in different risk groups of infants (Tables 5–9 and 5–10).

CENTRAL SLEEP APNEA

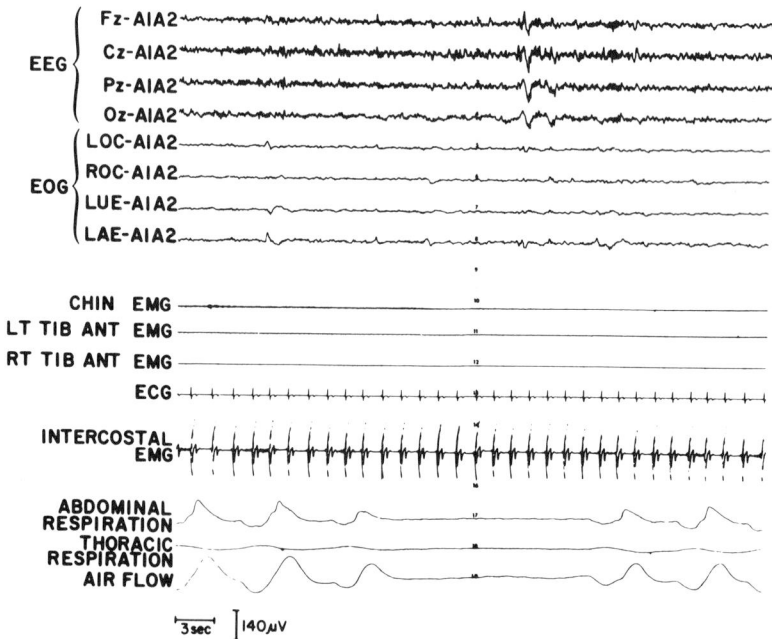

Figure 5–3. An example of polygraphic sleep study.

TABLE 5-9. PHYSIOLOGIC ABNORMALITIES IN INFANT APNEA SYNDROME

Prolonged sleep apnea
Frequent short apnea
Excessive periodic breathing
Depressed response to $\uparrow$ CO_2
Depressed response to $\downarrow$ O_2

An important question that has only recently been addressed is whether infants at risk for SIDS or future victims for SIDS could be identified on the basis of cardiac and/or respiratory abnormalities occurring prior to the SIDS event. Drs Southall, Richards, de Swiet, and Rhoden performed a multicenter prospective study that collected clinical and physiologic data on over 9000 infants with 24-hour tape recordings of electrocardiograms and breathing movements during the first 6 weeks of life. Included in these 9000 infants who were studied were 29 infants who subsequently died of SIDS. The authors had 40 recordings in these 29 infants, and these recordings were evaluated for episodes of prolonged cessation of breathing (20 seconds or more), ventricular pre-excitation, cardiac arrhythmias, bradycardia, and prolongation of the QT interval. The authors reported that none of the recordings obtained in the SIDS victims showed prolonged apnea or pre-excitation (Southall, Richards, Rhoden et al, 1982; Southall, Richards, de Swiet & Rhoden, 1983). Although the analysis of their data is far from complete, the results of this study give us two important pieces of data. First, the evaluation of normal, preterm or low birth weight infants during the first 6 weeks of life for the presence of cardiac or respiratory abnormalities when the infants have no symptoms cannot predict which infants will subsequently die of SIDS. Second, this study suggests that the apneas detected after a near-miss episode may be the consequence of the episode rather than the cause. Further evaluation of their data is underway to determine if there are any cardiac or respiratory abnormalities that may be predictive of the infant at risk for SIDS.

Slightly different results have been obtained by Shannon's group from the Massachusetts General Hospital, who reported in 1984 the re-

TABLE 5-10. THE SLEEP APNEA SYNDROMES

Central or neurogenic apnea
Obstructive apnea
Mixed apnea: central-obstructive
Convulsive apnea

sults of retrospective spectral analysis of pneumogram recordings obtained from eight infants at risk for SIDS, either because of previous apneas or a SIDS sibling, who subsequently died from SIDS and 22 age-matched control infants. These authors found that infants who subsequently died of SIDS had greater abnormal patterns of fluctuation of heart rate and respiratory activity as compared to retrospectively age-matched control infants (Gordon, Cohen, Kelly et al, 1984).

INDICATIONS FOR HOME APNEA MONITORING

Who then should be monitored at home with home apnea and brady-cardia monitoring (Table 5–11)?

From the standpoint of infants at risk for SIDS, the consensus opinion at this time is that there are two high-risk groups for whom home apnea and bradycardia monitoring should be considered (NIH Consensus Development Conference, 1987; Southall, 1983). The first are siblings of infants who have died of SIDS, and the second are infants who have had one or more episodes of prolonged apnea. It is important, however, to remember that very few SIDS victims have been observed to have prior warning episodes of prolonged apnea. Likewise, the occurrence of prolonged apnea in premature infants is common and yet is not predictive of SIDS. Most clinicians believe that the only way to manage SIDS until we better understand its etiology is to attempt to prevent it. Although it is uncertain whether stimulation during a spell of apnea can in fact prevent a sudden infant death, there is a certain imperative that it be attempted and there is some evidence to support the use of continuous monitoring of respiratory and cardiac activity in infants clearly thought to be at increased risk for SIDS. In one recently completed study of 34,865 live births from 1972 to 1977 in Onondaga, NY, in which an intensive apnea monitoring program was pursued, the death rate attributed to SIDS was compared with that occurring in 64,999 infant births over the pre-

---

TABLE 5–11. INDICATIONS FOR HOME CARDIORESPIRATORY MONITORING

Sibling or twin of SIDS* victim

History of severe or frequent apneic episodes

Polysomnogram or monitor documentation of apneas

Severe feeding difficulties with apnea and bradycardia

Pulmonary, cardiac, or neurologic disease

Infant with tracheostomy

Home ventilator patient

---

*SIDS = Sudden infant death syndrome.

ceding 7 years; there was a significant reduction ($p \leq 0.05$) in the incidence of SIDS during the monitoring period (Diagnostic and Therapeutic Technology Assessment, 1984). It is this author's contention that no other concept has shed so much light on SIDS and most probably no other concept with its consequence of continuous home monitoring has already salvaged so many babies as research into the different sleep apnea syndromes during infancy.

There are other disease states in which apnea is a common symptom in which home apnea monitoring is valuable and important. By definition, SIDS is not the diagnosis in patients with diseases that cause prolonged apnea and have been listed previously as disease states to be considered and ruled out when entertaining the diagnosis of infant apnea syndrome. Most investigators believe that infants who have apneas of at least 20 seconds duration deserve monitoring. In addition to infants at risk for SIDS, other infants in whom home apnea monitoring should be considered are premature infants with documented prolonged apneas whose breathing is still irregular but who are otherwise clinically well and who could be home with their parents if it were not for the occurrence of the apneas. This group would also include the infants with bronchopulmonary dysplasia who are candidates for home management of their chronic pulmonary disease. Various other disease states, including some congenital and acquired pulmonary diseases and various apneic encephalopathies and neuromuscular diseases, are prone to apneas, and home apnea monitoring may be considered for these patients. An additional group with which this author has had experience and believes should be considered for home apnea monitoring are infants with tracheostomies and infants on home mechanical ventilation. Because of the propensity for infant tracheostomies to become occluded rapidly with inspissated mucus or to become dislodged, this author feels that infants at home with tracheostomies should be monitored with a home apnea monitor whenever the parents are not in the room. Likewise, even though most ventilators have disconnect alarms, this author believes that any infant on home mechanical ventilation should have a separate home apnea monitor as a backup system to warn of problems whenever the parents are not in the room.

The duration of employment of home apnea monitoring varies from clinician to clinician. This author believes that infants who have been identified at risk for SIDS should be monitored at least until 6 months of age or until they have been 2 months without any documented apneic episodes. Infants with disease states that make them prone to apneas should be monitored until either the disease state is resolved or until the tracheostomy or home ventilatory care has been discontinued and the infant has been demonstrated to be free of apneas in disease states associated with apnea for a period of no less than 2 months.

THE PROS AND CONS OF HOME APNEA MONITORING

Three potential adverse affects of home apnea monitoring have been suggested. The first is that home monitoring has not yet been established as a preventive measure for SIDS. Almost all centers studying infant apneas and SIDS have experienced death from SIDS of infants on home apnea monitoring despite a functioning apnea monitor (Shannon et al, 1977). In rare instances the monitors failed to alarm, but in most circumstances the monitor has appropriately alarmed but the infant has failed to respond to appropriate cardiopulmonary resuscitation measures by parents, caretakers, and emergency medical services (Duffty & Bryan, 1982). The question has been appropriately raised that if an infant died while being monitored or after monitoring had been discontinued, there would be the possible enhancement of the family suffering (Wasserman, 1984). On the other hand, the incidence of SIDS has decreased in the last decade coincident with the use of home apnea monitoring in some babies, and some studies have shown a reduced death rate from SIDS with the use of home apnea monitoring compared retrospectively with historical controls. Still, it must be conceded that there is no proof that home apnea monitoring will prevent SIDS.

The second argument against the use of home apnea monitoring is its expense. The average cost for 6 months of home monitoring is approximately $1500 per infant, and the outright purchase of a home apnea monitor costs between $2000 and $3000. Most insurance companies and third-party payers will cover the rental of a home apnea monitor for infants who are legitimately at risk. Local chapters of the National Sudden Infant Death Syndrome Foundation also frequently can make available infant apnea monitors for families who cannot afford to rent or purchase them. The financial outlay for home apnea monitoring is small compared to the emotional trauma of losing a baby to SIDS.

The third criticism leveled against home apnea monitoring is the stress and anxiety that the home apnea monitoring creates (Ariagno, 1984). Most families in which there is an infant who is considered for monitoring are likely to have a high level of anxiety. In fact, in our experience, many parents have been taking turns staying up all night observing the infant when they are worried about SIDS or have noticed apneas in their infant. A monitor that reduces this anxiety, whether or not it protects the infant from death, is probably a good treatment. Unfortunately, benefit is often short-lived because alarms are inevitable and with the equipment available at present there is often no explanation for their origin; that is, many of the alarms are false alarms. This situation can result in increased anxiety and serves to consolidate parents' fears that their infant is at risk of dying, even though it is possible, if not probable, that many, if not all, the alarms were false (Table 5–12). Some authors have raised the question whether increasing anxiety in the par-

**TABLE 5-12. PROBLEMS COMMONLY ENCOUNTERED DURING
HOME APNEA MONITORING**

Inability to distinguish real alarms from false alarms

Increasing frequency of false alarms as infant matures and becomes more active

Monitor malfunction

Increased frequency of alarms during intercurrent illness, especially upper respiratory infections

Inability to find alternate caretakers (baby-sitters) for infants on home monitors

Skin irritation from electrodes

Significant life style changes including curtailed outside-of-home activities

Difficulty with finally deciding to discontinue home monitoring

ents might harm the baby (Smith, 1984). Observations that SIDS may occur at the time of increased stress in a family would support the possibility that in a predisposed infant anything that increases anxiety could be dangerous. Reinforcing the parents' belief that their baby might die may also result in a self-protective attempt to reduce the pain of impending death by withdrawing love or even rejecting the child. However, most studies that have attempted to look critically at this question have not found that apnea monitoring has resulted in reduced love or a predisposition to rejection of the child. In fact, the opposite has been found (Kahn & Blum, 1982). Likewise, the question has been raised as to whether monitoring adversely affects other family members or the cohesion of the family. Again, this question has been looked at in a few studies, and, again, the opposite has been found (Black et al, 1978; Cain et al, 1980). That is, home apnea monitoring has tended to increase the cohesion of the family and although there have been some problems in siblings, these problems were not different from the results of a new baby entering into any family. Many parents, although they report high rates of false alarms, still feel that the monitor has saved the baby's life and, when asked whether they would choose to monitor another baby or the same baby in the future, always choose the monitor over the alternatives of either continuous observation or taking the risk that the baby may have an apneic episode that is fatal. Recently there appeared a pertinent article by the mother of a previous SIDS victim describing the dilemma she faced in two subsequent babies, one of whom her physician recommended not be monitored and another whom her physician recommended be monitored. The conclusion of this mother who had experienced both a monitored and an unmonitored child after losing her first baby to SIDS was that she preferred the monitor (Silvio, 1984). She had learned that monitoring could be both very trying and costly but that it allowed her to enjoy her child's infancy in a more relaxed manner and that it provided her with the opportunity to save the baby's life if necessary, a chance she wishes she could have experienced with her first child, who died of SIDS. Our own experience with home apnea monitoring of approximately 300 babies has been quite similar. That is, many parents experience anxiety and stress from the use of the home apnea monitor but come to realize that the sensitivity of the monitor is such that it results in numerous false alarms but never fails to miss a true apnea. Each of the parents, when questioned, has stated that he or she would rather put up with the inconvenience and frustration of home apnea monitoring than risk the loss of a child to SIDS. Most parents feel that the home apnea monitoring at least permits them to sleep at night, no matter how interrupted their sleep may be by alarms. They come to realize that the alarms will interrupt their sleep, but they can sleep with the assurance that if an apnea does occur, the alarm will awaken them.

INFANT CARDIOPULMONARY RESUSCITATION

Critical to the management of any infant at risk for apneas with a home apnea monitoring program is the proper and thorough training of the parents, grandparents, and any other caretakers responsible for the infant in the techniques of infant cardiopulmonary resuscitation (CPR). Infant CPR differs from adult CPR, and one should not make the assumption that individuals who are certified in CPR know or have been trained in infant CPR (Table 5–13) (Orlowski, 1980; 1983).

The first step in approaching an infant who is believed to have had an apnea or who is triggering an apnea alarm on the monitor is to first assess the infant. This means turning on the lights if the room is dark and taking a few seconds to note the color and appearance of the infant and whether or not respiratory movements are visible. It should be noted mentally whether the infant is normal in color, pale, or cyanotic and whether the infant is flaccid, rigid, or normal appearing in tone or posture. If the infant appears not to be breathing, the next step is to gently stimulate the child. This stimulation can be picking up the infant, gently

TABLE 5–13. RESUSCITATION REQUIREMENTS DURING HOME MONITORING IN INFANTS WITH AND WITHOUT MULTIPLE EPISODES OF APNEA

	Infants with Multiple Episodes of Apnea*	Infants without Multiple Episodes of Apnea	Total
Infants requiring resuscitation	20	7	27
Infants not requiring resuscitation	16	43	59
TOTAL	36	50	86

*Babies with multiple episodes of prolonged apnea have an increased risk of requiring bag and mask resuscitation ($p \leq 0.001$).

stroking it, or rubbing its back or abdomen or head. The infant should not be shaken, slapped, or bounced. At this stage it should be clear whether the infant is breathing or not. If it is obvious that the infant is not breathing, the standard maneuvers of airway and breathing as the first steps in CPR should be undertaken: the infant should be properly positioned, the airway opened and cleared, and assessed by looking, hearing, and feeling for any spontaneous respiration with the airway maneuvers. If these maneuvers fail to induce spontaneous ventilation in the infant, the rescuers should proceed to mouth-to-mouth and nose ventilation. After four breaths the rescuer should then stop and assess further for the commencement of spontaneous ventilation and for the presence or absence of pulse. In regard to ventilation, three significant differences between infant and adult CPR should be emphasized. First, in the airway maneuver, the infant's head and neck should not be hyperextended but instead should be put into a sniffing position, with the occiput of the head just slightly off the surface of the bed and above the level of the shoulders. Second, when giving mouth-to-mouth and nose breaths to the infant, the breath should be gentle puffs from the mouth of the rescuer and not deep forced breaths from the rescuer's lungs. Third, the rate of ventilation should be faster than for the adult. That is, the ventilatory rate should be 30 to 40 breaths per minute. Enough air has been introduced into the infant's lungs when the infant's chest is seen to just begin to rise. Breaths to the infant are given with the rescuer's mouth over both the mouth and nose of the infant. When assessing the circulation, it is sometimes difficult to palpate pulses even in a normal, healthy, vigorous infant. Circulation is rarely interrupted in an infant who sustains an apnea and is reached quickly by the parents after the apnea monitor alarms. Therefore, in most circumstances circulation will be adequate and one needs only to breathe for the infant until spontaneous ventilation ensues. In order to not perform external cardiac massage in infants in whom circulation is normal, we stress that the circulation and pulses need to be checked for carefully in at least two sites. The sites that we stress are, in order of preference, brachial, femoral, and carotid pulses. If a pulse is felt in any of these areas, it should be assumed that circulation is adequate and external cardiac massage is not necessary. If pulses are absent and all sites have been checked, one should proceed immediately to combining external cardiac massage with mouth-to-mouth ventilation. We have the parents practice finding pulses on the infant so that they become comfortable with the sites for locating the pulse and how the normal infant pulse feels. The precordial site for locating pulses has been shown not to be good in the infant, although it certainly can be added as a fourth site for checking the pulse before proceeding to external cardiac massage. External cardiac massage should be performed over the lower one third of the sternum on the infant, with two fingers on the sternum, at a rate of 120 to 140 compressions per minute. The sternum should be depressed one third to one half of the anterior-posterior diameter of the chest, and care must be taken to not allow the fingers to wander off the sternum. One-rescuer CPR on the infant is best performed with a breath interposed between every five compressions, with the rescuer leaving the fingers on the infant's sternum and keeping their mouth over or near the infant's nose and mouth. Because of the small size of the infant, it is not necessary to change position between compressions and breaths. The parents should have the rescue squad's phone number readily visible at the phone, and in any circumstance where expired air ventilation or CPR has been necessary to restart the infant breathing, the emergency squad should be called and the infant should be immediately transported to the nearest hospital. Parents should keep not only the phone number of the rescue squad, but also their own address and phone number readily visible on the telephone because in an emergency, one cannot be expected to remember the emergency squad's phone number and frequently will not even be able to remember one's own address and phone number.

Home apnea monitoring and infant CPR are probably the two most important and most effective factors in the management of infants with recurrent apnea and infants at risk for SIDS.

A HOME APNEA MONITORING PROGRAM

The key to a successful home apnea monitoring program is proper preparation and positive reinforcement of parents and other caretakers. It is the responsibility of both the health-care professionals and the dealer supplying the equipment to provide these elements to the parents (Table 5–14).

The parents need to become familiar with the use and operation of the infant monitor, including the basic theory of its operation, all of its controls, wires, leads, and electrodes, and the methods of securing the monitor and lead wires. It is the author's experience that many parents are inherently frightened of using electrically operated equipment on their baby. Reassurance as to the safety and emphasizing that the construction of home monitors is governed by rigorous safety standards should be an important part of the educational program. Alternatively, and because many parents may wish to continue monitoring outside of the home (for example while traveling in a car or on camping trips) battery-operated monitors are gaining increasing acceptance. When recording equipment is also going to be employed, parents should be instructed in the proper modes for recording, how to load the paper into the recorder, how to troubleshoot any malfunction, and the proper disposition of the recorded data. An event log is an important adjunct to a home monitoring program, and many dealers supply event logs as part of their monitoring program.

TABLE 5–14. EVALUATION OF READINESS OF PARENTS TO ACCEPT HOME APNEA MONITORING

Demonstrates knowledge of CPR*

Demonstrates understanding of common terminology: apnea, bradycardia, tachycardia, monitor

Demonstrates understanding of alarm and monitor placement to assure loudest signal

Demonstrates understanding of internal and external alarm settings

Demonstrates use of detachable cord or battery charger

Demonstrates knowledge of use and duration of battery

Demonstrates use of ON–OFF power supply

Demonstrates understanding of respiratory light indicator

Demonstrates understanding of respiratory alarm light indicator and reset function

Demonstrates understanding of cardiac light and reset function

Demonstrates use of electrode lead wires

Demonstrates understanding of electrode placement

Demonstrates understanding of "loose wire" alarm light and reset function

Demonstrates ability to perform lead wire "loop test"

*CPR = Cardiopulmonary resuscitation.

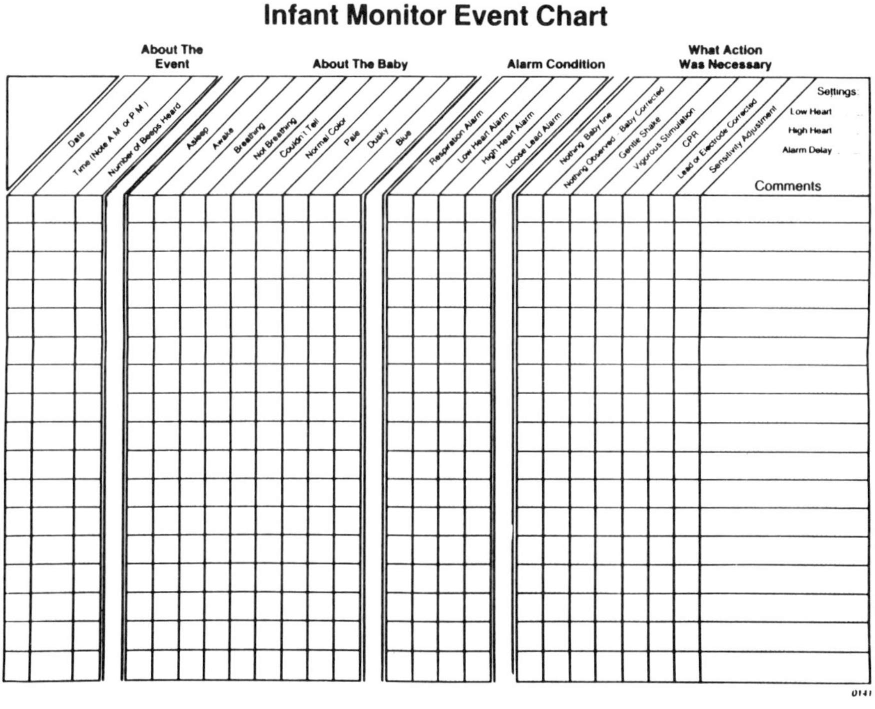

Infant Monitor Event Chart

Figure 5–4. An event tracking chart for parental use at home.

Parents should be instructed in what data to record and what action is to be taken when certain patterns begin to emerge (Fig 5–4).

The methods of responding to alarms need to be reinforced and tested. We recommend the use of mock alarm drills using an infant mannequin to reinforce the desired actions on the part of the parents and other caretakers.

Home apnea monitoring requires various adjustments in daily living routines, and we like to emphasize to the parents that home apnea monitoring is only tolerable and effective when the responsibilities are shared. We make various recommendations to parents on sharing these responsibilities but allow the parents to work out the final arrangements. We also point out that elimination of extraneous noise while the monitor is in use is an important but sometimes neglected aspect. We emphasize that it is important that relatives, friends, and other caretakers be trained in the use of the monitor so that the parents may go out on occasion and live as normal a life as possible.

Critical to any successful home monitoring program is 24-hour availability of a doctor, nurse, or technician who can troubleshoot problems and make available repair or replacement service when needed. Psychosocial support is also important, and we put parents into contact with social workers, visiting nurse service, other monitoring parents, and regional support groups for parents of babies on monitors, such as local chapters of the National Sudden Infant Death Syndrome Foundation. Suppliers of home apnea monitors should be encouraged to maintain stock levels of monitors and all other necessary supplies to make available both rental and purchase options for the equipment, to provide direct billing service to insurance companies or other third-party payers, and to encourage third-party payers to consider the cost-saving aspects of home apnea monitoring as compared to prolonged hospitalization or institutionalization of children with recurrent apneas.

On the other side of the coin, we deplore the unethical principle of contacting all parents of newborns or pregnant mothers and apprising them of the availability of home apnea monitoring when the infant has no risk factors for apneas.

PSYCHOLOGICAL ASPECTS OF SUDDEN INFANT DEATH

There is no more frustrating and devastating occurrence than the loss of an infant, and this is even worse if the infant was being monitored in the hope of preventing such an occurrence. Once a baby is pronounced dead, the parents should be offered the opportunity to say good-bye to their baby and encouraged to hold and fondle their child in the utmost privacy during this terribly difficult time (Orlowski, 1984). Not all parents want to see or hold their baby after its death, but they should have the opportunity and possibly be encouraged, because contact aids in the grieving process. Parents who have lost a baby to SIDS need a great deal of support, counseling, and sympathetic understanding (Zebal & Woolsey, 1984). Social workers, psychiatrists, and clergy can play an invaluable role during this difficult time. Parents will typically demonstrate disbelief, guilt, or anger at the sudden loss of a previously healthy child or a child who is being monitored in order to prevent death (Smialek, 1978). They may search for something they should have seen or recognized that would have prevented the death or they may strike out at the pediatrician or family physician who had given the child a clean bill of health or recommended home apnea monitoring to prevent SIDS. It is important to emphasize to the parents that a physician cannot predict or prevent SIDS and that in some cases even home apnea monitoring and cardiopulmonary resuscitation cannot prevent SIDS. Parents will also appreciate hearing that there does not appear to be any suffering in SIDS and that the death appears to occur very rapidly and is not due to suffocation or struggling to breathe. It is also important to emphasize that SIDS is not contagious and that even though a minor viral infection or upper respiratory infection may have preceded the death, there is no evidence of a killer virus that threatens other family members or neighbors. The baby has not been the victim of a freakish disease; as many as 7000 infants die as a result of SIDS each year in the United States. What the parents need most, however, is someone who will sit with them, answer any questions, and be receptive and sympathetic. Parents are frequently reluctant to express guilt outwardly for fear that they may be blamed for the death of the child. Guilt in the parents can be uncovered by offering the parents the statement: "Parents often blame themselves when their baby dies like this" and then being receptive to their response (Bergman, 1974). Guilt can be the most destructive emotion impeding the grieving process, and it should be dealt with immediately and any misconceptions clarified (Mandell et al, 1980).

It is important also to emphasize that parents who have just suffered the catastrophic loss of their child should not be questioned by police, physicians, or other personnel about the possibility of child abuse or infanticide. It is the coroner's responsibility to determine if homicide is involved (Bass et al, 1986).

We recommend that a follow-up counseling session be scheduled for the family of a SIDS victim 4 to 6 weeks after the death. At this time parents and other family members should be encouraged to discuss any questions that may continue to haunt them or have been raised by friends or relatives. Inadequate or inappropriate grief reactions may require further appropriate counseling or support services. The family should also be put in contact with the local chapter of the National Sudden Infant Death Syndrome Foundation if such contact had not already been previously established (Gould & James, 1979). The services of this organization can be invaluable in helping parents to cope with the sudden loss of their child and to know that they are not alone in having experienced such a loss (Bergman, 1979).

REFERENCES

Ambler MW, Neave C, Sturner WQ: Sudden and unexpected death in infancy and childhood. *Am J Forensic Med Pathol* 1981; *2*:23.

Ariagno RL: Evaluation and management of infantile apnea. *Pediatr Ann* 1984; *13*:210.

Bass M, Kravath RE, Glass L: Death scene investigation in sudden infant death. *N Engl J Med* 1986;*315*:100.

Beal SM: Some epidemiological factors about sudden infant death syndrome (SIDS) in South Australia, in Tildon T, Roeder LM, Steinschneider A (eds) *Sudden Infant Death Syndrome*. New York: Academic Press, 1983: p 15.

Beckwith JB: *The Sudden Infant Death Syndrome*. US Department of Health, Education, and Welfare publication No. 76–5137. Government Printing Office, 1976.

Bergman AB: Psychological aspects of sudden unexpected death in infants and children, review and commentary. *Pediatr Clin North Am* 1974;*21*:115.

Bergman AB: The sudden infant death syndrome: What can you do? *Medical Times*, April 1979.

Black L, Hersher L, Steinschneider A: Impact of the apnea monitor on family life. *Pediatrics* 1978;*62*:681.

Brooks JG: Apnea of infancy and sudden infant death syndrome. *Am J Dis Child* 1982;*136*:1012.

Cain LP, Kelly DH, Shannon DC: Parents' perceptions of the psychological and social impact of home monitoring. *Pediatrics* 1980;*66*:37.

Diagnostic and Therapeutic Technology Assessment (DATTA): Questions and answers: Apnea monitoring for newborns at risk of sudden infant death syndrome. *JAMA* 1984;*251*:531.

Duffty P, Bryan MH: Home apnea monitoring in "near-miss" sudden infant death syndrome (SIDS) and in siblings of SIDS victims. *Pediatrics* 1982;*70*:69.

Froggatt P, Lynas MA, MacKenzie G: Epidemiology of sudden unexpected death in infants ("cot death") in Northern Ireland. *Brit J Prev Soc Med* 1971;*25*:119.

Gordon D, Cohen RJ, Kelly D, et al: Sudden infant death syndrome: Abnormalities in short term fluctuations in heart rate and respiratory activity. *Pediatr Res* 1984;*18*:921.

Gould JB, James O: Management of the near-miss infant: A personal perspective. *Pediatr Clin North Am* 1979;*26*:857.

Irgens LM, Skjaerven R, Peterson DR: Prospective assessment of recurrence risk in sudden infant death syndrome siblings. *J Pediatr* 1984;*104*:349.

Kahn A, Blum D: Home monitoring of infants considered at risk for the sudden infant death syndrome. *Eur J Pediatr* 1982;*139*:94.

Kleinberg F: Sudden infant death syndrome. *Mayo Clin Proc* 1984;*59*:352.

Mandell F, McAnulty E, Reece RM: Observations of paternal response to sudden unanticipated infant death. *Pediatrics* 1980;*65*:221.

Merritt TA, Valdes-Dapena M: SIDS research update. *Ped Ann* 1984;*13*:193.

Naeye RL: The sudden infant death syndrome: A review of recent advances. *Arch Pathol Lab Med* 1977;*101*:165.

Naeye RL: Sudden infant death. *Sci Am* 1980;*242*:56.

National Institute of Health Consensus Development Statement: Infantile Apnea and home monitoring. *Pediatrics* 1987;79:292.

Nickerson BG: Terminology: Near-miss SIDS, letter to the editor. *Pediatrics* 1982;*69*:386.

Orlowski JP: Cardiopulmonary resuscitation in children. *Pediatr Clin North Am* 1980;*27*:495.

Orlowski JP: Pediatric cardiopulmonary resuscitation. *Emerg Med Clin* 1983;*1*:3.

Orlowski JP: Critical care aspects of the sudden infant death syndrome, in Shoemaker NC, Thompson WL, Holbrook PR (eds): *Textbook of Critical Care*. Philadelphia, Saunders, 1984, chap 13.

Peterson DR, Chinn NM, Fisher LD: The sudden infant death syndrome: Repetitions in families. *J Pediatr* 1980;97:265.

Quattrochi JJ, Baba N, Liss L, et al: Sudden infant death syndrome (SIDS): A preliminary study of reticular dendritic spines in infants with SIDS. *Brain Res* 1980;*181*:245.

Schulte FJ, Albani M, Schnizer H, et al: Neuronal control of neonatal respiration—sleep apnea and the sudden infant death syndrome. *Neuropediatrics* 1982;*13*:3.

Shannon DC, Kelly DH, O'Connell K: Abnormal regulation of ventilation in infants at risk for sudden-infant-death syndrome. *N Engl J Med* 1977;297:747.

Silvio KT: SIDS and apnea monitoring: A parent's view. *Pediatr Ann* 1984;*13*:229.

Smialek Z: Observations on immediate reactions of families to sudden infant death. *Pediatrics* 1978;*62*:160.

Smith JC: Psychosocial aspects of infantile apnea and home monitoring. *Pediatr Ann* 1984;*13*:219.

Southall DP: Home monitoring and its role in the sudden infant death syndrome. *Pediatrics* 1983;72:133.

Southall DP, Richards JM, Rhoden KJ, et al: Prolonged apnea and cardiac arrhythmias in infants discharged from neonatal intensive care units: Failure to predict an increased risk for sudden infant death syndrome. *Pediatrics* 1982;70:844.

Southall DP, Richards JM, de Swiet M, et al: Identification of infants destined to die unexpectedly during infancy: Evaluation of predictive importance of prolonged apnea and disorders of cardiac rhythm or conduction. *Br Med J* 1983;286:1092.

Summary of Proceedings: Second International Conference on Causes of Sudden Infant Death, Seattle, 1969. National Institutes of Health, publication No. 1746-0007. National Institute of Child Health and Human Development, 1971.

Valdes-Dapena MA: Sudden unexplained infant death 1970 through 1975: An evolution in understanding. *Pathol Annu* 1977;*12*:117.

Valdes-Dapena MA: Sudden infant death syndrome: A review of the medical literature 1974–1979. *Pediatrics* 1980;*66*:597.

Wasserman AL: A prospective study of the impact of home monitoring on the family. *Pediatrics* 1984;*74*:323.

Zebal BH, Woolsey SF: SIDS and the family: The pediatrician's role. *Pediatr Ann* 1984;*13*:237.

6

Sleep Apnea

KEVIN J. GRADY, MD
JOSEPH A. GOLISH, MD
ATUL C. MEHTA, MD

VENTILATION DURING SLEEP

Sleep alters ventilatory function in virtually everyone. In respiratory patients, this dysfunction can have adverse physiologic effects. In 1% of the population, complete cessation of breathing occurs periodically during sleep, so-called sleep apnea. Snoring during sleep and daytime hypersomnolence are the principal symptoms, but cardiopulmonary sequelae can occur. Various therapeutic approaches are available, including several respiratory therapy modalities applied in the lung. Nasal continuous positive airway pressure (CPAP) is the most exciting and promising of these techniques.

Sleep is not a uniform state but in fact a heterogeneous cyclic progression of several different stages. The three main stages are (1) waking or arousal; (2) non-rapid eye movement (REM) sleep; and (3) REM sleep. Each stage can be recognized on the basis of electroencephalogram (EEG), electro-oculogram (EOG), and electromyogram (EMG) patterns during polysomnography. Non-REM sleep, or "quiet" sleep, displays high-voltage slow-wave EEG patterns, whereas active sleep (REM) shows a low-voltage mixed-frequency EEG pattern. Non-REM sleep consists of four different stages: stages 1 and 2 are transitions between arousal and deep sleep; stages 3 and 4 are the deepest levels of sleep. There is orderly progression through the four stages of sleep into REM sleep. REM sleep consists of two phases, one associated with phasic movements, such as REM, and the other lacking these phasic movements.

Control of respiration during wakefulness and during sleep differs. Even within sleep there is a variation in non-REM and REM ventilatory stimuli. During non-REM sleep the major factor affecting breathing is metabolic homeostasis of carbon dioxide. The level of carbon dioxide is the main stimulus to breathing. During REM sleep, especially during the phasic period, breathing movement is not controlled by carbon dioxide levels but appears to subserve nonrespiratory requirements. During both REM and non-REM sleep, hypoxemic ventilatory responsiveness remains intact.

Mechanisms that can lead to hypoxemia and oxygen desaturation with sleep are multiple. During early non-REM sleep there is unstable, periodic breathing; in later stages, decreased carbon dioxide sensitivity and possibly changes in carbon dioxide threshold lead to increasing carbon dioxide and decreasing oxygen levels. With REM sleep there is a loss of metabolic stimulus (i.e., carbon dioxide) to ventilatory drive; therefore, there is chaotic respiratory movement. Furthermore, during phasic REM sleep intercostal muscle paralysis can further increase carbon dioxide levels and decrease oxygen saturation.

Patients with normal lungs usually do not have significant changes in Po_2 and Pco_2 levels during sleep. However, certain lung diseases such as chronic obstructive pulmonary disease (COPD), asthma, kyphoscoliosis, and pulmonary fibrosis are associated with decreased respiratory function during sleep. Sleep-related breathing disturbances should be suspected in these patients if there is any evidence of inappropriate polycythemia or pulmonary hypertension for a given waking state oxygen level, if sleep fragmentation is present, and if patients are at high risk, such as being male, obese, or hypoxemic. One proposed mechanism for worsening hypoxemia in COPD patients is a change in chest wall and diaphragmatic mechanics. During REM sleep, and particularly during phasic portions when intercostal muscle paralysis occurs, the diaphragm is called upon to supply a larger percentage of tidal volume. In COPD patients with hyperinflation and flattening of diaphragms, there is a resultant decrease in tidal volume and worsening of hypoxemia and hypercarbia. Decreased ciliary function during sleep may also be involved in worsening ventilation–perfusion mismatches and hypoxemia. Finally, base line hypoxemia leads to greater oxygen desaturation with a given change in Po_2 because of the sigmoidal configuration of the oxyhemoglobin desaturation.

SLEEP APNEA SYNDROME

Sleep apnea syndrome, once considered rare, is an important sleep-related breathing disorder. Apnea is defined as a complete absence of air flow for 10 seconds or more. Hypopnea is defined as a marked reduction of air flow for more than 10 seconds. A sleep apnea index is defined as the number of respiratory events per hour of sleep. Sleep apnea syndrome is defined as an apneic index greater than five with apneic episodes occurring in both non-REM and REM sleep. Sleep apnea is divided into three main categories: central, obstructive, and mixed. Central apnea is defined as cessation of both air flow and respiratory effort. Obstructive apnea is the termination of air flow that is associated with continued or possibly increased respiratory drive. A mixed sleep apnea episode begins as a central apnea and concludes with an obstructive apnea.

Pathophysiology

The pathophysiology of central sleep apnea is still poorly understood but is thought to be related to failure of the respiratory control center to adequately adjust ventilation. A decrease in neural stimuli to the respiratory muscle results in cessation of muscular activity. On polysomnography, episodes of no air flow and no thoracic or abdominal motion are noted. The resulting physiologic changes of hypoxemia and arousal lead to sporadic respirations and can lead to a clinical picture of sleep apnea. Central sleep apnea occurs much less frequently than the obstructive variety. The hypoxemia is less in degree, as are the resulting hemodynamic sequelae.

The events that lead to obstructive sleep apnea are dynamic and are related to the imbalance between upper airway neural activity and diaphragmatic neural activity. In the waking state, there is synchrony between the motor activity of the upper airway musculature, including the genioglossus muscle and the lateral pharyngeal wall musculature, and the diaphragm and intercostal muscular activity. With this synchronicity present, pharyngeal negative pressure does not exceed airway support, and no airway occlusion occurs. This balance is lost in obstructive sleep apnea and leads to obstruction, hypoxemia, and hypercarbia. Hypoxemia then leads to arousal, with eventual reestablishment of ventilation. Conditions such as obesity, myxedema, cranial abnormalities, and acromegaly predispose to this dynamic obstruction by narrowing the pharyngeal anatomy in a fixed fashion. Alcohol and sedatives may further decrease neural activity and increase the likelihood of obstruction. The end result of either central or obstructive apnea is nocturnal fluctuating respiration, arousal, hypoxemia, and hypercarbia. These changes lead to the clinical picture of sleep apnea.

Diagnosis

The patient's history plays a very important part in the diagnosis of sleep apnea syndrome. Three main categories of symptoms are seen in sleep apnea syndrome: nocturnal symptoms, daytime behavioral symptoms, and those symptoms related to cardiovascular sequelae. Nocturnal symptoms are best described by the patient's spouse. Historical information usually includes complaints of loud snoring as far back as the teenage years. Frequently, nocturnal respiratory pauses are noted followed by very loud respiratory surges. Automatic behavior, nocturnal enuresis, and insomnia are also noted. The daytime symptom of hypersomnolence is almost always present. Progressive intellectual and personality changes may be described by both patient and family. Morning cloudiness, headaches, and sexual impotence may also be presenting symptoms.

Physical examination may be normal in sleep apnea patients. However, clinical evidence of cardiopulmonary dysfunction such as hypertension, cor pulmonale, polycythemia, and left ventricular dysfunction may be presenting manifestations. Approximately 60% of patients with sleep apnea are obese; approximately 5% to 10% of these are morbidly obese. Otolaryngological examination may show evidence of deviated nasal septum, micrognathia, or retrognathia. The patient should be examined for evidence of endocrine abnormalities such as myxedema and acromegaly.

Polysomnography is the key test in the diagnosis and evaluation of sleep apnea syndrome. The duration and time of day of polysomnography continues to be a controversial matter. Daytime screening polysomnography is probably sufficient to evaluate severe sleep apnea, but in mild to moderate cases nocturnal recordings may be needed. Nocturnal polysomnography is more likely to include REM sleep and therefore to detect oxygen desaturation and the incidence of severe cardiac arrhythmias. Oximetry alone, even at home, can be used to screen patients for sleep apnea or to document the efficacy of therapy.

The parameters recorded during nocturnal polysomnography usually include an EEG, the EOG, the chin EMG, and the ECG. EEG, EOG, and EMG are utilized to determine the stage of sleep. Additional techniques may be included: ear oximetry to measure oxygen saturation; impedance plethysmography to allow calculation of tidal volume; nasal and buccal thermistors to measure air flow; and chest and abdominal strain gauges to evaluate paradoxical respiratory movement and help differentiate between mixed obstructive and central sleep apneas. More invasive hemodynamic monitoring, including systemic arterial blood pressure monitoring and pulmonary artery pressure (PAP) monitoring, can be done. By analysis of nocturnal polysomnography, the frequency and duration of apneic episodes can be determined and classified into three subsets of sleep apnea: central, obstructive, and mixed. This information can be helpful in determining further medical and surgical management.

In the patient with obstructive sleep apnea syndrome (OSAS), several methods are available to evaluate the anatomic structures of the upper airway. These include xerograms, CT scan, and fiberoptic nasal pharyngoscopy during the awake and sleep state. CT imaging allows a static rather than dynamic evaluation of the upper airway structures. Diminished cross-sectional areas of the nasopharynx, oropharynx, and hypopharynx appear to correlate with a vulnerability to functional obstruction. By detecting structural abnormalities in the upper airway, CT scanning may suggest benefit of surgical therapy in OSAS; the lack of such abnormalities may lend support to medical management. Since uvulopalatopharyngoplasty (UPP) appears to be more effective in nasopharyngeal and oropharyngeal obstruction, CT scanning may be helpful in defining the level of obstruction.

Fiberoptic nasopharyngoscopic visualizing of structures obstructing the upper airway during the waking and sleep states may, like the CT scan, favor surgical management of obstructive sleep apnea. Fiberoptic evaluation should include examination of the nasopharynx, the oral pharyngeal inlet, the hypopharynx, and the supraglottic larynx during quiet forced inspiration and expiration and also during the Müller maneuver.

Other tests that may be helpful in the evaluation of patients with sleep apnea include blood levels of thyroid-stimulating hormone (TSH) for detection of possible hypothyroidism, which can cause or worsen sleep apnea. Twenty-four-hour Holter monitoring may be suggestive of OSAS if the classic pattern of bradycardia followed by tachycardia is detected. The usefulness of Holter monitoring as a screening modality, however, is questionable. Spirometry and resting arterial blood gas determinations may be useful in ruling out associated respiratory disorders such as COPD, neuromuscular disease, and central alveolar hypoventilation. The carbon dioxide stimulation test can identify those patients with sleep disorders associated with daytime alveolar hypoventilation.

Initial studies suggest that flow-volume loops may be helpful in identifying patients with obstructive sleep apnea. The presence of inspiratory "sawtoothing" or variable extrathoracic obstruction was thought to be a sensitive and specific marker of upper airway obstruction. A recent study has questioned that premise.

Management of Obstructive Sleep Apnea

Some patients with OSAS by sleep laboratory criteria are identified during evaluation for problems such as impotence and insomnia. If there is no other clinical evidence of obstructive apnea, the best approach is observation with serial follow-up sleep studies. The medical management of clinically significant obstructive sleep apnea has to be viewed on several levels including (1) reversal of factors that worsen airway obstruction; (2) pharmacologic therapy; and (3) mechanical or nonsurgical airway support.

Removal of Airway Obstruction. For the obese patient with obstructive sleep apnea, an important therapeutic modality should be sustained weight reduction. The beneficial effect of weight loss is most likely secondary to an increase in the upper airway cross-sectional area. In addition, central chemosensitivity to carbon dioxide may be increased.

There are several endocrine diseases associated with obstructive sleep apnea syndrome, including hypothyroidism, acromegaly, and Cushing's syndrome. Acromegaly probably causes obstructive apnea secondary to an enlarged, thickened tongue. Similarly, Cushing's syndrome may increase pharyngeal fatty tissues that can lead to obstructive apnea. Treatment of these endocrine abnormalities frequently reverses the obstructive sleep apnea.

Both alcohol and respiratory depressants alter upper airway muscle activity and may lead to or worsen preexisting occlusive apnea. Elimination of these agents will improve the nocturnal respiratory pattern. Avoidance of smoking, industrial irritants, and treatment of allergic or chronic rhinitis with the nonsedating H_1 receptor blocker, terfenadine (Seldane), or topical steroids may also lessen occlusive apneic episodes.

Pharmacologic Therapy. Initial studies on the use of supplemental oxygen in obstructive sleep apnea suggested that it might be deleterious, since individual apneic episodes may be prolonged. A recent study by Smith et al (1984) demonstrated that low-flow continuous nocturnal oxygen may be beneficial in patients with obstructive sleep apnea and daytime hypersomnolence. Smith showed that low-flow oxygen increased base line oxygen saturation, decreased sleep disorders during non-REM sleep, and significantly reduced the percentage of central and mixed sleep disorder events.

Pharmacologic manipulation of obstructive sleep apnea has met with a variable degree of success. The use of the tricyclic antidepressant protriptyline (Vivactil), which is nonsedating, seems to improve clinical symptoms of upper airway obstruction in some patients. Protriptyline decreases the number of apneic episodes through its established effect of decreasing the percentage of REM sleep. Many patients on protriptyline have improved weight reduction while on the drug, which may be an additional mechanism to explain the improvement in clinical symptoms. The major side effects of protriptyline are due to its anticholinergic action, including urinary retention, arrhythmias, and orthostatic hypotension. The starting dosage is usually 5 to 10 mg one hour before bedtime and can be increased to a maximum dose of 30 mg.

Progestational agents have been shown to improve waking arterial oxygen concentration but have no significant effect on the incidence, duration, and rate of occlusive apneic episodes in most cases. Variable results have been seen with other drugs such as thyroxine, nicotine, and theophylline.

Mechanical Airway Support. Mechanical modalities for reversing the episodes of obstructive apnea have recently come into vogue. These include nasal CPAP and tongue-retaining devices. Nasal CPAP may function as a "pneumatic splint" by reducing the net negative oropharyngeal pressure generated by inspiratory effort. Other possible mechanisms for the beneficial effect of nasal CPAP include increased neural drive of the oropharyngeal muscles secondary to increased stimulation of the upper airway receptors or reduced upper airway resistance from dilation of the airway column. Studies by Sanders (1984) showed nasal CPAP to be well tolerated in a majority of patients and successful in reducing the frequency of both occlusive and mixed obstructive patterns. Long-term efficacy of nasal CPAP has yet to be shown. Unlike protriptyline, nasal CPAP does not decrease duration and frequency of REM sleep and therefore restores normal sleep architecture.

Unfortunately, the earlier mechanical devices needed to deliver nasal CPAP were cumbersome, and therefore compliance was a problem. The system included a blower or condenser flow generator system, conduit, a nasal delivery port, and a positive end-expiratory pressure (PEEP) valve. Newer nasal CPAP systems have been shown to be well-suited for both hospital and home care use. With the exception of the "custom-fitted" nasal masks, these systems are available as professional home care material. The monthly rental charge for the equipment varies from $150 to $250 and is covered by most third-party payers. At present an FDA-approved CPAP system is available from Respironic.

Included in the original Respironic system (Fig 6–1) is a blower air source and a PEEP valve that is built into the nasal mask, which eliminates the additional expiratory conduit. The newer version of the device has moved the PEEP valve to the blower to minimize noise to the patient. Three standard nasal masks are available: small, medium, and large. For patients who experience facial pressure sores caused by improperly fitting

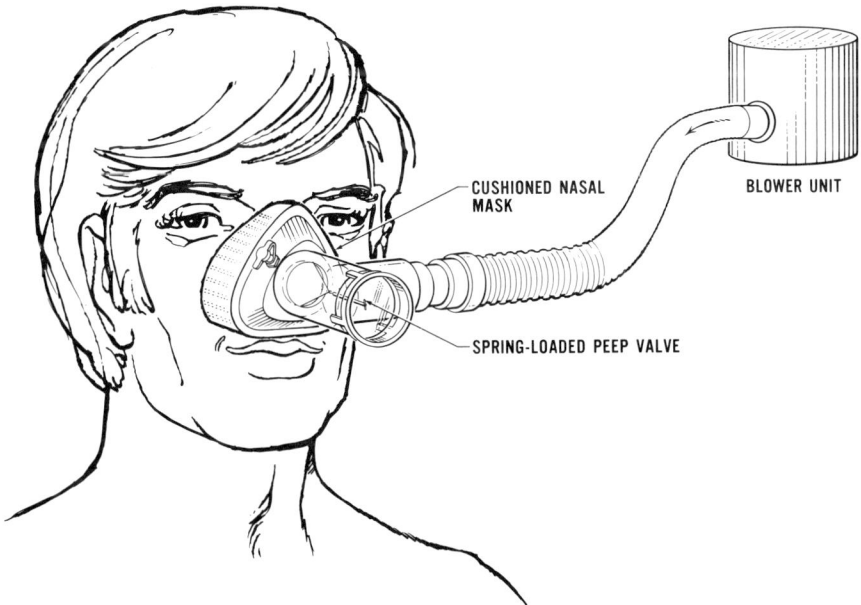

Figure 6–1. Diagram of a nasal CPAP apparatus.

masks, fitted masks can be made from plastic molds. If needed, nasal cannulas can be modified to provide an adequate seal without using a mask. These are not yet commercially available, however.

Several levels of PEEP valves are available. Optimal PEEP can be determined by recording oxygen desaturation during polysomnography using different levels of PEEP. The amount of PEEP that shows the least degree of desaturation should be used on the CPAP system (Fig 6–2). Two basic air sources are available: blower systems or condensers. Condenser systems usually deliver air flow of lower relative humidity and

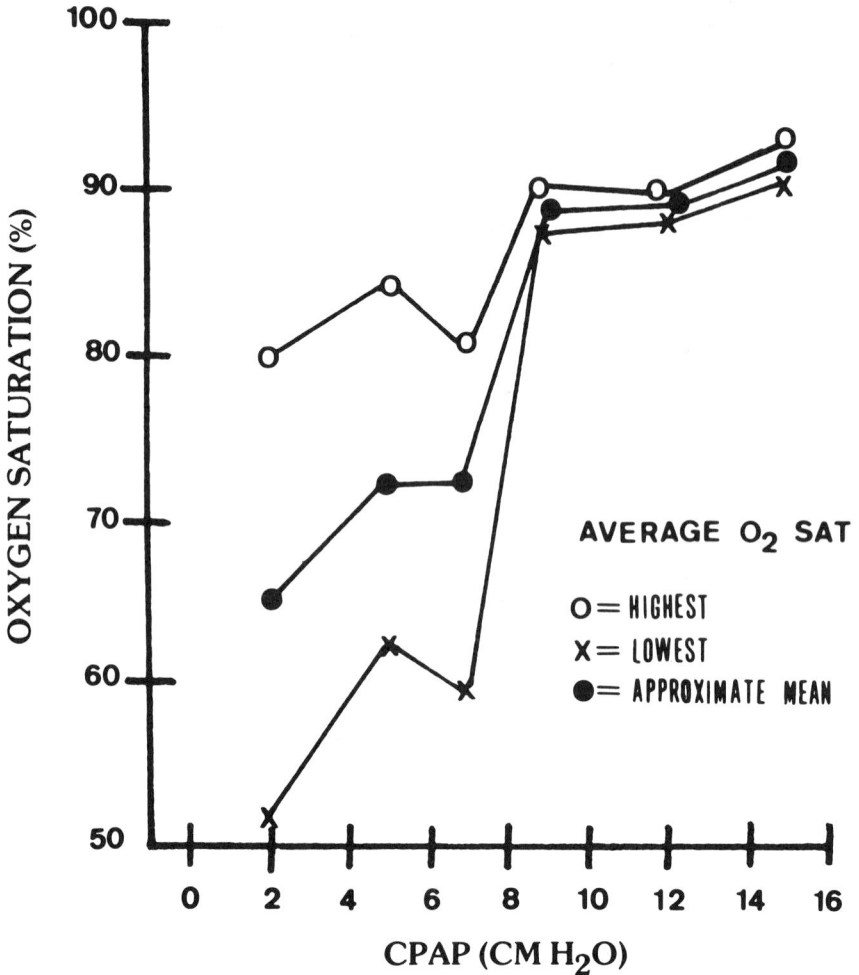

Figure 6–2. Titrated CPAP levels and corresponding oxygen saturation measured while patient was asleep and using nasal CPAP system with custom-fitted mask. *(Reproduced with permission from Sleeper GP, Strohl KP, Armeni MA:* Nasal continuous positive airway pressure for at-home treatment of obstructive sleep apnea: A case report. *Respir Care 1985; 30:93.)*

temperature than that of the blower systems. There is a higher incidence of nasal mucosal irritation, epistaxis, and sore throats with lower humidity air sources. This complication can usually be alleviated by the use of a blower system or by the addition of a heated, humidified cascade system to a condenser air source.

Complications of nasal CPAP include pressure necrosis from improperly fitting nasal masks and conjunctivitis from air leaks around loosely fitting masks. Both problems can be minimized by a properly fitted mask. Gastric distension, as seen with full-face CPAP masks, has fortunately not been a problem to date. The noise produced by CPAP systems can limit sleep in some patients, especially once obstructive apnea improves and hypersomnia dissipates. Because of these complications, compliance with nasal CPAP still appears to be a limiting factor to its routine use in obstructive sleep apnea patients.

An alternative to nasal CPAP, in those patients who do not tolerate it, is the use of continuous nasal air flow delivered through nasal prongs. This method is not as effective as nasal CPAP or nasal cannula CPAP but may provide some clinical improvement in mild to moderate obstructive sleep apnea.

Samuelson designed and patented a tongue-retaining device (TRD) to increase the dimension of the nasal-breathing passage during sleep (Cartwright & Samuelson, 1982). The TRD was designed to hold the tongue away from the posterior pharynx by means of negative pressure applied to the lingular component of the device. Clinical trials using polysomnography showed a substantial reduction in the frequency and duration of obstructive apnea. The TRD appears to be a viable alternative in patients with mild to moderate obstructive apneas whose anatomic and functional lesions appear predominantly in the proximal oropharynx. The limitation to the use of the TRD again appears to be patient compliance.

Surgical Procedures. Surgical procedures for the treatment of obstructive sleep apnea are divided into two main categories: (1) indirect methods, such as surgery for obesity control and tracheostomies; and (2) direct methods such as UPP, surgical repair of nasal septal deviations, adenoid and lingular tonsil removal, craniofacial skeletal adjustment, and excision of pharyngeal space-occupying lesions.

Despite numerous medical and surgical alternatives in the treatment of obstructive sleep apnea, tracheostomy remains the modality most likely to succeed in providing consistent long-term benefit. Tracheostomy bypasses the critical level of obstruction, i.e., the oropharynx. It is the only reliable immediate treatment of obstructive sleep apnea; therefore, it is recommended for all patients with life-threatening obstructive apnea in the absence of another surgically treatable anatomic upper airway obstruction. High-risk patients with OSAS who should be treated initially with tracheostomy include those with incapacitating daytime hypersomnolence, severe oxygen desaturation with saturation levels less than 45%, significant hypertension with apneic episodes, and serious cardiac arrhythmias. In the appropriate setting, reversal of symptomatology of hypersomnolence and cardiopulmonary sequelae can be obtained in virtually all instances.

The two main techniques for tracheostomy placement are the standard tracheostomy and the skin-flap-constructed tracheal fenestra technique. Because the standard tracheostomy's higher incidence of prolonged healing time and infected granulation tissue may lead to stomal obstruction and perichondritis, the skin-flap-constructed tracheal fenestra has become increasingly popular. Silver fenestrated tracheostomy tubes or newer Silastic tracheostomy tubes are usually used. At some centers, customized fenestrated tubes are used, especially in the obese patient with a short, stubby neck. The use of "button tracheostomy" can be complicated by obstruction during sleep as a result of enlarged soft tissue of the neck and should be avoided.

Tracheostomy leaves the patient aesthetically disfigured; therefore it is critical that both patient and family take part in an intensive education program. This incorporates social and psychologic evaluation along with discussion of tracheostomy hygiene and care. It is important that this training be done before the tracheostomy is performed for maximum success.

Since patency is needed only during sleep in most patients, the tracheostomy tube may be plugged during the day and covered. Obese patients with obstructive sleep apnea often are able to lose weight after tracheostomy even though they were unable to do so before the procedure. In this group of patients, the tracheostomy stoma may be closed at a later date.

The second approach to the anatomic problem of obstructive sleep apnea is surgical enlargement of the pharyngeal airway by removal of redundant pharyngeal mucosa (UPP). In some centers, tracheostomies are also placed at the time of UPP because transient worsening of sleep apnea may occur secondary to edema. The success of UPP has been variable, and this may be related to the selection of patients and differences in surgical technique. At present, it appears that most patients have decreased symptoms, and approximately 50% of patients have a 50% or greater decrease in their apneic index. UPP appears to decrease the number of apneic episodes by transforming them to hypopneic episodes.

A report by Heimer et al (1983) showed clinical improvement along with diminution in the number and duration of occlusive episodes after the repair of a deviated nasal septum. Improvement may be related to reversing high nasal resistance. Similar clinical improvements have been noted in surgical removal of lingular tonsils. Obstructive sleep apnea patients with adenotonsillar enlargement can at times be cured with surgical correction, as may patients with micrognathia or retrognathia by means of mandibular osteotomies.

A rational approach to the management of obstructive sleep apnea

(Table 6–1) should include an initial trial of weight reduction followed by a 1- to 2-month trial of protriptyline at the usual starting dose of 5 to 15 mg one hour before bedtime, which can be adjusted upward in 5- to 10-mg increments. A maximum daily dose of 30 mg is suggested. For those patients without subjective or polysomnographic improvement and whose airway anatomy shows obstruction by endoscopic or cephalo-metric measurements, UPP with or without tracheostomy should be considered. Continuation of weight reduction and pharmacologic manipulation after UPP may facilitate early decannulation. Noninvasive techniques such as nasal CPAP or tongue-retaining devices can be tried before surgery in compliant patients desiring a nonsurgical approach. For patients with severe obstructive sleep apnea, tracheostomy remains the initial procedure of choice.

Management of Central Apnea

Treatment of central apnea is basically the same as for alveolar hypo-ventilation. Weight reduction plays an important part, as it does in ob-structive sleep apnea. Low-flow oxygen can be beneficial in some patients by preventing oxygen desaturation during sleep. Improvement in hypo-ventilation may be due to reversal of the brainstem depression by hy-poxemia. It is important that all patients started on oxygen be carefully monitored subsequently during sleep to prevent paradoxic worsening of the PCO_2 level and worsening hypoxemia secondary to increased duration and frequency of apnea.

Pharmacologic therapy of central apnea has been less encouraging than that of obstructive sleep apnea. Medroxyprogesterone, a respiratory stimulant, has been beneficial in treating some patients with central apnea and hypoventilation. The usual dose is 20 mg by mouth three times daily. If no improvement in central apnea is noted with the above measures, support with a respirator, cuirass, or a rocking bed can be considered. A cuirass is a negative-pressure ventilator that functions similarly to an "iron lung." The major drawback of the cuirass is difficulty in fitting obese patients properly. The rocking bed takes advantage of gravity to effect

TABLE 6–1. TREATMENT MODALITIES OF OBSTRUCTIVE SLEEP APNEA

Mechanical	Removal of Contributing Factors
Low-flow oxygen	Obesity
Tongue-retaining device	Endocrine abnormalities
Nasal prong CPAP*	Alcohol or sedatives
Nasal mask CPAP	**Pharmacological**
Surgical	Protriptyline
Correction of anatomic	Thyroxine
abnormalities	Theophylline
Deviated septum repair	Nicotine
Uvulopalatopharyngoplasty	
Tracheostomy	

*CPAP = Continuous positive airway pressure.

respirations. By changing the level of inclination, the tidal volume can be adjusted to some degree. The respiratory rate is controlled by adjusting the rocking bed oscillating rate. For patients with persistent hypercarbia during daytime, techniques of voluntary ventilation, such as hypnosis, can be tried.

A more invasive option for patients with central apnea or hypoventilation who have persistent hypercarbia and polycythemia is diaphragmatic pacing. This technique involves placement of electrodes on both phrenic nerves.

SUMMARY

Sleep apnea is a disorder that has been recognized only in recent years. It is characterized by a disorder of sleep architecture resulting from disturbance of respiratory control and airway patency. Hypersomnolence, snoring, and pulmonary hypertension are the cardinal manifestations. Various management strategies including pharmacologic, surgical, and mechanical approaches have been devised. The newest and most exciting of these is the in-home application of nasal CPAP, which maintains airway patency in obstructive sleep apnea and restores normal sleep patterns. Other mechanical modalities can be used to support ventilation in central sleep apnea and alveolar hypoventilation.

REFERENCES

Cartwright RD, Samelson CF: Effects of a nonsurgical treatment for obstructive sleep apnea: The tongue-retaining device. *JAMA* 1982;*248*:705.

Heimer D, Scharf SM, Lieberman A, et al: Sleep apnea syndrome treated by repair of deviated nasal septum. *Chest* 1983;*84*:184.

Sanders MH: Nasal CPAP effect on patterns of sleep apnea. *Chest* 1984;*86*:839.

Sleeper GP, Strohl KP, Armeni MA: Nasal continuous positive airway pressure for at-home treatment of obstructive sleep apnea: A case report. *Respir Care* 1985;*30*:90.

Smith PL, Haponik EF, Bleecker ER: Effects of oxygen in patients with sleep apnea. *Am Rev Respir Dis* 1984;*130*:958.

7

Adjunctive Respiratory Modalities and Techniques

JEFFREY LUCAS, RRT

Respiratory home care has grown dramatically within the past 5 years. Almost every category of pulmonary disease has been treated at home in some way or another. Therefore many types of therapies and treatment modalities have been transplanted from the hospital to the private home. Many, if not all, of these regimens have had to be rethought and reimplemented to allow for effective use in the hands of the lay caregiver or patient. Not only have established therapies been reintroduced to the home care area but totally new techniques and equipment have been created by the needs of this new and growing field.

The purpose of this chapter is to provide an overview of a number of the more commonly used treatments, techniques, and equipment found in respiratory home care today. The major areas of adjunctive therapy that will be discussed here will include patient and family training and their introduction to home care in general. Ideas on follow-up care and routines will be presented, along with certain self-help programs that can be useful to the patient and easily implemented at home. Finally, a few types of equipment that are less commonly used (but are nice to have available) will be covered.

It was felt that the adjunctive modalities to be discussed in this chapter were important enough to be included within this book but that they did not quite fit anywhere else; therefore this "miscellaneous" chapter was conceived.

PATIENT AND FAMILY TRAINING

This section of the chapter is meant to offer certain methods by which the patient and family can: (1) best use their new equipment and (2) function most effectively and comfortably within their new life styles at home with some form of medical therapy.

Patient and family training is a most important aspect of successful respiratory home care.

Each piece of equipment or therapy modality that is required to treat the patient at home obviously requires teaching the users in some manner.

The medical personnel involved with patient discharge planning should keep in mind that this patient and family are returning home to a new environment and changed life style that has been brought about by the introduction of new equipment, care routines, people (home care personnel), and financial responsibilities they have never lived with before.

These changes in life style can add to the anxiety, fear, and resentment that already accompany chronic illness. Proper education and introduction to these changes can minimize their untoward effects and enhance successful home care experience.

Patient and family training should include a number of elements to alleviate apprehension and promote a successful hospital-to-home transition. These factors include:

1. *Predischarge familiarization with new techniques and equipment use.* Ideally, the same type of equipment that is to be used at home should be introduced to the patient and family days before actual discharge. This can reduce the apprehension about dealing with a completely new modality when seen for the first time at home. Initial instruction on its use and maintenance in the hospital will allow better compliance with its use in the home (Figs 7–1 and 7–2). The home care personnel have the burden of introducing and explaining new equipment and methods of oxygen therapy to the patient and family for the first time. The day of discharge is not the best time to be introducing new equipment and tasks to a family. It must also be remembered that very often the personnel may be dealing with an elderly patient and spouse who may not comprehend new material as readily as the younger patient and family. By allowing the patient to actually use the equipment in the hospital before discharge, a smoother hospital-to-home transition should result (Table 7–1). If training can be accomplished before discharge, the arrival of home care personnel on the day of discharge can be used as reinforcement and reassurance rather than initial training in a very hectic atmosphere.

2. *Predischarge determination of insurance coverage.* The issue of financial responsibility for the equipment and services placed in the home is also frequently left for the home care personnel and is usually discussed, along with new equipment, on the day of discharge. This again adds to the anxiety of the first day at home with a new life style. The insurance verifications for payment should be made in the hospital before discharge. This allows time for explaining how the insurance company will reimburse and for

NORTHCOAST OXYGEN COMPANY, INC.
12710 TRISKETT ROAD
CLEVELAND, OHIO 44111
PHONE: (216) 267-0033

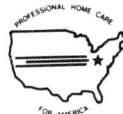

INSTRUCTIONS FOR OXYGEN CONCENTRATOR THERAPY

PRESCRIBED LITER FLOW: _____

PRESCRIBED DURATION: _____

DELIVERY DEVICE: _____

IMPORTANT!
NO SMOKING AND STAY AT LEAST 5 FEET FROM OPEN FLAMES WHILE USING YOUR OXYGEN. (CANDLES, FLAME ON GAS STOVE, ETC.)

1. Connect your humidifier to the screw on adaptor on the front panel of the concentrator.

2. Fill ½ full with distilled water.

3. Connect your nasal cannula or oxygen mask (whichever was prescribed) to the humidifier. Extension tubing can be added to allow for mobility away from your unit.

4. Keep your concentrator at least 6 inches from walls or curtains. Do not allow inlet filter to become blocked. Keep your concentrator away from heaters or heating ducts.

5. Plug the concentrator into 110V electrical outlet. It ideally should not be on the same circuit with other major household appliances.

6. Turn the concentrator on and be sure your flow indicator reads _____ liters per minute.

IMPORTANT!
OXYGEN IS A DRUG. USE IT JUST AS IT WAS ORDERED BY YOUR PHYSICIAN. TOO MUCH OR TOO LITTLE CAN BE HARMFUL.

7. Wash your inlet filter on your concentrator every 3 days in warm, mild detergent water. Rinse well, pat dry, and replace it immediately.

8. If you are using long connecting tubing, condensed water may accumulate in your tubing. This is to be expected. When this happens, empty your humidifier and replace it. Run the concentrator with your dry humidifier until the water evaporates from your tubing. You can wear it as you do this. When tubing is dry, replace distilled water in your humidifier.

9. You may not "feel" the oxygen entering your nose. This is normal at times. If you do not think you are getting oxygen, follow these steps:
    1. Be sure all connections are tight where your humidifier screws onto your unit, and be sure the top and bottom of the humidifier are screwed on straight and tight.
    2. Look for bubbling in the water in the humidifier.
    3. Place nasal cannula in glass of water and watch for bubbles.
    4. If you have performed all the above and still you have a problem, call your North Coast Oxygen therapist.

10. If you have an electrical power failure, turn your unit off, this will shut off the alarm and use your back-up oxygen cylinder as instructed. **BE SURE YOUR UNIT IS PLUGGED IN!**

Figure 7–1. This instructional form is designed to be a *guide* for inclusion of certain points during patient and family training. This guide can be adapted to fit the needs of the locality.

NORTHCOAST OXYGEN COMPANY, INC.
12710 TRISKETT ROAD
CLEVELAND, OHIO 44111
PHONE: (216) 267-0033

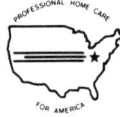

INSTRUCTIONS FOR AEROSOL MEDICATION THERAPY

PRESCRIBED MEDICATION: _____

PRESCRIBED FREQUENCY: _____

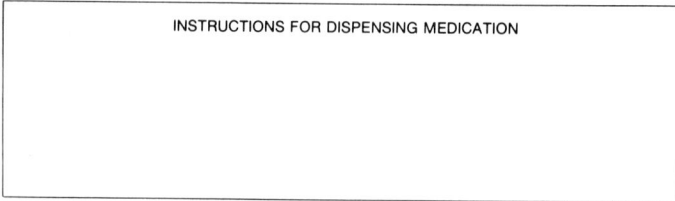

> INSTRUCTIONS FOR DISPENSING MEDICATION

1. Take your treatment until your medication runs out to be sure you get your proper dosage.

2. While taking your treatment sit upright in a comfortable chair or sit up in your bed.

3. Take **slow** deep breaths and hold your breath for a second during each inhalation of your medication.

4. Exhale normally. Do not breathe fast and deep you may become dizzy and feel numbness and tingling in your face and hands. If this happens stop your treatment and relax until these feelings are gone. Begin again but remember **slow** and deep.

5. After each treatment take your nebulizer apart and rinse in distilled water. Allow to air dry between treatments.

6. Every 3 days wash your nebulizer in mild detergent water and rinse well.

7. Follow by soaking in a 1 part white vinegar and 3 parts water solution for 20 minutes. Rinse well and allow to dry. Store in clean plastic bag after dry if you are not going to use it soon.

8. If you are hospitalized for a lung infection, let us know. We will sterilize your unit and return it when you come home.

9. Keep your medications in the refrigerator.

PRECAUTIONS

Stop Treatment If:
1. Numbness and tingling is felt in face, hands or feet. Relax and slow your breathing down.
2. If you feel your heart racing or pounding, or if your pulse rate increases by more than 20 beats per minute, stop your treatment and try again later. If you experience the same problem, call your doctor or let us know at North Coast Oxygen Company.

Figure 7–2. This instructional form is designed as a guide for inclusion of certain points during patient and family training. This guide can be adapted to fit the needs of the locality. **Note:** The blank box on this form is to allow space for drawing pictures of medication eye droppers or syringes, etc. This serves as a guide for using the correct increments for medication dosage.

TABLE 7–1. BENEFITS ASSOCIATED WITH PREDISCHARGE TRAINING

The patient and family will be more comfortable with the unit at home for the first time

The patient has time to formulate questions on his or her own in the hospital, before being left alone with the unit at home

The family will have time to decide where the equipment is best placed in the home before the patient arrives

Fears concerning oxygen use in the home can be discussed and minimized in the hospital

Predischarge training allows the home care personnel to use the day of discharge as reinforcement and reassurance

how much. The patient and family should also know what personal financial responsibility they have toward their equipment and services. Most people would not want to buy or rent services from anyone without prior knowledge of the cost or the opportunity to shop for price and service. Why should the patient accept service before knowing the cost? The home care company should be involved as early as possible during these discharge plans. This helps in formulating an early relationship between the patient and family (consumer) and the company that many times will be a close working relationship in the future.

3. *At-home reinforcement of therapy and equipment operation on the day of discharge.* Again, this is not the day to be introducing new equipment, new procedures, new personnel, and new financial burdens to the patient and family. The patient and family, by this time, should be familiar with what is going to happen, and when the home care personnel arrive this period can now be used to adapt the equipment use to the individual's home and life style. Options for the patient to consider can also be introduced. If the patient's condition or need changes, he or she may then be aware of what is available to fit these new need(s). Predischarge training helps the hospital-to-home transition immensely. A phone call on the day after to ask if the first night alone went well adds to the patient's security, knowing that he or she can depend on someone in the community for help if need be.

4. *Introduction of home care supplier to the patient and family.* Once the patient and family have returned home, the home care supplier begins to play an important role in promoting a functional life style within the patient's new environment. On (or preferably before) the day of discharge the patient and family should be "introduced" to the home care company via the company's own personnel. This introduction is very simple, but important, and should relate key points of information the family will need to know in the near future (Table 7–2).

TABLE 7–2. KEY POINTS OF INFORMATION THE FAMILY NEEDS TO KNOW ABOUT THEIR HOME CARE SUPPLIER

Normal operating hours. The family should be aware of normal operating hours Monday through Friday and weekend hours if available. These are times when personnel are available for questions, deliveries, and replenishment of supplies

Emergency after-hours calls. Family should be aware that in the event of an emergency (equipment malfunction, oxygen replenishment, etc) they can reach company personnel 24 hours per day, seven days per week. Make this emergency phone number readily available if different from the regular number

Provisions for other technical services or equipment. Family should be aware of all that is available to them. In the event the patient's needs change, they will be familiar with options and can stay with one supplier

Billing procedure. Explain the procedure (do you fill out and send claim forms; what will the patient be billed for and why)

Follow-up services. If follow-up personnel are to be visiting the home in the future, state this to the family. When that individual calls for an appointment the family need not be as concerned about the person's identity and will be expecting him or her

Proper instruction offered to the patient and family results in more than knowing how to operate the equipment and perform the therapies. A thorough knowledge of the equipment and therapies should result in enhanced confidence levels for the patient and family. The patient should not be allowed to live with apprehension regarding the use of the equipment, therapies, or oxygen itself. The patient and family members should be fully aware of all the options currently available to aid patient mobility and conserve oxygen product, and of the avenues of travel open to them.

Once the patient has returned home, follow-up visits should begin. The person at home requiring continual medical therapy remains a patient, and that patient's condition, care routines, needs, and concerns continually change. Follow-up care is an integral portion of respiratory home care.

FOLLOW-UP CARE AND HOME VISITS

Home care follow-ups can offer many advantages to the patient and family (Table 7–3). Many instances occur where the shut-in or severely disabled patient cannot visit the physician's office for regular checkups. The ventilator-dependent patient and family often rely heavily on the availability of home care personnel to offer assistance and relay information to the physician. Figure 7–3 is an example home care follow-up form. By employing the home care personnel as liaison between patient and physician, important care plan decisions can be made rapidly, unnecessary calls are placed to the physician less frequently, and the patient and family are satisfied with prompt responses to their problems.

As the patient readjusts and becomes oriented to the new environ-

TABLE 7–3. ADVANTAGES TO RESPIRATORY HOME CARE FOLLOW-UPS

Home care personnel act as liaison between patient and physician

Follow-up visits offer a convenient source of information for the patient about the therapy regimen and equipment use

Patient compliance with ordered therapy and rehabilitation protocols are monitored

Home care personnel can keep patient and family abreast of new developments that can be of benefit

Emergency assistance is available in the event of exacerbations or equipment failures

Prophylactic maintenance of equipment is performed to minimize interruptions in therapy

Follow-up visits offer the patient and family a sense of security through knowing someone in the community is available as resource or help

ment, many questions may arise about equipment use during travel, problems associated with mobility around home, etc. In many instances the patient is unwilling to contact the physician about these "small" matters but does feel very comfortable discussing these points with the follow-up personnel in the home surroundings. Thus the regular visits become a convenient source of information gathering.

Regular home care visits are very beneficial in maintaining patient compliance with ordered therapy. For example, many patients feel there is a physiologic dependence if they "overuse" oxygen. Thus the patient who is prescribed oxygen 24 hours per day may not use it. The patient who has been discharged with orders to continue the pulmonary rehabilitation program that was started in the hospital may not do so, because he or she has not experienced immediate benefits from the prescribed diet, exercise routine, and guidelines on work simplification. The visiting therapist can assess these problems and ensure that the patient follows orders. The hour meter on the oxygen concentrator will indicate whether the patient is using oxygen as prescribed. If the patient is on liquid or compressed gas cylinders (CGCs), the number of deliveries will indicate the amount of oxygen the patient is using. Pulmonary rehabilitation techniques many times become tedious and boring. The key to success with these prescribed therapies is persistence, regularity, and documentation of improvements. The visiting therapist becomes an incentive and watchdog of performance for the patient. Various equipment types require regular maintenance and prophylactic care to maintain proper function and uninterrupted service for the patient. These minor maintenance routines and performance checks can also be performed by the therapist.

The rapidly changing and growing field of respiratory home care has spawned a tremendous growth in new products and technology. It is impossible for the patient to know all that is available to him or her. Visiting home care personnel can suggest new items and self-help strategies available to enhance comfort, improve mobility, conserve oxygen product, and heighten the patient's self-image.

NORTH COAST OXYGEN COMPANY, INC.

12710 Trisket Rd.
Cleveland, Ohio 44111
Phone: (216) 267-0033

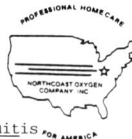

PROFESSIONAL HOMECARE

NORTHCOAST OXYGEN COMPANY INC

NAME: Mr. Bill Jones
ADDRESS: 123 Main Street
PHONE: 456-7897
PHYSICIAN: Dr. John Bauer
CATEGORY #: Two

DX: Emphysema, chronic bronchitis FOR AMERICA
RX: oxygen 2 LPM continuously
aerosol with 0.3cc alupent in 3.0cc saline
EQUIPMENT: oxygen concentrator, aerosol qid
SERIAL # 123

PHYSIOLOGICAL PARAMETERS
ASSESSMENT

BP	140/80
PULSE	89
RR	30

- Auscultation
- Observance of accessory muscle use
- Visual clinical assessment of:
  Dependent edema   Shortness of breath
  Neck vein engorgement   Pursed lip breathing
  Color

EQUIPMENT

HOURS	2620
calculated usage	480 hrs./mo
LPM	2 LPM
FIO 2	92%

- Is it cleaned and maintained?
- Does it meet the patient's present requirements?
- Does it function properly?
- Does it allow for patient activity?

MEDICATION: AMOUNT/FREQUENCY

BASELINE SAO 2	80%
with O2	87%
without O2	81%
SAO 2 AT REST	
with O2	86%
without O2	81%
SAO 2 DURING A.D.L.	
with O2	85%
without O2	79%
SAO 2 DURING EXERCISE	
with O2	n/a
without O2	n/a

0.3cc alupent in 2.5cc saline qid
Mylanta II 10cc Q4H prn
Lasix 40 mg Q AM

FAMILY SUPPORT/ENVIRONMENTAL CONDITIONS

Patient lives alone but son and daughter visit frequently
and provide outings. Apartment needs cleaning along with
equipment. Mentioned to family; they offered to provide
assistance in this area.

THERAPIST COMMENTS

HOSPITAL DATES	last hospitalized 6 mos. ago 9/9/86

I feel Mr. Jone's level of activity outside the home has
continually progressed with the insistence of his children.
More instructional time will be spent on pursed lip breathing
and energy conserving tips around the home during A.D.L.

EQUIPMENT: CLEANING AND FREQUENCY

Mr. Jones must be reinforced in the area of disinfecting
medication nebulizers as previously instructed. No obvious
signs of respiratory tract infection.

DATE/TIME: _____

PATIENT SIGNATURE: _____   THERAPIST: _____

Figure 7–3. This follow-up form was designed for communicating with the referral source or the physician or both. Simple checklists do not lend themselves to individualized observations.

ADJUNCTIVE EQUIPMENT AND TECHNIQUES

The following ancillary equipment types and self-help techniques have been demonstrated to be effective and beneficial for many patients. The adjunctive modalities have become popular as patient aids and may be suggested during regular home care visits.

Nasal Oxygen Administration Aids

While using oxygen for months and possibly years via the nasal cannula, many patient frequently complain about painful, dry, and inflamed nostrils. The constant irritation of the plastic prongs within the patient's nose can make continuous oxygen use very uncomfortable. Under these conditions it is easy to realize why many individuals do not use their oxygen as prescribed. A sensible alternative to the nasal cannula is the Bi Flo Nasal Oxygen Mask (Fig 7–4). There is no plastic placed directly into the nares and only slight pressure is placed on the patient's upper lip (Fig 7–5). The nasal oxygen mask has been a great help to many patients.

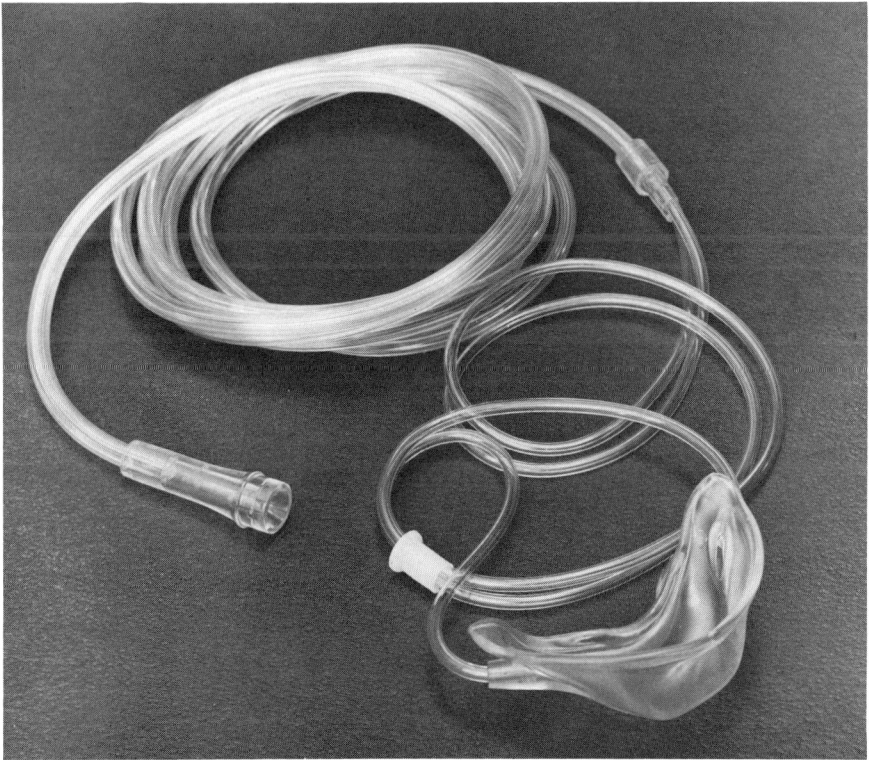

Figure 7–4. The Bi Flo Nasal Oxygen Mask. *(Courtesy of Intec, Blue Springs, Mo.)*

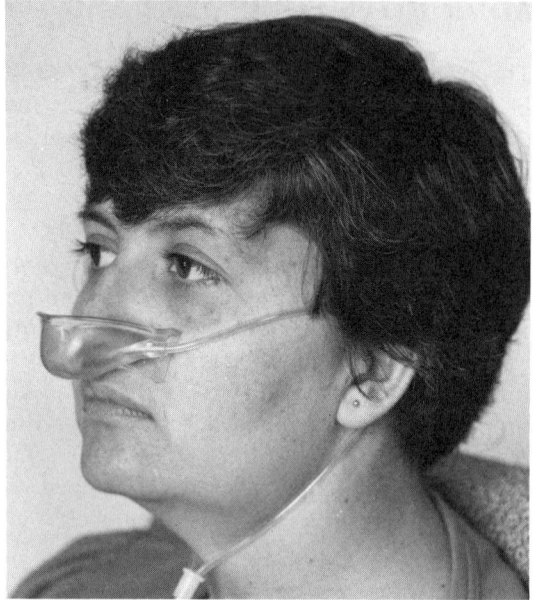

Figure 7–5. The Bi Flo Nasal Oxygen Mask reduces the irritation and inflammation at the nostrils that can be caused by the conventional prong-type nasal cannula.

The conventional nasal cannula can cause many problems for the continuous oxygen user.

These problems include:

1. Soreness over the ears and on the face.
2. Soreness and irritation under and around the nostrils.
3. Displacement during sleep.
4. Obvious presence of the device on the patient's face.

A product called Oxy–Ears has dealt with the problem of soreness over the patient's ears from continuous use of lariat-style nasal cannulas (Fig 7–6). They are small, soft, foam cylinders that fit over the cannula at the point at which it rests on the ears. This product can add considerable comfort to the continuous oxygen user.

Engineered Specialty Products, Inc., has designed three separate nasal cannula types in an attempt to alleviate some of the common oxygen administration problems identified above. These cannulas are called the Oxy–Frame, the nocturnal cannula, and the head cannula (Fig 7–7).

The three cannulas each have a specific purpose. The Oxy–Frame cannula conceals the oxygen tubing within a pair of eyeglass frames that can be fitted with prescription lenses or clear lenses. The typical pressure and irritation points caused by the conventional cannula have been eliminated.

The nocturnal cannula incorporates a soft headband and secures the

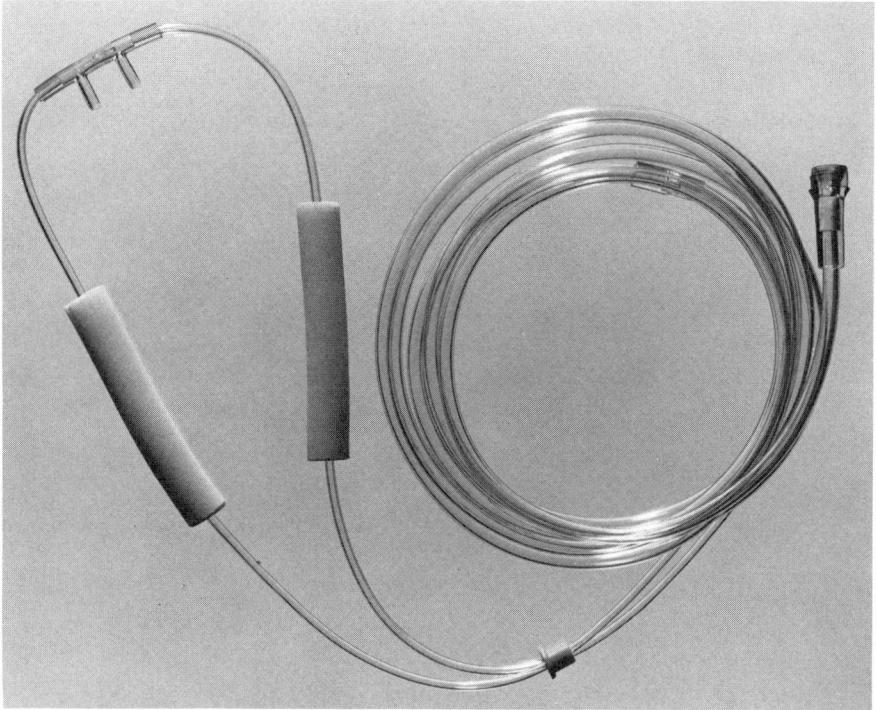

Figure 7–6. Oxy–Ears. *(Courtesy of American Medical Products, Phoenix, Ariz. Photo by Conley Photography, Inc., Tempe, Ariz.)*

oxygen delivery tubing to the nose, which prevents it from being displaced during sleep.

The head cannula is secured at the forehead, again eliminating the common irritation sites at the nostrils, cheeks, and ears. This device can be used as an alternative cannula, allowing healing to occur at the normal irritation points.

Another useful oxygen administration aid is a new product called Air Lift. Air Lift is a lightweight backpack device designed to carry a liquid oxygen portable container on the patient's back (Fig 7–8). This backpack-type carrier uses a nonflammable mesh pouch, which allows adequate ventilation for the enclosed liquid portable. The Air Lift backpack carrier offers a number of specific advantages for the oxygen user, which include:

1. Facilitates normal activities of daily living by freeing both hands and keeping the oxygen portable secure and out of the way of whatever activity the patient may be performing.

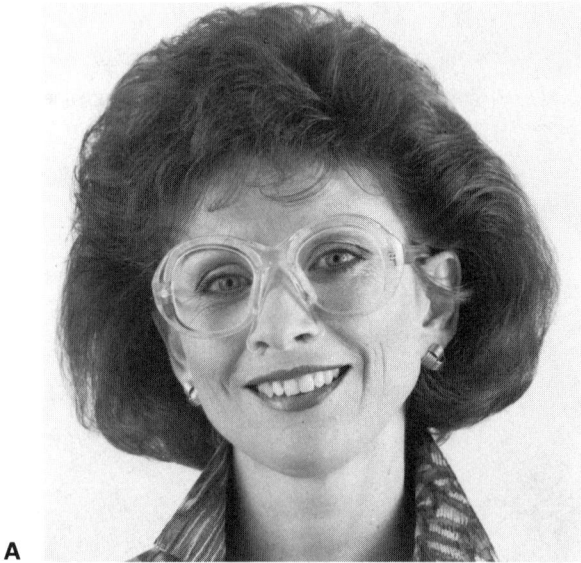

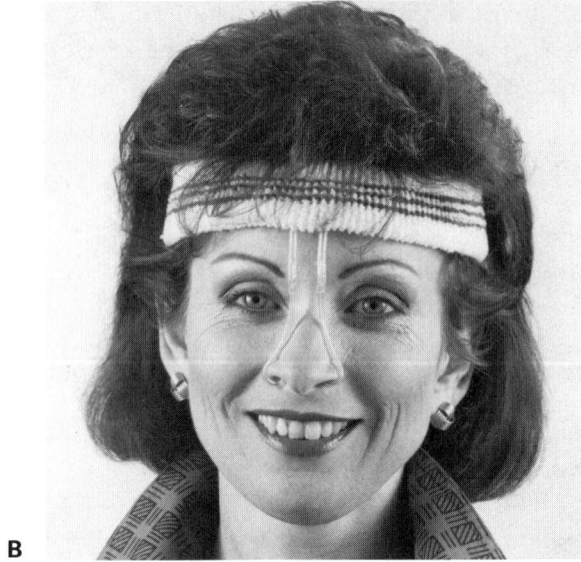

Figure 7–7. A. The Oxy–Frame cannula conceals the tubing within eyeglass frames. **B.** The nocturnal cannula incorporates a soft headband and secures the tubing to the nose.

C

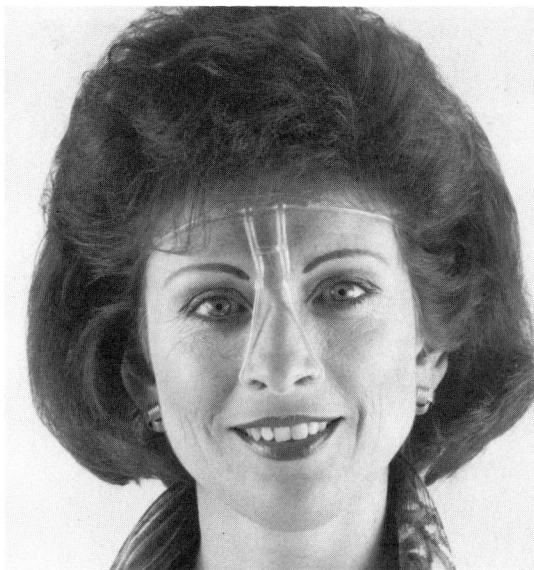

Figure 7–7. (cont.) C. The head cannula is secured at the forehead. *(Courtesy of Engineered Specialty Products, Inc., Sarasota, Fla.)*

2. Benefits parents of babies requiring oxygen therapy. Again both hands are free for holding the infant, feeding, etc.
3. Provides greater recreational mobility and can serve well during the exercise sessions of pulmonary rehabilitation programs.

Continued surveillance and follow-up visits in the home for patients requiring oxygen therapy can obviously be beneficial to the patient and family. Many helpful suggestions can be offered to assist the patient in using his or her oxygen properly and comfortably, along with adapting its use to fit each individual's life style.

The proper use of oxygen in the home must be continually evaluated. Depending upon the patient's diagnosis and condition at hospital discharge, the use of oxygen at home can change over time.

The pulse oximeter is a convenient, noninvasive monitoring tool that has allowed home care personnel to simply and reliably document the patient's proper use of oxygen at home (Fig 7–9). The pulse oximeter quickly and accurately measures arterial blood oxygen saturation (Sao_2) levels rather than the partial pressure of oxygen in the arterial blood (Pao_2). There are many benefits to the use of oximetry for at-home monitoring; it should not, however, be used as the only determining parameter for adjusting oxygen therapy (Table 7–4). Oximetry is best used to monitor *trends* in the patient's oxygenation status over time and during various levels of activity (Kochansky, 1984). Once a trend has been identified (either toward progression or regression in the patient's performance), further clinical and laboratory evidence should be compiled before a significant change in therapy can be ordered. As simple, easy, and avail-

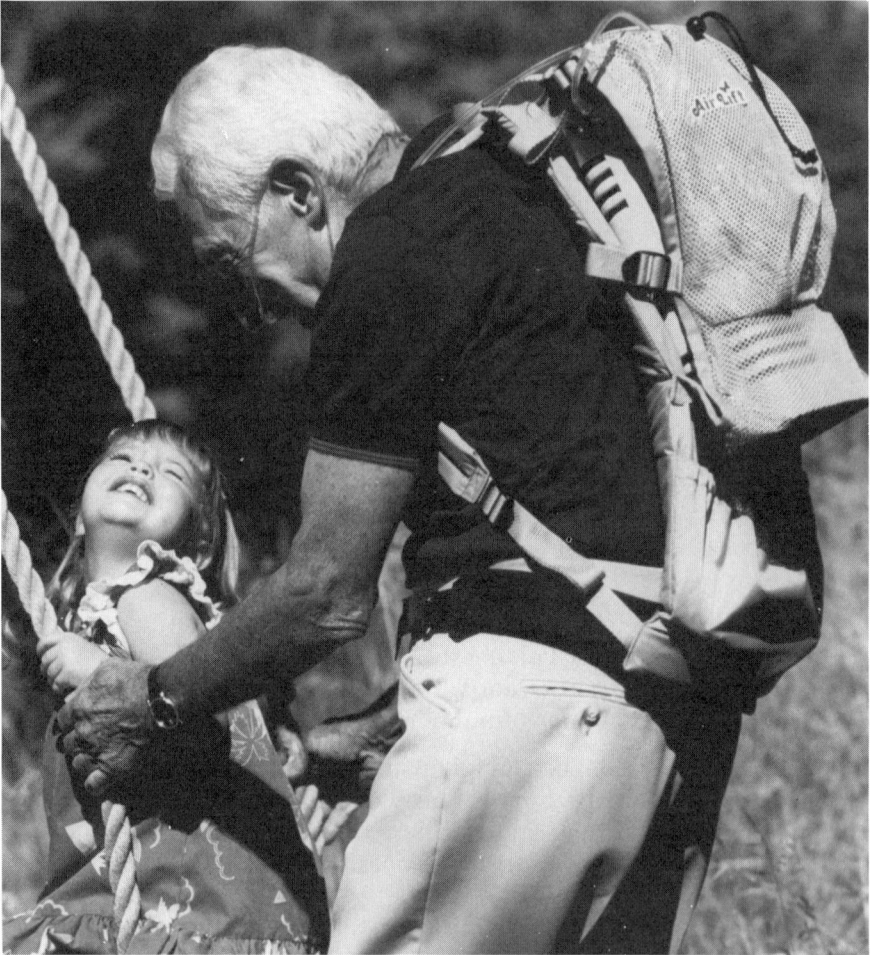

Figure 7–8. Air Lift, a backpack-style device for carrying a liquid oxygen portable. *(Courtesy of Air Lift Unlimited, Inc., Golden, Colo.)*

able as oximetry has become, its disadvantages must also be realized (*see* Table 7–4).

The introduction of this type of monitoring equipment to the practice of respiratory home care has added new dimensions to the concept of follow-up care in the home.

Aerosol Therapy Aids

The active, traveling patient requiring regular aerosol therapy now has a versatile medication compressor available. The Travelneb compressor incorporates many desirable features within one unit (Fig 7–10). This compressor operates on 110-volt AC, 12-volt DC via cigarette lighter adapter,

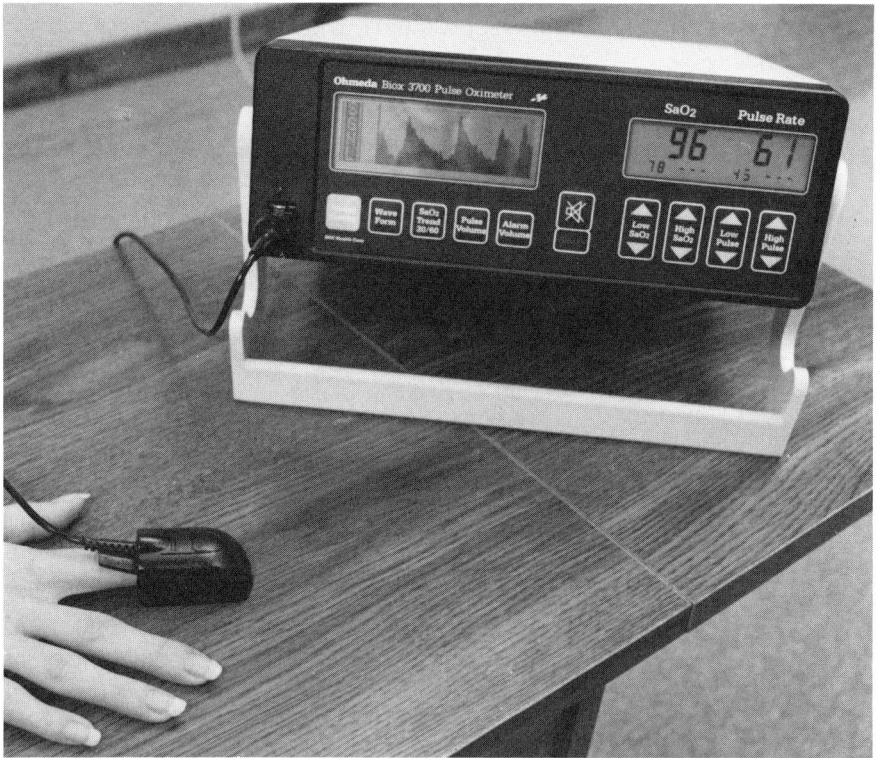

Figure 7–9. The pulse oximeter enables home care personnel to quickly and reliably document the patient's oxygenation status at home.

TABLE 7–4. ADVANTAGES AND DISADVANTAGES TO USING THE OXIMETER WHEN EVALUATING HOME OXYGEN THERAPY

Advantages	Disadvantages
The units have been proven accurate when used properly	Units are relatively expensive and the testing is not universally reimbursed
Enables physician and home care personnel to evaluate objectively the patient's oxygenation status over time, allowing therapy regimens to be tailored to coincide with changes in patient condition	Improper technique can result in false readings; excessive room light entering the probe will hamper testing
Permits physician and home care personnel objective evaluation of the patient's oxygenation status during various levels of activity (i.e., at rest, during sleep, during activities of daily living, etc)	The presence of abnormal hemoglobin types will result in inaccurate readings. Elevated carboxyhemoglobin (HbCO) may cause falsely high readings
Can offer quick and easy base-line data (Sao_2) before discharge that will add clinical relevance to subsequent testing in the home	Hemoglobin oxygen saturation levels by themselves indicate very little about the patient's overall pulmonary condition
Noninvasive	Hemoglobin saturation measurements can be affected by a host of other contributing factors. These can include changes in body temperature, blood pH, arterial carbon dioxide tension, etc

157

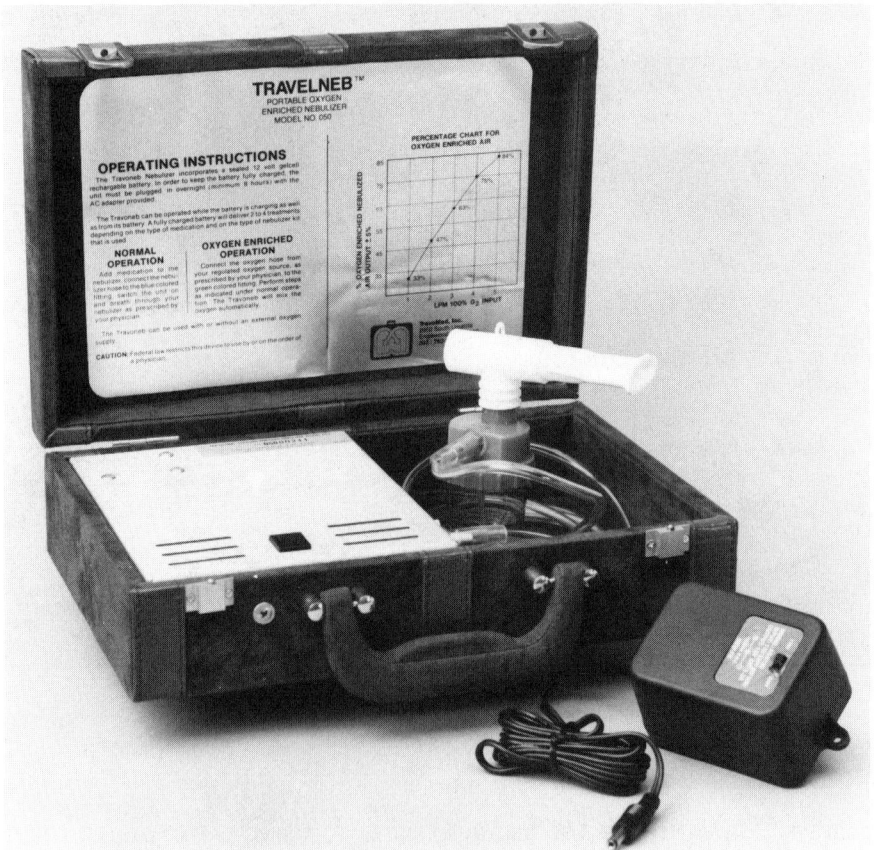

Figure 7–10. The versatile Travelneb aerosol compressor. *(Courtesy of Travomed, Inc., Englewood, Colo.)*

and 12-volt DC via its own self-contained nickel-cadmium battery. The 110-volt power cord (which is detachable) is also the internal battery charger. A small switch on the battery charger allows 220-volt operation, which is very common overseas. The compressor also incorporates an oxygen inlet that allows for oxygen administration during aerosol therapy, if desired. This is a popular compressor for those patients continuing employment as truck drivers, police, etc. Overseas travel is also simplified with this unit.

Individuals requiring aerosol therapy over prolonged periods frequently ask if they can make their own normal saline solution at home as a diluent for their medications (Table 7–5). Indigent patients and those on fixed incomes can also benefit by making their own saline solution.

TABLE 7–5. HOMEMADE SALINE SOLUTION*

1. Add ¼ teaspoon of noniodized salt to 1 cup of distilled water in a small jar with screw-on lid
2. Place lid on jar loosely
3. Place jar in a pan of water. (Water level in pan should be at least three quarters of the height of the jar)
4. Cover pan. Bring water to a boil and continue to boil for 25 minutes. Allow to cool. Remove jar and tighten lid
5. Store saline solution in the refrigerator. **Note:** Make fresh solution every week. Do not make more than you will use in a week
6. Discard any solution that has become discolored or cloudy

*One half teaspoon of solution is approximately equal to 2.5cc.
Adapted from Self Help: Your Strategy for Living With COPD. *Published by The Christmas Seal League, Pittsburgh.*

The visiting therapist usually offers these suggestions if the need is obvious.

A useful assessment device for the asthmatic patient requiring aerosol therapy at home is the peak flowmeter. Peak-expiratory flow rates (PEFR) have been shown to be an effective index for evaluating bronchodilator therapy (Van As, 1982; Williams, 1979).

This small, inexpensive flowmeter simply requires the patient to provide a forced maximal expiratory effort through the device to measure PEFR. This author has been using the Assess Peak Flow Meter for patients in the home (Fig 7–11). The use of a peak flowmeter at home is beneficial for a number of reasons.

1. By performing a PEFR test before and after bronchodilator therapy at home, the patient can actually visualize the benefits of therapy. This can enhance patient compliance with ordered therapy and improve long-range treatment objectives.
2. Bronchodilator therapy can be tailored to fit the individual's needs. Medication dosage can be altered by the physician to achieve maximum results or therapy can be discontinued if no improvement with therapy can be documented.
3. Regular measurements of PEFR by the patient during outdoor activities can aid in determining early onset of exercise or cold-induced bronchospasm.

The follow-up therapist is instrumental in teaching the patient and family how to use this device to its optimal potential.

The metered-dose inhaler (MDI) has gained immense popularity as an affordable, convenient form of inhaled medication therapy for the treatment of asthma and other bronchospastic disorders (Fig 7–12). Since

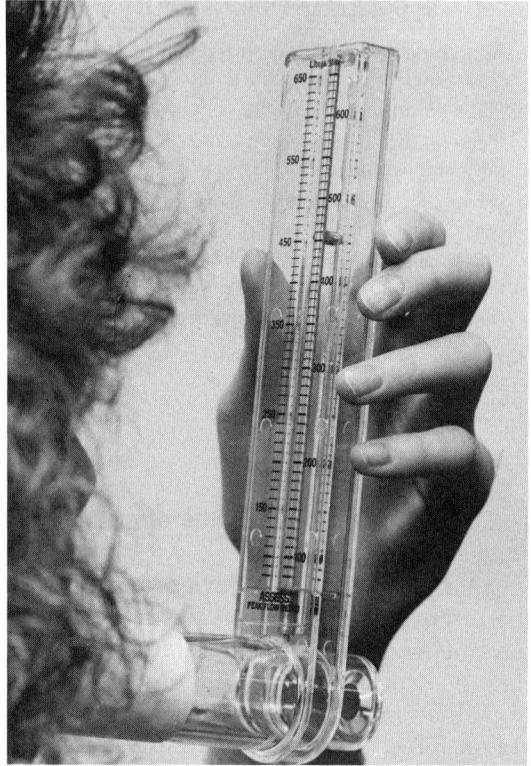

Figure 7–11. The Assess Peak Flow Meter. *(Courtesy of Health Scan Products, Inc., Cedar Grove, NJ.)*

the MDI basically administers undiluted medication to the patient, one to three puffs per treatment is normally adequate to supply the required dose. The MDI can only be effective if used properly. The follow-up personnel should periodically review administration technique with the patient during regular visits. (Table 7–6 can be used as a basic procedural review for patients using the MDI.)

A reservoir aerosol delivery system (RADS) can be added to the MDI if the patient demonstrates difficulty in coordinating delivery technique with the inhaler. The RADS will accumulate the aerosolized medication in the reservoir for inhalation in the event the patient does not inhale as soon as the MDI is compressed (Fig 7–13).

In many instances the patients using the MDI may not know how much medication is left in the canister. There is no volume indicator incorporated in the device. To prevent waste or running out at an inopportune time, the chart depicted in Figure 7–14, can help the patient estimate how much medication is remaining and allow him or her to refill the prescription before running out.

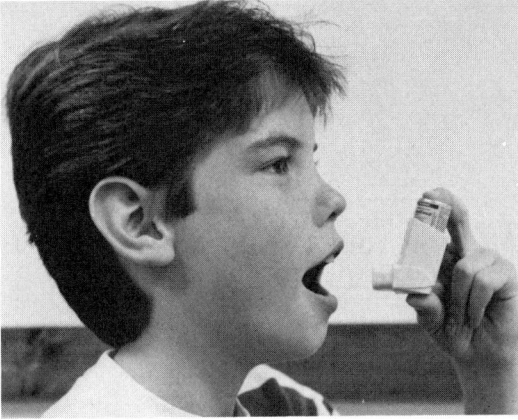

Figure 7-12. A patient using a typical metered-dose inhaler (MDI) for convenient relief from bronchospasm.

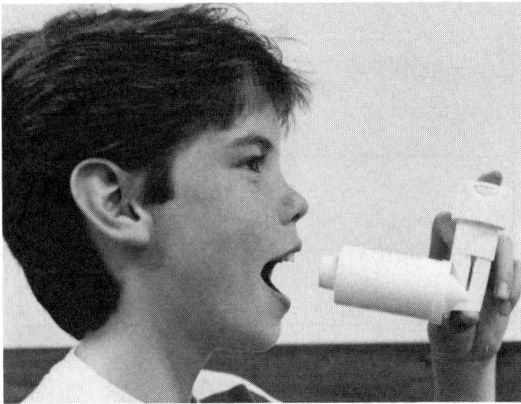

Figure 7-13. The MDI used with a reservoir, as shown. Many types of reservoir applications exist on the market today.

TABLE 7-6. HOW TO USE THE METERED DOSE INHALER

1. Shake the inhaler well and remove the protective cap. The metal canister should be on top

2. Hold the inhaler properly by placing your index finger on the top of the metal canister and your thumb on the bottom of the plastic mouthpiece

3. Exhale completely

4. Place the inhaler about 1 to 1½ in in front of your open mouth

5. Begin to breathe in deeply through your mouth; press the canister down with your index finger. Continue to breathe in very deeply to carry the medication into your lungs

6. Hold your breath for a second before exhaling through pursed lips

7. Your doctor may have prescribed more than one puff per treatment; if so, wait one minute before the next puff or as the package directions indicate. Do not exceed the dosage prescribed by your physician

8. Replace cap on inhaler. Rinse mouthpiece and cap daily

9. Rinse mouth with water after each treatment

10. Do not puncture or burn your inhaler; its contents are under pressure

REFILL YOUR PRESCRIPTION FOR YOUR INHALER WHEN IT IS <u>ONE-QUARTER FULL</u>.

This chart shows an easy method for *estimating the contents of your inhaler*. Simply place your canister in a bowl of water and compare its position with the chart below.

Empty

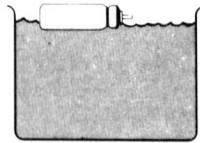

¼ Full (50 puffs)

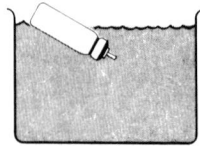

½ Full (100 puffs)

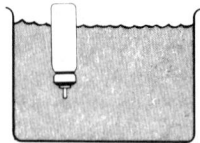

¾ Full (150 puffs)

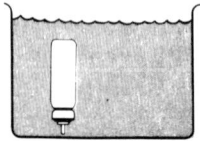

Full (200 puffs)

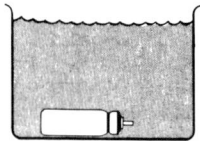

Figure 7–14. Monitoring the contents of the metered dose inhaler (MDI). *(Reprinted from* Self-help: Your strategy for living with COPD. *The Christmas Seal League, Pittsburgh, PA.)*

EQUIPMENT CLEANING TECHNIQUES

Patients receiving various forms of respiratory home care (i.e., aerosol therapy, mechanical support of ventilation, oxygen therapy, etc) are required to clean their equipment periodically. To date, there exists no uniform method or substance agreed upon by the majority of caregivers to be the most universally accepted cleaning method. Traditionally a white-vinegar-and-water solution has been the most popular form of in-home disinfecting. Depending upon the volume of equipment to be cleaned, white vinegar has the potential to become very expensive with prolonged use; consequently a number of cold chemical disinfectants have come into use, particularly the double and triple quaternary ammonium chloride compounds. These require the mixing of 1 oz/gal of water, and this solution can be reused by the patient for a period of 7 to 14 days. The vinegar-and-water mixture should be discarded after each use. The cleaning and disinfecting of equipment at home is covered in detail in Chapter 8.

A multitude of new and useful equipment aids and techniques exist on the market today. We will continue to see new product lines being developed. Patients at home can benefit from these products only if the home care service continues to monitor their needs and introduce the new products. There is no evidence to suggest that oxygen use and other respiratory therapy modalities at home will significantly decline in the near future. Therefore, we must make every effort to provide these therapies in private homes as efficiently and economically as possible.

REFERENCES

Kochansky M: Ear oximetry as a method of determining home oxygen prescriptions. *Resp Care* 1984;29:1211.
Williams MH: Evaluation of asthma. *Chest* 1979;76:3.
Van As A: The accuracy of peak expiratory flow meters, editorial. *Chest* 1982;82:263.

8

Ventilator Care at Home

JEFFREY LUCAS, RRT

Mechanical ventilation in the home has recently gained vast popularity. A variety of influences have been responsible, the most prominent being:

1. Committed physicians and health-team members offering appropriate supportive and rehabilitative care to the chronically disabled, making it possible for the patient needing mechanical life support to live at home.
2. Early diagnosis and treatment of debilitating pulmonary disorders, resulting in increased longevity that necessitates extended care and thus alternative site requirements.
3. Socioeconomic stresses demanding reductions in costs placed on the health-care industry.
4. Concerned family members wanting greater access to the institutionalized family member.
5. Recent technologic advancements offering portability, simplicity, versatility, compactness, and enhanced safety to the homebound ventilator-dependent patient and the patient's caregivers and environment.

Caring for the ventilator-dependent patient at home is being accomplished on a large scale quite successfully all over the world (Goldberg, 1983; Goldberg & Faure, 1986; O'Ryan & Burns, 1986). This patient population will continue to grow as the general medical community and third-party payers come to realize the benefits and observe the rewards offered by this alternative.

The goal of this chapter is to outline the major processes necessary to provide a successful hospital-to-home transition for the ventilator-dependent patient and his or her family. This chapter will also examine assessments of the patient as a prime candidate for home ventilation, the family as "primary caregivers," and a physical view of the home as well as equipment selection and routine care, regular patient follow-up, and various cost analyses for this type of care.

IDENTIFYING THE PRIME CANDIDATE FOR HOME MECHANICAL VENTILATION

The majority of patients managed most successfully in the home environment can be identified as those patients clinically unable to support the necessary ventilatory requirements to sustain life in the absence of acute pulmonary dysfunction, significant oxygenation disorders, or contributing multiple-organ-system failure. In other words, the patient's day-to-day cardiopulmonary status must be relatively stable without wide fluctuations that could only be treated by aggressive in-hospital modalities.

Patients meeting this criterion offer minimal management problems on a day-to-day basis, which in turn will lessen stress on the patient and the primary caregivers.

Three profiles have emerged from the population of ventilator-dependent patients studied by this author to date:

1. The patient who is unable to maintain adequate spontaneous ventilatory function over prolonged periods.
2. The patient who exhibits stable ventilatory failure with a prognosis of extended longevity but requires continuous mechanical support.
3. The newly diagnosed terminally ill patient who demonstrates stable ventilatory failure with a prognosis of minimal longevity.

Table 8–1 lists the disorders grouped in each profile.

TABLE 8–1. PATIENT PROFILE TYPES REQUIRING ASSISTED VENTILATION IN THE HOME

	Group Description	Diseases Involved
Profile 1	Mainly composed of neuro-muscular and thoracic wall disorders; particular stage of disease process allows patient certain periods of spontaneous breathing time during the day; generally require only nocturnal mechanical support	Amyotrophic lateral sclerosis (early stage) Multiple sclerosis Kyphoscoliosis and related chest-wall deformities Diaphragmatic paralysis Myasthenia gravis
Profile 2	Requires continuous mechanical ventilatory support, associated with long-term survival	High spinal cord injuries Apneic encephalopathies Late-stage muscular dystrophy
Profile 3	Usually returns home at request of patient and family; disease is terminal, life-expectancy is short, patient and family wish to spend remaining time at home; patients may pose significant management problems at home as a result of rapidly deteriorating condition	Lung cancer End-stage chronic obstructive pulmonary disease (COPD) Amyotrophic lateral sclerosis (end stage)

TABLE 8–2. SUMMARY OF FUNDAMENTAL ASSESSMENT CRITERIA RELATED TO SUCCESSFUL VENTILATOR CARE

Competent, trainable family, live-in friend, or dependable professional staff possessing the ability to take over in the absence of family and willing to spend the time required for proper training

Patient willing to go home

Family fully understands diagnosis and prognosis

No evidence of acute underlying pulmonary abnormalities

Patient's clinical pulmonary condition stable and free of contributing multi-organ system failure

Family aware of their financial responsibilities

Psychologic consultation requested at inception of discharge planning

Home environment suitable for returning patient

Electrical facilities at home adequate to safely operate all equipment

Patient environment controlled, avoiding drafts during winter months and ensuring proper ventilation in warm seasons

Substances that may produce allergic responses are removed or controlled

Adequate equipment cleaning and storage space provided

This is by no means an attempt to pigeonhole prime candidates for mechanical ventilation in the home; it must be stressed that each patient and supporting family should be viewed independently. Many other factors will play a role in the final decision-making process. These will be discussed later.

At the time a patient is initially considered to be a candidate for going home, the plan should immediately be presented to the family for open discussion. Input from the physician, patient, and family at the beginning of the decision-making process can clarify the fears, responsibilities, and expectations of those who will be involved in the undertaking. All three parties must explore the implications of changing family life styles, continuous care, and financial responsibilities, as well as the ultimate course of the disease process. A united decision must be made at this time before the next step in the process of going home can be initiated.

Once the physician, patient, and family have decided that the return to home is feasible, an overall assessment of the patient and home is initiated. This will include a summary of the patient's present clinical state, an assessment of family as primary caregivers, and a look at the physical layout of the residence to ensure a safe and efficient environment. Table 8–2 summarizes the primary points that must be assessed.

Suitable primary caregivers in the home generally can be competent, enthusiatic, trainable family members but can also be live-in friends or hired professional personnel. Whatever the case, they must be aware that their services will be required on a 24-hour, seven-days-per-week schedule if the patient is in need of continuous mechanical ventilator

ventilator support. For the patient requiring only nocturnal support, the primary caregiver must still be available at all times. This is an enormous undertaking; therefore, plenty of backup professional help must be available before home ventilator care is instituted.

HOME CARE TEAM MEMBERS

Several key health-care professionals are important in the successful management of the ventilator-dependent patient at home. The professional staff involved in the plans for going home and the patient's continued care should include the following:

- *The primary physician.* He or she will receive regular input from the primary caregivers and the professionals involved in the continuing care, enabling him or her to decide on care-plan changes (e.g., changes in medication usage, ventilator settings, etc). The physician should also be involved in the discharge instructions and planning in order to be familiar with all aspects of the patient's circumstances. If the primary physician is not a pulmonary specialist, one should be involved on a consultation basis.
- *The psychologic consultant.* It is imperative that the patient, and the family as well, have access to the services of a psychologic consultant. Some patients and their families cope exceedingly well with the changes imposed on their life styles. However, others do not, and professional psychologic help can relieve intrafamily conflicts, guilt, and other problems arising from their new responsibilities as the caretakers of a handicapped family member. It is easy to sympathize with the lay person who, within the time frame of approximately 1 month, has moved from the role of visitor in a completely unfamiliar environment to one offering the complete care and responsibility for a family member on mechanical life support. This emotional and physical stress will dramatically affect the lives of those involved with the day-to-day care of the ventilator-dependent patient.
- *The respiratory therapist.* The therapist should be involved as the instructor, follow-up person, and consultant on a continuing basis. It is preferable that the same therapist instruct the primary caregivers on ventilator and circuit function, tracheostomy tube care, suctioning, etc. In many instances one therapist with experience in this area will be asked to coordinate and implement the entire process of going home, from initial assessment and instruction to transporting the patient home and providing the follow-up. Maintaining the involvement of the same personnel from start to finish is important. This continuity allows the patient and family to gain confidence and improves communications with all involved.

- *The nurse.* Primary nursing should be instituted at the time the patient is selected as a candidate for home ventilator care. This will ensure continuity of care and also offer another consultant to the family over the course of in-hospital training and preparation. The nurses assigned to the patient on a regular basis should either attend all family instructional sessions or actively participate in the instruction so that the family is not given conflicting information. The key to a rapid and successful training program for the lay individual is (1) keep it *simple*; (2) *rehearse*; and (3) *reinforce*. This can only be accomplished when all personnel involved are on the same track. The nurse is helpful in providing suggestions to ease daily care routines, skin care, vital sign records, medication usage and effectiveness, and acting as liaison to the primary physician.
- *The discharge planner or social service staff member.* This person is a very important member of the home care team. Arrangements with a reputable home care and equipment supplier must be made; the financial burden of equipment and professional personnel (if needed) can be lessened dramatically by the discharge planner who investigates all avenues of financial aid to the family. The discharge planner can also arrange for needed community services to be made available to the patient and family. These services may include providing transportation, visiting nurses, occasional meals, socializing, or whatever the particular situation may require to lessen the burden on the primary caregivers.
- *The home care and equipment supplier.* The supplier must be a reputable firm that employs trained respiratory therapists who can advise the home care team as to what type of oxygen system (if needed) will be most efficient, economical, and safe for the particular mechanical ventilator being used. The vendor must also be a full-service company, able to supply and service all of the patient's equipment needs (e.g., mechanical ventilator, tracheostomy dressings, oxygen supply, etc). This will relieve the family of any further confusion from having to call more than one supplier when a piece of equipment needs service or supplies need replenishing. The home care supplier must have respiratory therapists on staff who are on call 24 hours a day, seven days a week, to respond to any mechanical or oxygen system failure that may have to be repaired or replaced. Costs vary widely among home equipment suppliers and this should be a consideration; however, it should not preclude the prerequisite of good service performed by qualified personnel.

Indeed, it is important that all personnel involved in the initial instruction, discharge planning, and continuing follow-up be knowledgeable, qualified individuals in the aspects of home care and mechanical ventilation relative to their responsibilities.

PRIMARY CAREGIVERS: THE FAMILY

Ideally there should be more than one person in the family designated as the primary caregiver; this will allow family members to break from the routine and stress of caring for the patient. The patient on mechanical support of ventilation in the hospital, specifically in critical care units, experiences sleep and sensory deprivation and may also suffer from poor nutritional support (Schraeder, 1979). In the home, the same problems can occur if there is not sufficient help to allow the primary caregivers personal time off. It is important that these conditions be monitored during regular follow-up visits, and that the caregivers are given time to attend to their own personal needs.

Not all ventilator-dependent patients at home require 24-hour support or care. A large percentage require only nocturnal support and lead very active, relatively normal daytime lives; for the most part they care for themselves and their own equipment. Even in the case of nocturnal-only ventilator support, however, family members should still attend instructional sessions. They will then be able to provide effective assistance in case of an emergency or if the patient requires help during an exacerbation. This home-ventilator patient–family relationship is the ideal one. This group of patients usually experiences few or no management problems, family stress and anxiety is at a minimum, and the patient can continue with daily living almost totally unencumbered. These patients are examples of those described in profile 1 (Table 8–1).

Patients described in profiles 2 and 3 (Table 8–1) will require much more time and effort and will encounter many more problems.

The patient profiled in the third category can provide an exhaustive task for the caregivers. In certain instances, as in the case of the older person with terminal, end-stage lung cancer, the family may wish to bring the patient home for what time is remaining, no matter what the cost in terms of time and money. The initial assessment may reveal that this patient is not the ideal candidate for home ventilator care, but how does one deny the family's wishes? Do we as providers of health care and services even have the legal right to say no? At times this patient group will tax the resources of every member of the health team involved. Here it must again be emphasized that the success of the home situation rests on complete and thorough in-hospital preparation.

The family must also completely understand the patient's diagnosis and prognosis. If the family is not fully aware of the patient's limitations and the probability (depending upon the disease entity) of continued deterioration of physical state, false hopes, despair, and depression may occur. This may result in resentment toward the entire situation and all participating members of the team. In situations such as this, the family may also spend a great deal of money on unnecessary accessory equipment, such as exercise bicycles, treadmills, and the like. The fire of resentment is fueled when excess expenses are incurred fruitlessly in an already expensive undertaking.

CLINICAL PROFILE OF THE IDEAL HOME VENTILATOR PATIENT

A very important aspect of the initial assessment is to determine the patient's clinical stability. It is difficult to define clinical stability in a patient requiring life support for a progressive disease. However, most successful home management situations have involved the following pre-discharge characteristics:

1. Relatively unchanging ventilatory parameters for 2 to 4 weeks, resulting in minimal fluctuations of acid-base and blood gas status.
2. Minimal demonstrable shunt (requiring a fractional inspired oxygen concentration [F_IO_2] of 35% to 40% or less to correct) for 2 to 4 weeks.
3. Nondeteriorating spontaneous ventilatory parameters (tidal volume, spontaneous ventilatory frequency, minute volume, vital capacity, negative inspiratory force) for 2 to 4 weeks.
4. Minimal use of diuretics, chronotropic or ionotropic agents, afterload reduction agents, or vasopressors (extreme in-home management problems can arise as a result of multi-organ-system failure).
5. No evidence of acute underlying pulmonary abnormalities, i.e., infection, pleural effusions, atelectasis, etc.
6. Last, but not least, proper tracheostomy tube cuff maintenance procedures should be closely observed. Tracheal-esophageal fistulas resulting from improper cuff care present the same inordinate management problems in the home that they do in the hospital. Food and medication aspiration and aerophagia resulting in abdominal distension are recurrent hazards that can sorely disrupt an otherwise successful in-home course.

COST CONSIDERATIONS

As early as possible during the in-hospital assessment routine, the family must be apprised of the costs of home ventilator care. This point should actually be discussed during the early decision-making process with the physician, patient, and family. Financial obligations will definitely play a major role in determining the feasibility of the project. Table 8–3 shows an in-home versus in-hospital cost comparison. Regardless of what the insurance reimbursement may be for the patient, it is a rare instance in

TABLE 8–3. HOME VERSUS IN-HOSPITAL COST COMPARISON FOR VENTILATOR CARE*

| | Average Monthly Cost | | Average Daily Cost |
	Home Care† ($)	In-Hospital‡ ($)	In-Hospital‡ ($)
Patient A	875	21,461	715
Patient B	1013	23,353	778
Patient C	1175	27,950	932
Patient D	1004	21,397	713
Patient E	892	17,370	579

*All costs calculated from actual patient billing statements of expenses incurred between March 1979 and October 1982. Only 5 of 25 patients reported here because of extreme similarities in charges.
†Figures represent total cost of replenishable medical supplies such as gloves, suction catheters, and oxygen plus rented equipment (e.g., ventilator, wheelchair, bedside commode, etc). Expenditures not consistent from family to family, such as hired nursing care or physician visits, are not reported.
‡Hospital room charge (ward and nursing services) plus respiratory therapy costs (ventilator, oxygen, arterial blood sampling, bronchopulmonary hygiene, and aerosol therapy if itemized). Figures do not include physician or procedure charges for services such as radiography, laboratory, etc.
Reproduced with permission from O'Ryan JA, Burns DG: Pulmonary Rehabilitation: From Hospital to Home. *Chicago, Year Book, 1984, p 218.*

which the third-party payer will pay 100% of the expenses incurred. The family is almost always responsible for a portion of that cost, which can be staggering, depending upon insurance coverage.

A close approximation of the actual financial outlay that will be required of the patient and family should be determined before any further steps are taken in the process of bringing the patient home. It is not realistic to believe that third-party payers will reimburse most of the cost. The burden of paying the portion of expenses not covered by the third party varies from family to family, but it can be assumed that it will be of serious importance to most families. Actual figures, reimbursement, and cost commitments from third-party payers and suppliers should be obtained and presented to the family at the very beginning, before any actual home care arrangements are made.

The home-equipment supplier or vendor must also be very much aware of reimbursements when accepting a ventilator-dependent patient. There are many services supplied by the vendor that are not yet recognized or paid for by most insurance carriers.

Medicare classifies medical-equipment vendors as suppliers of equipment. The vendor is reimbursed by Medicare for equipment rentals only. Many ventilator-dependent patients are at home today because of the early efforts of certain medical equipment suppliers who have on staff highly trained and dedicated medical professionals, such as respiratory therapists and nurses, who made it possible to move a patient from the acute-care facility to the private home. Most of the family training and discharge planning was performed by the staff of the equipment vendor.

This situation can be termed a vendor-based home ventilator program, in contrast to one that is initiated through the hospital, which is identified as a hospital-based home ventilator program.

All of the considerations concerning home ventilator care identified in this chapter must be organized, planned, and followed through to ensure that home ventilator care will be successful. These considerations include:

1. Evaluating the patient as proper candidate for home ventilator care.
2. Predischarge planning with the medical care team members.
3. Selecting and training the primary caregivers.
4. Communicating with the insurance carriers.
5. Evaluating the home.
6. Selecting and placing primary and ancillary equipment.
7. Custom installations if necessary, i.e., piped-in oxygen system.
9. Follow-up and continuing care.

All of these functions are accomplished today by either the hospital-based program or the vendor-based program. If the program is a vendor-based one, who will reimburse for the staff-hours spent in training, planning, and assessing? Because Medicare (and other carriers as well) will only reimburse a *portion* of the equipment *rentals*, not all ancillary services are reimbursable. Table 8–4 indicates the nonreimbursed predischarge time investments that can regularly occur in a vendor-based home ventilator program (Lucas, 1987). To keep nonreimbursed expenditures to a minimum, the vendor must preplan, coordinate, and execute the discharge plan rapidly and efficiently. There also exist postdischarge time requirements and services, which are not reimbursed, that are virtually necessary to ensure a successful hospital-to-home transition for the patient and family. These postdischarge time investments and related services are outlined in Table 8–5 (Lucas, 1987).

It is obviously very costly and time-consuming to move a ventilator-dependent patient from hospital to home. As important as the patient's and family's awareness of their financial responsibilities in this endeavor, the vendor must also be aware of the total cost to perform this service, in which the following factors must be considered: (1) inadequate Medicare (and other carriers') reimbursements for equipment rentals; (2) total lack of reimbursements for selected services and vendor functions; and (3) the very long time vendors must wait to receive payment. The vendor's home-ventilator patient population must survive 14 months before that account can begin to show a profit. Although this statement sounds cold and impersonal, it is an unavoidable fact that if the accounts do not become profitable, ventilator-dependent patients will not be able to come home in the future.

This author believes that at the present standards of government

TABLE 8–4. NON-REIMBURSED PREDISCHARGE TIME INVESTMENTS* FOR THE HOME-BOUND VENTILATOR-DEPENDENT PATIENT IN A VENDOR-BASED PROGRAM

Service	Time Investment (hours)
Planning with physician	½–1
Planning with discharge planner	2–3
Planning with nursing staff	1–2
Planning with respiratory therapy staff	1–2
Communication with insurance company	½–1
Visits to patient's home	2–3
Travel time	variable
In-office planning	2–3
Setup time	2–3
Family or lay caregiver training	12–18
Home nurse training (if used)	2–3
Custom installation of oxygen piping system (if necessary)	5–10†
Total time requirements	25–40
or	
with custom piping installations	30–50
THUS	
Average time requirements	37 hours
Respiratory therapist's rate of pay	$10.00–$17.00/h
Range of time invested in dollars	$370.00–$629.00
Average predischarge cost investment that is not reimbursed	$500.00

*All figures are based on averages experienced with this author's association with 43 home-going ventilator-dependent patients. Dollar figures and time requirements will vary from region to region.
†Includes planning, equipment gathering, staff-hours during installation.

reimbursement, the medical equipment company choosing to perform mechanical ventilation in the home is performing a community service, rather than engaging in a sound business enterprise.

EVALUATION OF THE HOME

Once the patient assessment has been completed, an evaluation of the home is performed. The electrical facilities are evaluated to determine their adequacy for safe operation of all equipment that will be placed in the home. Table 8–6 lists common electrically operated medical equipment and its amperage requirements. A number of the items listed in Table 8–6 may be operating simultaneously, which means that the household electrical circuitry must be adequate to supply the necessary amperage at peak use periods. Another requirement is that all grounded

TABLE 8–5. POSTDISCHARGE TIME INVESTMENTS AND SERVICES FOR THE HOME-BOUND VENTILATOR-DEPENDENT PATIENT*

Service	Time/Cost
First Month	
Day of discharge	3–6 h
Initial family support visit	2–3 times/wk for first 2 wk (4–12 h)
Formal first month follow-up visit (submit reports to referral personnel and physician)	2 h
Average first month nonreimbursed time investments	14.5 h, $195.75
Subsequent Months	
Follow-up personnel per visit (1/mo)	$30.00–$50.00, plus mileage
One visit per month for changing tracheostomy tube	(1 h plus travel) $30.00–$50.00
Average 1–2 visits per month for miscellaneous reasons	2–4 h, plus travel
Summary	
Over first 6 months	Average $1200.00
The second 6-mo period	Average $850.00
Full year	Approximately $2000.00–$3000.00

*The reported figures are averages relative to this author's experience. Costs and services will vary from region to region.

electrical outlets that are to be used for any of the medical devices be placed on specially designated 15- to 20-amp-rated circuits with their own fuse box or circuit breaker. This will prevent any power overload or outages on that circuit from overused or faulty household appliances.

Observation of the patient's room and other general care areas where the patient may be is important to determine ideal placement of electrical outlets, space requirements for equipment and supply storage, and ease of movement for the patient and family.

Often dining rooms or living rooms are converted to patient-care areas in the home. Equipment needs will play a large role in determining space requirements. The complete patient management system should be envisioned at this time. Will one H-cylinder of oxygen be sufficient to supply the patient's needs over an appropriate time period, or will the patient require a large 180-L liquid reservoir with five manifolded H-cylinders as emergency backup? Where will the oxygen be stored? From which entrance will it be delivered? Where will the gas connections for the primary and backup ventilators be installed? Will the patient need

TABLE 8–6. AMPERAGE REQUIREMENTS FOR COMMONLY INSTALLED HOME CARE EQUIPMENT

Equipment (Manufacturer)	Amperes
Bennett MA–1 Ventilator (Puritan–Bennett Corporation)	4.5
PLV–100 Ventilator (110 volt operation) (Lifecare)	1.25
Medimex MVP–1500 E Ventilator (Medimex, Inc)	1.0
Mobilaire III Oxygen Concentrator (Invacare Corporation)	3.5
DeVo44 Oxygen Concentrator (Devilbiss Corporation)	5.0
Cascade I Humidifier Heater (Puritan–Bennett Corporation)	1.2
Pulmoaide Aerosol Compressor (Devilbiss Corporation)	1.3
Timeter PCS–4 Air Compressor (The Timeter Group)	5.5
Semi-Electric Hospital Bed (Invacare Corporation)	2.0
Suction Machine (Intermittent) (American Caduceus Industries Inc)	6.0
Beta Bed Air Mattress Pump Model HM90 (Huntleigh Group Inc.)	0.5

an electrically operated hospital bed, a bedside commode, or a walker? These are only a few examples of questions that must be answered. Substances that may produce allergic responses from the patient must be removed or effectively controlled. The room or care area that has been selected must be draft-free during the winter months, while provisions for proper ventilation and air conditioning in warm seasons must be ensured. Adequate areas for equipment processing must be identified. These areas should have some degree of counter space for disassembling and reassembling the equipment that requires disinfection and reuse. Drying and storage areas for processed tubing and miscellaneous parts will also be needed. The home should be inspected for proper screening to limit invasion of houseflies, mosquitoes, and other insects that may contaminate clean equipment or infect or annoy the patient.

Once the patient has been identified as a home-going candidate, the caregivers chosen, and the home inspected, training sessions can be introduced.

INSTRUCTION

Thorough training for the family is essential to produce successful home care and management. The training period offers the opportunity for the family to build self-confidence. They must be assured they can accomplish the tasks and correct commonly encountered problems on their own. Most patients and their families approach the early instruction with fear and anxiety. This can be alleviated by keeping the instructions simple and concise. The first meeting should consist of an organized breakdown of the entire program. Reference and summary material should be given to the caregivers at the beginning of instruction. This will tell what will be expected of them throughout and offer an opportunity to discuss and review the material in private. Table 8–7 shows a sample outline of one training session. Outlines of all training sessions are presented to the family in advance. Each one is designed to describe what is important about that particular session and includes a number of performance objectives that must be completed before they move on to the next topic. This particular program incorporates six sessions that are entitled: I. the ventilator, control panel, and alarms; II. tubing circuitry, humidifier, and cleaning procedure; III. secretion removal and suctioning the airway; IV. tracheostomy tube and stoma site care; V. taking vital signs; VI. medication dispensing.

A participatory, hands-on approach to the equipment from the beginning can be an effective means of tempering apprehension. Allow one day (if possible) between each scheduled training period. This will give the family time to assimilate and practice the new techniques presented to them. Each successive meeting should begin with a practical review of the techniques and information given during the previous session. Family training should be conducted at the patient's bedside. Training periods occurring here allow the patient to become familiar with his or her own equipment and care routines. The patient also gains confidence in the family members as caregivers when he or she can visualize the daily progress being made.

The hospital nursing staff should be kept abreast of the family's progress so they may allow them to perform those care duties in the hospital when they come to visit. Allowing the caregivers to participate in the care routine provides continuing reinforcement and practice of skills and offers an opportunity for the family to gain confidence and experience in managing the various problems that may arise. Whenever possible, the family should be given the actual equipment to take home with them so they may practice assembling and operating such items as tubing circuitry, suction machines, tracheostomy tubes, and tracheostomy-tube-care kits.

The caregivers should be trained to change the tracheostomy tube

TABLE 8–7. EXAMPLE OF TOPICS COVERED DURING ONE FAMILY TRAINING SESSION

Session Topic:	Tubing Circuitry, Humidifier and Cleaning Procedure
Description:	This presentation will be concerned with assembling, disassembling, and troubleshooting the tubing circuitry and humidifier. The proper cleaning and disinfecting procedure will also be covered, along with how to recognize common signs of pulmonary infection at home.
End-of-session objectives:	The following objectives are goals that should be accomplished before the next session is begun. The family or caregiver(s) should be able to:

1. State the basic importance of the humidifier as it applies to the person with an artificial airway
2. Trace the pathway of inspired and expired gases through the tubing circuitry
3. Completely disassemble and reassemble the tubing circuitry and humidifier without errors
4. Completely disassemble and reassemble the spirometer (if used) without errors
5. Indicate all areas of the circuit and humidifier that may be the origin of a gas leak
6. Test for circuit integrity before the circuit is placed on the patient
7. Recite the method and frequency of circuit cleaning, disinfection, and storage
8. Discuss the importance of hand washing before the circuit or airway is handled
9. Recite five common signs of impending pulmonary infection

TRAINING CHECKLIST   **NOTES**

____ Gas pathway through circuit
____ Function of exhaust valve manifold
____ Disassembly of humidifier
____ Disassembly of spirometer
____ Check for circuit integrity
____ Cleaning procedure
____ Family to reassemble total
       circuit and humidifier
____ Family to troubleshoot circuit
       with malfunctions
____ Common signs of pulmonary
       infection

whenever necessary. By doing so, expensive trips to the hospital, out-patient facility charges, and the unwieldy task of transporting the patient for what is actually a relatively quick and simple procedure can be eliminated. The family should also be able to place a new tube in the event of an airway emergency.

Avoid setting a mandatory discharge date toward which to work; to ensure adequate preparation, the in-hospital instruction should not be hurried. Ideally, when the instructional routine is completed, a 24- to 48-hour period is arranged so the family may live in with the patient at the hospital. During this time the family should be permitted to offer complete, around-the-clock care for the patient. This experience gives the patient and family a good overall perspective on their recently acquired abilities as well as the opportunity to resolve any final questions or concerns.

Final procedural assessments are performed by the prescribing physician, respiratory therapist, and nurse to determine the caregivers' skill in equipment troubleshooting and patient-care regimen. These assessments will offer a comprehensive view of the family's abilities.

ANCILLARY EQUIPMENT SELECTION

The task of selecting the appropriate equipment for the patient is not difficult if one is simply listing supply needs for the home that parallel in-hospital supplies. Generally speaking, what the patient is using daily in the hospital is what will be needed at home. However, situations and supplies *not* seen daily in the hospital will often pose logistic problems in the home. For instance, if the patient is ambulatory and does not require continous mechanical support, there may be a need for a portable ventilator with a self-contained or portable external power source. Will the patient be spending extended periods of time away from home? If so, he or she may require a portable suction unit with battery- or manually operated capabilities. Oxygen systems, when required, pose a number of logistic questions. What type of oxygen system must be installed to meet the patient's needs? How and where will the oxygen system be placed? How will the oxygen and humidity be provided from room to room when the patient is off the ventilator? The qualified and experienced home care and equipment supplier is best suited to offer solutions to these questions. These situations must be presented to the supplier early to allow for sufficient preparation time.

The family should be given a complete listing of all the equipment and supplies that will be placed in the home so provisions for proper storage can be made before the patient goes home. Table 8–8 is an actual equipment and supply listing. Although this listing appears lengthy, it is by no means extraordinary for the homebound ventilator-dependent patient.

VENTILATOR SELECTION

In this author's experience with 45 home ventilator patients, many types of ventilators have been employed for home use. Most have been volume- or time-cycled positive-pressure units that require attachment to the pa-

TABLE 8–8. TYPICAL DISCHARGE EQUIPMENT AND SUPPLY LISTING

A. Primary ventilator

1. Type and brand
2. Manual resuscitator
3. Disposable or permanent ventilator circuits
4. Replacement ventilator filters
5. Extra humidifier (cascade or condenser type)
6. Daily flow sheets
7. External 12-volt battery
8. 12-volt battery power cord

B. Emergency backup ventilator

1. Type and brand of pneumatically operated unit
2. Backup ventilator circuits
3. Manifolded compressed gas cylinders as power source
4. Test lung
5. Humidifier for backup ventilator

C. Suction equipment

1. Primary 120-volt suction machine
2. Spare collection bottle
3. Extension suction tubing
4. Suction catheters
5. Clean gloves
6. Backup manually operated or 12-volt suction unit
7. Yankauer suction catheters

D. Tracheostomy supplies

1. Spare tracheostomy tubes
2. Tracheostomy dressings
3. Sterile trach-care kits
4. Sterile water-soluble lubricant
5. Syringes
6. Sterile gloves (for changing trach tube)
7. Povidone-iodine ointment or equivalent
8. Trach tube ties
9. Sterile cotton swabs

E. Oxygen source

Depending upon each patient's situation, the oxygen source may be compressed gas cylinders (CGCs), an oxygen concentrator, or liquid oxygen (LOX) reservoirs. Dictates of the patient-care requirements at home may also necessitate a combination of these systems

F. Supplemental airway humidity

1. Type and brand of portable or mobile heated humidifier or external condenser-type humidifiers
2. Twenty- or fifty-ft lengths of oxygen connecting tubing
   Note: If 50-ft connecting tubing is used, pressure-compensated flowmeters are recommended
3. Air compressor
4. Oxygen source (if necessary)
5. Tracheostomy humidity or aerosol collars
6. Large-bore aerosol tubing
7. Condensation drainage bags

TABLE 8–8. (cont.)

G. Solutions

  1. Large-volume saline
  2. Unit-dose saline
  3. Distilled water
  4. Hydrogen peroxide
  5. Povidone-iodine or equivalent
  6. Enteral feeding
  7. Germicide

H. Miscellaneous durable medical equipment (DME)

  1. Hospital bed
  2. Overbed table
  3. Trapeze
  4. Patient communication aid
  5. Bedside commode, urinal, or bedpan
  6. Walker
  7. Wheelchair
  8. Stethoscope
  9. Sphygmomanometer
 10. Air mattress and pump

I. General miscellaneous

  1. Emergency phone number listing
  2. Plastic bag lined, covered waste receptable
  3. Equipment instructions

tient via an artificial airway. Others are finding similar success using negative-pressure ventilators, which do not require attachment to artificial airways (Alexander et al, 1979; Holtackers et al, 1982). The use of the negative-pressure ventilator, however, is restricted to patients with little intrinsic pulmonary involvement and relatively normal chest wall configurations.

A large number of important variables must be considered when choosing a ventilator for home use. Some of the major considerations include the following:

1. *Safety*. The ventilator must be mechanically dependable over long periods of time. It should be UL-approved (or equivalent) and safe to operate in an oxygen-enriched environment. The controls should be tamper proof so that children that may live in or visit the patient's home cannot alter the settings, and the machine must incorporate alarm systems appropriate to the situation.

2. *Reliability*. The preset parameters should not fluctuate over a prolonged operating period or change as a result of extraneous influences, such as circuit type, patient positioning, varying lung compliance, or chest wall configurations.

3. *Power source*. If the ventilator is pneumatically driven, it must be remembered that gas sources in the home—unlike in the hospital—are not limitless, as they are sometimes thought to be

and as they are used. If the unit is electrically operated, the rate of power consumption should be known. This can be very important when determining battery life when away from a continuous power source. Depending upon the circumstance, arrangements may have to be made for either a backup ventilator or standby power source in the event of a mechanical or electrical failure.

4. *Ease of operation.* An excess of alarms and controls can confuse the patient and family. The controls should be well marked and calibrated; if not, a simple problem may become difficult to correct by telephone and may add complexity to the initial training sessions. All filters that are to be changed on a regular basis must be easily accessible, and the patient circuit should be simple, lightweight, and easy to troubleshoot.

5. *Versatility.* As mentioned previously, in situations in which the patient does not require continuous ventilatory support, the ventilator should be able to travel with the patient. The travel could be in anything from a wheelchair to a commercial airliner. The unit must also offer appropriate ventilatory modes to meet with changing patient support and comfort requirements.

6. *Cost.* Exotic critical care capabilities (that may be unnecessary for in-home ventilator use) or excessive gas use will certainly increase the cost of the unit. However, an inexpensive ventilator may actually become less cost-effective if it requires additional operating or monitoring equipment. If the ventilator is carefully chosen to fit the specific needs of each patient, the cost factor will usually be found justifiable for that application.

The decision to place a backup ventilator in the home will be based upon the individual patient's requirements, because not all patients will require an emergency unit. Remember also that Medicare will not reimburse for any emergency backup equipment. This is not always the case with private insurance carriers.

Patients are generally set up with a secondary unit if it is believed the patient would be in danger in case of electrical failure or malfunction of the primary unit. To assess for this need, a number of factors are considered, including: (1) the number of hours per day on ventilatory support; (2) the inspired oxygen concentration; (3) the availability and response time of the local emergency squad or ambulance service; and (4) the distance from the nearest hospital and equipment supplier.

Arrangements should be made with the local power company for emergency restoration of power. Figure 8–1 is an example form letter used for this purpose. Figure 8–2 shows an example of a backup ventilator with a reserve compressed-gas power source for the unit. The primary ventilator in Figure 8–2 is a LIFECARE PLV–100, which incorporates its own internal battery for short operating periods (1 to 1½ hours) during power outages or short outside trips. This does not prevent mechanical failures of the unit, hence the need for the secondary compressed-gas-powered ventilator.

Proper equipment selection and advanced planning for emergencies will decrease or eliminate unnecessary trips to the home for minor problems or last-minute deliveries. This can also immeasurably add to the

---

PROFESSIONAL HOME CARE

NORTHCOAST OXYGEN
COMPANY, INC

FOR AMERICA

Dear Sir:

MR. JOHN SMITH whose address and phone number is:

123 MAINSTREET

ANY WHERE , U.S.A

_123 - 4567_ is a patient of ours requiring a mechanical life support system. This life support system is a ventilator which completely supports the patient's ventilatory needs.

The Electric Company's support to the patient and family is urgently needed. In the event of a power failure this person's life is in danger. All of the families at home utilizing this type of life support system are also supplied with a manually operated resuscitator, which will enable the family to assist the patient for short periods.

We urge the names of these families be placed on a priority list for restoration of electricity. Also, if there is a forewarning of a power failure, please notify these families so that proper arrangements can be made.

Thank you for your cooperation in this matter. If we can be of any further assistance, please call us. We will be forwarding you the physician's prescription, validating the patient's diagnosis and subsequent need for mechanical life support.

Sincerely,

Jeff Lucas

Jeff Lucas, R.R.T.
President

NORTH COAST OXYGEN CO., INC.
12710 TRISKETT RD.
CLEVELAND, OHIO 44111
(216) 267-0033

Figure 8–1. Form letter requesting emergency power restoration.

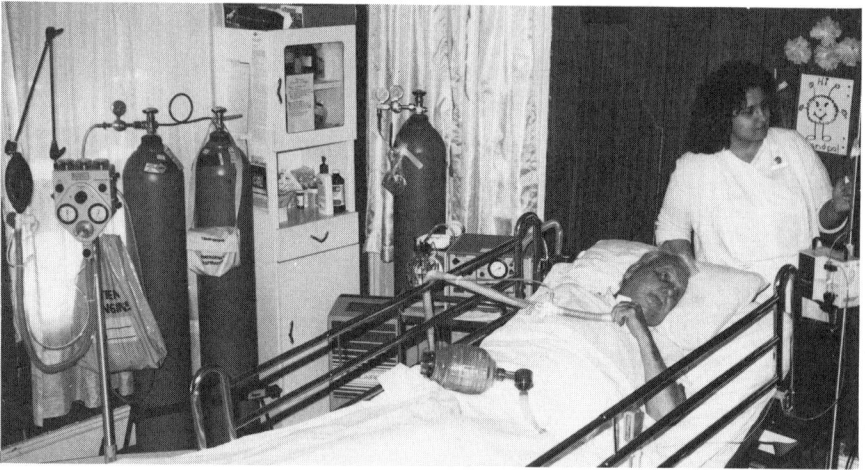

Figure 8–2. A patient at home requiring mechanical life-support for 24 hours per day needs a backup ventilator with compressed-gas power source.

family's confidence, knowing they are equipped and able to manage most unexpected situations.

Types of Home Care Ventilators

Quite a number of ventilators on the market today have been designed for home care use (Kacmarek & Spearman, 1986). Most home care ventilators have been designed for compactness, portability, and ability to be operated with various power sources. The typical positive-pressure-type home ventilator can be operated continuously on 120-volt AC house current, for short periods (one to two hours) on its own internal 12-volt DC battery, or for longer periods (2 to 20 hours) with an external 12-volt DC battery, depending on the manufacturer.

Each home ventilator has its specific drawbacks, some more serious than others. Since this patient population has grown so dramatically in the past five years, the Food and Drug Administration (FDA) is keeping very close watch on quality control standards in manufacturing, service, and repair of these units.

Again, the home ventilator is not designed to support the critically ill patient, and many of the advanced features found on hospital-type ventilators are not incorporated.

All things considered, the "typical" and most popular home ventilators in use today are safe and reliable if used as the manufacturer intended. A few of the commonly used home ventilators will be surveyed here to offer a comparative analysis of common features at present incorporated within these units.

LIFECARE Ventilator Model PLV–100. The PLV–100 ventilator is a microprocessor-controlled home ventilator whose use and operation is relatively easy for lay caregivers to understand (Fig 8–3). Most controls are calibrated for easy reference and a number of the important ventilatory functions are digitally displayed, which simplifies trouble shooting in the home. Table 8–9 provides a listing of the operational and design features for the PLV–100 ventilator.

LIFECARE Ventilator Model PLV–102. The PLV–102 ventilator is a recently released upgraded model of the PLV–100 ventilator (Fig 8–4). The majority of the features that have been added (along with the additional cost) make it difficult to classify it as a home ventilator per se.

The added features include: sigh breath capabilities, 50-psi oxygen source inlet allowing for continuous F_IO_2 adjustment between 21% and 90%, an in-line oxygen sensor, 30-second alarm silence capability, the ability to maintain oxygen concentrations during spontaneous breathing in the synchronized intermittent mandatory ventilation (SIMV) mode, and an option to attach a computer terminal and printer and an optional remote alarm.

With its added features, the PLV–102 is an ideal transport ventilator for the critically ill, a possible backup ventilator for the intensive care unit, and in limited specific circumstances for use as a home ventilator.

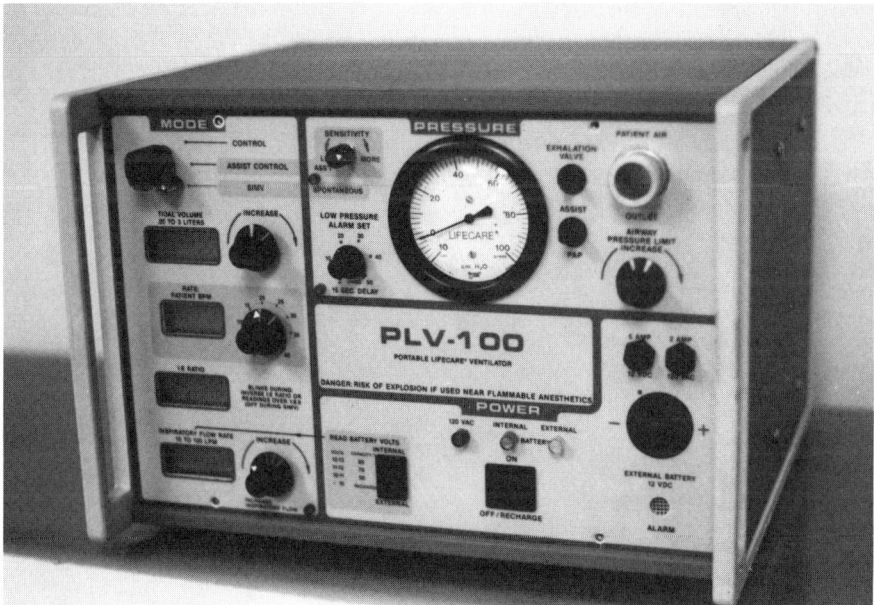

Figure 8–3. The PLV–100 ventilator by LIFECARE.

TABLE 8-9. LIFECARE PLV-100 FEATURES

Front Panel Controls

Mode selector	Control, Assist/Control, SIMV*
Tidal volume	50 cc–3000 cc
Breath rate	2–40 bpm*
Inspiratory flow rate	10–120 lpm*
Battery test switch	Indicates voltage for internal or external battery
Main power switch	ON-OFF/recharge battery
5-amp circuit breaker	Protects 12-volt power circuit
2-amp circuit breaker	Protects 120-volt power circuit
Airway pressure limit	5–90 cmH$_2$O
Sensitivity control	+3 cm H$_2$O to −6 cmH$_2$O Pressure
Low-pressure alarm	2 cmH$_2$O–50 cmH$_2$O
Marked exhalation valve supply line	
Marked proximal airway pressure supply line	
Marked patient air outlet	

Available Power Sources

120-volt AC 50/60 HZ
220-volt 50/60 HZ for foreign use
12-volt DC internal battery
12-volt DC external battery

Front Panel Visual Indicators

Tidal volume	Digital display
Breath rate	Digital display
I:E ratio	Digital display
Inspiratory flow rate	Digital display
Increase inspiratory flow	Red light
120-volt AC power	Green light
Internal battery use	Amber light
External battery use	Yellow light
Pressure manometer	−10 cmH$_2$O–100 cmH$_2$O
Patient assist	Green light
15-s delay for low-pressure alarm	Green light

Unit Alarms

Low pressure	Visual/Audible
High pressure	Audible
Apnea	Visual/Audible
Inverse I:E ratio	Visual
Increase inspiratory flow	Visual
Low internal battery	Visual/Audible
Low external battery	Visual/Audible
Reverse battery connection	Audible
Power failure	Audible
Unit malfunction	Audible
Change of power source	Audible

Physical Dimensions

Height	9.0 in
Width	12.25 in
Depth	12.25 in
Weight	28 lb

*bpm = breaths per minute; lpm = liters per minute; SIMV = synchronized intermittent mandatory ventilation.

186

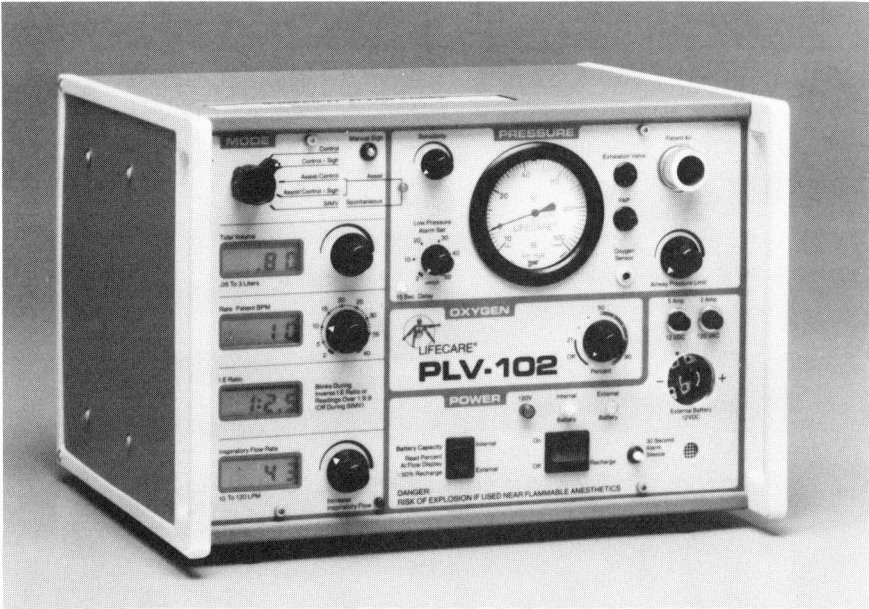

Figure 8–4. The PLV–102 by LIFECARE.

Table 8–10 indicates the specific functional differences that have been incorporated in the PLV–102 as compared to the PLV–100.

Aequitron LP6 Ventilator. The Aequitron Medical LP6 Ventilator is also a microprocessor controlled home ventilator incorporating a number of unique details and operational characteristics (Fig 8–5). Some of these features include differentiating audible alarms indicating life-threatening and nonlife-threatening occurrences. An optional printer that will record ventilator performance at preset intervals or on demand, and locking calibrated control knobs. The Aequitron LP6 also offers an 18 month service warranty. Table 8–11 provides a comparative listing of the operation and design features for the Aequitron LP6 Ventilator.

Puritan–Bennett Ventilator Companion 2800. Puritan–Bennett has for years been a leader in manufacturing the hospital and critical care type of ventilator. Their relatively recent acquisition of the Thompson line of the home ventilators and the production of the Companion 2800 has provided them with a significant entry into the home ventilator market.

The Companion 2800 incorporates all the significant features common to most home ventilators (Fig 8–6). This is also a microprocessor-controlled unit with clearly marked and calibrated controls. Some of the features unique to this unit include: adjustable volume control for alarms,

TABLE 8–10. LIFECARE PLV–102 FEATURES IN ADDITION TO THOSE OF PLV–100

Front Panel Controls	
Mode selector	control & sigh
Sigh volume	150% of set tidal volume
Sigh frequency	1 sigh breath every 100 tidal breaths
Manual sigh	Push to activate one breath
Oxygen percent control	Adjust from 21%–90%
Oxygen sensor	Plug in to activate
30-s alarm silence	Push to activate
Available Power Sources	
Same as PLV–100	
Front Panel Visual Indicators	
Manual sigh	Yellow light
Oxygen percent	50% and greater marked red
30-s alarm silence	Yellow light
Alarm code display (in flow window)	Digital display
Unit Alarms	
Oxygen (source inlet pressure)	Audible
Physical Dimensions	
Same as PLV–100	

a simple oxygen accumulator for easy adjustment of oxygen concentration, expanded ventilatory rate capabilities to 69 per minute, an optional patient call switch, and remote alarms. Table 8–12 provides a listing of the operation and design features for the Companion 2800 ventilator.

Medimex MVP–1500E Ventilator. The Medimex MVP–1500E home ventilator is a new addition to the market (Fig 8–7). This ventilator was

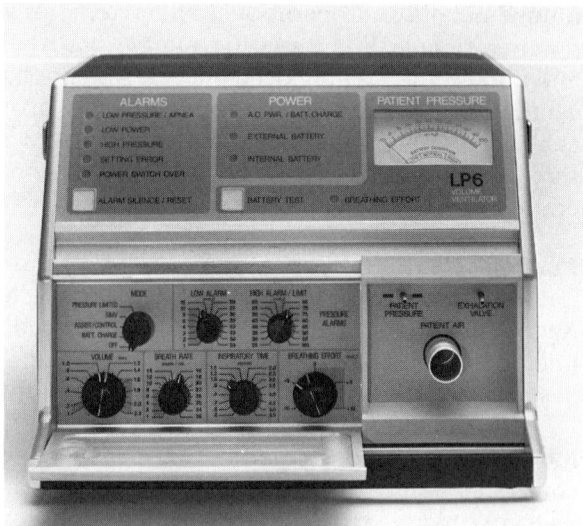

Figure 8–5. The Aequitron Medical LP6 Ventilator.

TABLE 8–11. AEQUITRON LP6 FEATURES

Front Panel Controls

Mode selector—Off, Battery charge, Assist/Control, SIMV, Pressure limited	
Low alarm	$1CMH_2O$ − 55CM H_2O pressure
High alarm/Limit	25 CMH_2O − 100 CMH_2O pressure
Volume	100 CC − 2,200 CC
Breath rate	1–38 bpm
Inspiratory time	0.5 − 5.5 seconds
Breathing effort	$-10CMH_2O$ −
	+ 10 CMH_2O pressures
Marked patient pressure supply line	
Marked exhalation valve supply line	
Marked patient air outlet	
Alarm silence/Reset/Test	60 second silencing
Battery test	Charge level indicator for internal
	and external battery

Available Power Sources   **Physical Dimensions**

120-Volt AC 50/60 HZ		Height	9¼ in
220-Volt AC 50/60 HZ		Width	12½ in
12-Volt DC internal battery		Depth	13½ in
12-Volt DC external battery		Weight	32 lbs

Front Panel Visual Indicators

Low pressure/Apnea	Red light
Low power	Red light
High pressure	Red light
Setting error	Red light
Power switch over	Red light
AC power/Battery charge	Green light
External battery	Amber light
Internal battery	Flashing amber light
Patient pressure scale	$-10CMH_2O$ −
	+ 100 CMH_2O pressure
Battery condition	Low, normal, high
Breathing effort	Green light

Unit Alarms

Low pressure/Apnea	Visual/Audible-Dual tone alarm
Low power	Visual/Audible-Dual tone alarm
High pressure	Visual/Audible-Single tone alarm
Setting error	Visual/Audible-Single tone alarm
Power switch over	Visual/Audible-Single tone alarm
Internal battery use	Visual/Audible-Every
	5 min reminder tone alarm
Activation of accessory printer	Audible-Single reminder tone
Microprocessor error	Visual/Audible-All alarms

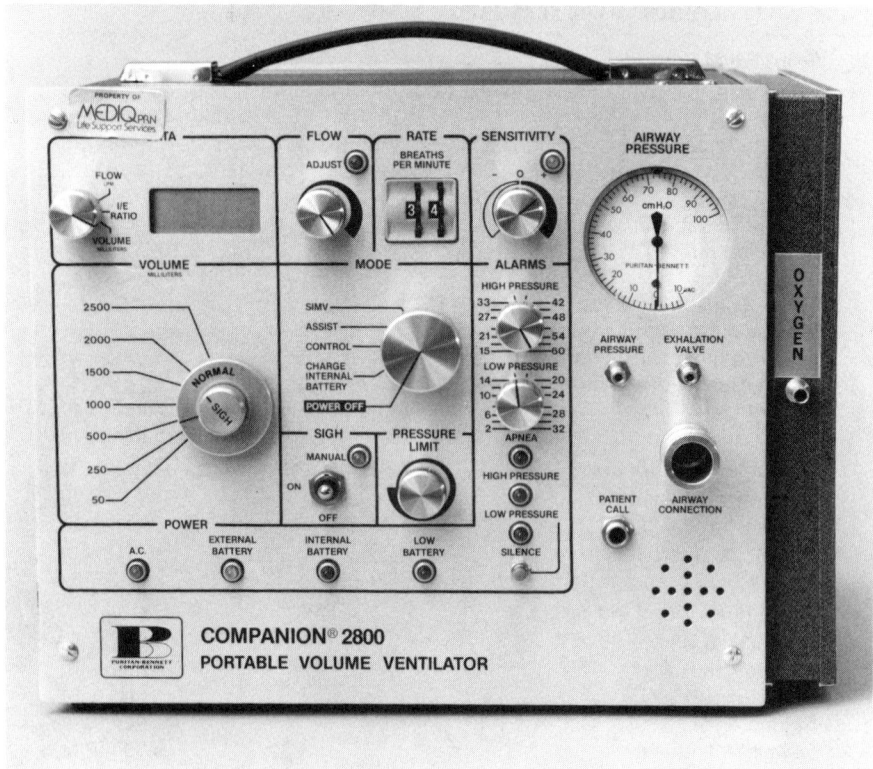

Figure 8–6. The Puritan–Bennett Companion 2800.

designed to be a low-cost, low-frills unit that can be serviced at the bedside and incorporates the features necessary to support the majority of home ventilator-dependent patients.

The MVP–1500E claims its internal battery will offer up to six hours of function under proper conditions. Almost every portion of this ventilator (including the motor brushes) can be repaired or replaced by the dealer. This feature is significant because down time is cut dramatically and the number of spare units that must be stocked can be significantly reduced.

This unit includes most of the same popular operating features as its competitors, including: 120-volt AC, 12-volt internal battery, and 12-volt external battery capabilities, remote alarms, portability, assist and intermittent mandatory ventilation (IMV) modes of ventilation, and all necessary alarms. Table 8–13 lists the operation and design features for the MVP–1500E ventilator.

Porta–Lung. The Porta–Lung negative-pressure ventilating chamber is a new design for an old ventilatory concept (Fig 8–8). This fiberglass and clear acrylic ventilating chamber can be considered a second generation

TABLE 8-12. PURITAN-BENNETT COMPANION 2800 FEATURES

Front Panel Controls

Data Switch	Provides for digital display of peak flow I:E ratio, and tidal volume
Flow control	40 lpm–125 lpm*
Rate control	1 bpm–69 bpm*
Sensitivity control	-5 cmH$_2$O– $+15$ cmH$_2$O
High-pressure alarm control	$+15$ cmH$_2$O– $+60$ cmH$_2$O
Marked proximal airway pressure supply line	
Marked exhalation valve drive line	
Marked patient air outlet (airway connection port)	
Low-pressure alarm control	$+2$ cmH$_2$O– $+32$ cmH$_2$O
Patient call receptacle	Plug-in
Supplemental oxygen accumulator	
Alarm silence switch	60 s delay
High-pressure limit control	$+10$ cmH$_2$O– $+70$ cmH$_2$O
Mode selector switch	Selects: Control, Assist SIMV*, Battery Recharge, and OFF
Sigh switch	Controls manual sigh or regular interval sigh
Normal volume control (tidal volume)	50 cc–2800 cc
Sigh volume control	125 cc–2800 cc

Available Power Sources

120-volt AC 50/60/HZ
220-volt AC
12-volt DC internal battery
12-volt DC external battery

Physical Dimensions

Height	10 in
Width	11⅜ in
Depth	12 in
Weight	33 lb

Front Panel Visual Indicators

Pressure manometer	-10 cmH$_2$–100 cmH$_2$O
Apnea alarm indicator	Red light
High-pressure alarm indicator	Red light
Low-pressure alarm indicator	Red light
Low-battery indicator	Red light
Internal battery indicator	Red light
AC power indicator	Green light
External battery indicator	Amber light
Flow rate	Digital display
I:E ratio	Digital display
Tidal volume	Digital display
Sigh indicator	White light

Unit Alarms

Flow (inverse I:E ratio)	Visual/Audible
Low pressure	Visual/Audible
High pressure	Visual/Audible
Apnea	Visual/Audible
Low battery	Visual/Audible
Power switchover	Audible
Ventilator malfunction	Audible

*bpm = breaths per minute; lpm = liters per minute; SIMV = synchronized intermittent mandatory ventilation.

191

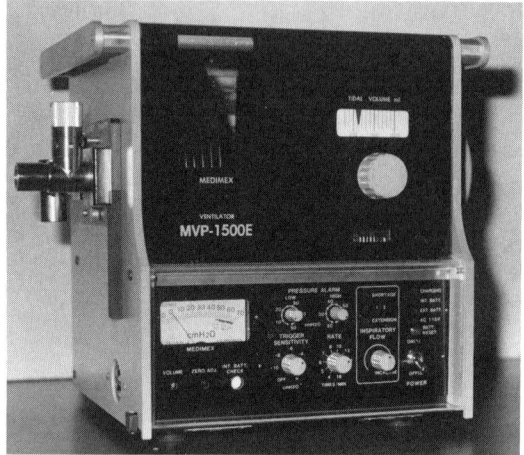

Figure 8–7. The MVP–1500E by Medimex.

"iron lung." It weighs approximately 100 lb (as compared to the 800-to-900-lb iron lung) and has offered a new dimension of portability to the previously stranded patient using the iron lung. The Porta–Lung must be used in conjunction with a mechanical negative-pressure generator such as the **LIFECARE 170C** shown in Figure 8–8. This negative pressure chamber has the following advantages above that of the iron lung:

- Very light and protable.
- Greater negative ventilating pressures.
- Low maintenance costs.
- Can be used in vans and motor homes.
- Better aesthetic quality.

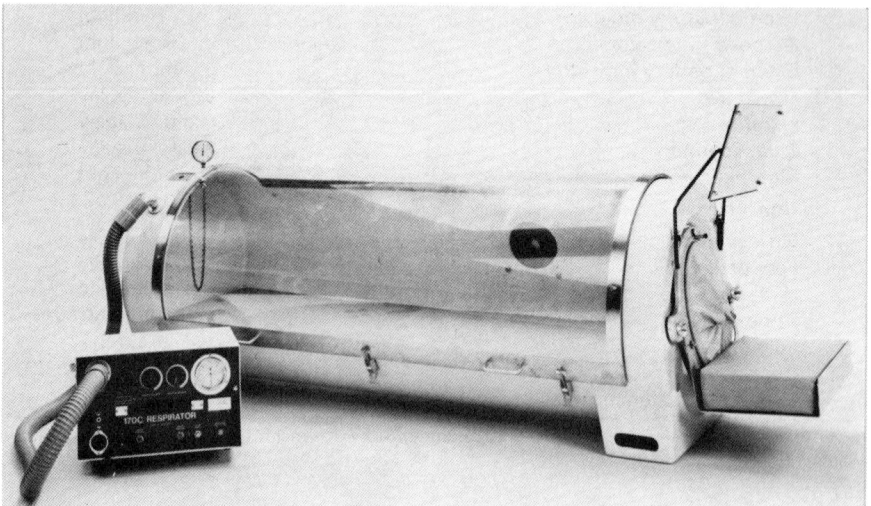

Figure 8–8. The Porta–Lung Negative-Pressure Ventilating Chamber for adults.

TABLE 8–13. MEDIMEX MVP–1500E FEATURES

Front Panel Controls

Tidal volume	300 cc–1500 cc
Hour meter	0–5000 h
ON/OFF switch	
Inspiratory flow control	Noncalibrated
Rate control	4 bpm to 18 bpm*
Trigger sensitivity	0 cmH$_2$O– –10 cmH$_2$O
Zero adjust	Adjusts pressure gauge
Volume control	Adjusts alarm volume
Low-pressure alarm	10 cmH$_2$O–50 cmH$_2$O
High-pressure alarm	20 cmH$_2$O–60 cmH$_2$O
Internal battery check button	

Available Power Sources

115-volt AC
12-volt DC internal battery
12-volt DC external battery

Front Panel Visual Indicators

Tidal volume	Calibrated scale
Hour meter	Calibrated scale
115-volt AC power	Green light
External battery	Green light
Internal battery	Red light
Battery charging	Green light
Flow rate shortage	Red light
Flow rate 1:2	Green light
Flow rate extension	Amber light
High pressure	Red light
Low pressure	Red light
Trigger sensitivity	Amber light

Unit Alarms

High pressure	Visual/Audible
Low pressure	Visual/Audible
Inverse I:E ratio	Visual/Audible
Low battery	Visual/Audible
Power source changeover to 12-volt	Visual/Audible

Physical Dimensions

Height	12 in
Width	13 in
Depth	12 in
Weight	50 lb

*bpm = Breaths per minute.

The Porta–Lung is being manufactured in two sizes, adult and pediatric, and will soon be available in an infant model also.

The medical equipment supplier is faced with a difficult decision when determining what type(s) of ventilator to purchase. Many factors must be considered in the purchase of this high capital expense item.

These decisions continue to become more difficult as the ventilator-dependent patient population grows and third party reimbursement stagnates. It is to be hoped that future product development will enhance ventilator reliability and long-term function and that it will become accepted that alternate-site care for this patient population is economically feasible and deserves further financial support.

EQUIPMENT DECONTAMINATION AND INFECTION CONTROL

Decontamination of respiratory therapy equipment and careful adherence to infection control procedures are vital aspects of mechanical ventilation in the home. Although no hard data exist, it is logical to assume that a patient is at less risk from infection at home than while hospitalized. Nosocomial pneumonia is the third most common nosocomial infection and is the most frequent death-related infection occurring in the hospital (Simmons & Wong, 1982). Because a large percentage of these infections can be linked to cross-contamination, a well-managed patient at home should be able to avoid such infections. When proper procedures and decontamination techniques are followed, the incidence of rehospitalization for pulmonary infection can be minimized. Table 8–14 illustrates the fact that proper training and strict adherence to the decontamination routine will prove effective in preventing pulmonary infections at home.

The areas of infection control that are of prime concern for any ventilator-dependent patient can be roughly categorized into two areas: (1) aseptic procedural techniques, which include tracheostomy tube care, stoma care, and suctioning; and (2) decontamination of such equipment items as humidification systems, patient circuits, and the ventilator itself. The majority of airway procedures, such as tracheostomy tube cleaning, stomal cleaning, and suctioning, are taught as clean techniques, rather than sterile techniques. The practice of thorough hand washing and the use of clean gloves before any airway manipulation occurs are taught to the family. The use of sterile gloves is unnecessary and expensive. Sterile disposable suction catheters are required for use during each suctioning attempt. Sterile and draped conditions are mandated only during tracheostomy tube changing procedures in the home. Cleansing of the inner cannula of the tracheostomy tube is also performed as a clean technique, and the solution used is one of 1:1 hydrogen peroxide and distilled water, yielding a 50% solution. Distilled water is also required as a suction catheter rinse and for use in all humidification devices.

Decontamination of all reusable respiratory therapy equipment, such as ventilator circuitry, aerosol tubing, nebulizers, and humidifiers is performed every three days with an initial washing in a non-residue-forming household detergent, then a thorough rinsing, followed by soaking in a 2% white vinegar and distilled water solution (a 1:3 dilution). There has been some controversy in the literature regarding the effectiveness of vinegar for use as a disinfecting agent in the home (Assembly for Com-

TABLE 8–14. COMPARISON OF TOTAL DAYS SPENT ON MECHANICAL VENTILATOR AT HOME VERSUS NUMBER OF HOSPITAL READMISSION DAYS EXPERIENCED FOR TREATMENT OF ACQUIRED PULMONARY INFECTION*

Patient	Total Home Care Days	Total Hospital Readmission Days
A	405	8
B	133	0
C	1284	0
D	20	0
E	227	13
F	716	15
G	725	0
H	210	0
I	329	0
J	507	0
K	134	11
L	164	0
M	137	0
N	313	0
O	283	0
P	1144	0
Q	245	0
R	457	0
S	466	17
T	188	0
U	782	0
V	43	0
Total	**8912**	**64**

*Figures shown represent an average 0.7% hospital readmission rate for treatment of pulmonary infection acquired at home.
Reproduced with permission from O'Ryan JA, & Burns DG: Pulmonary Rehabilitation: From Hospital To Home. *Chicago, Year Book, 1984, p 228.*

prehensive Respiratory Care; Flieg, 1982). Although in this author's experience it has worked well for the patients sent home, recently the use of a double-quaternary ammonium compound that has become increasingly popular and available for the home patient has been recommended. In a very recent study by Chatburn, Kallstrom, and Bajaksouzain (1988) a 1.25% white vinegar solution was compared with a commercially available double quaternary as a disinfectant for handheld nebulizers. They concluded that the 1.25% white vinegar solution (1:4 dilution) was as effective as the double quaternary for single use. This author continues to recommend the double quaternary compound as a disinfectant in the home where large volumes of equipment must be disinfected on a regular basis. The double quaternary solution can be reused for 10 to 14 days, whereas the vinegar solution must be replaced for each cleaning.

The exterior surfaces of the ventilator can be kept clean with a commercially available broad spectrum germicide or a 70% ethyl alcohol solution. All filters are to be changed at the frequency recommended by the manufacturer. The family is taught to recognize the early signs and symptoms of a respiratory tract infection; if such a situation arises, the physician is contacted immediately. A sputum sample is obtained for culture and sensitivity, and the appropriate antibiotic is prescribed (if necessary) and administered at home.

Keeping equipment regularly cleaned and properly stored in the home is not at all a difficult task, but if not performed properly or at the prescribed intervals, the result may be recurrent hospitalizations.

COMMUNITY SERVICES

A multitude of community services are available to the patient and family. The services appropriate to the patient's and family's needs should be investigated and made use of.

Before the patient is discharged, the family should communicate with their local power company, emergency squad or ambulance service, and the fire department. The power company will appropriate priority service in the event of a power failure to the home patient requiring life-support equipment. Those services can range from supplying a portable generator for restoring temporary power to awarding rate discounts. The nearest ambulance service or community rescue squad should be notified before the patient returns home. At this time, arrangements should be made for them to visit the home the day the patient returns to visualize the physical layout of the home, the patient's condition (e.g. bed-confined, tracheostomy tube, need for suction equipment, etc), various equipment being used, and the oxygen system and its location in the home. By actually visiting the home and observing the patient's environment, the emergency service personnel and fire department can best tailor their response and services to any potential crisis.

In many instances, because of the nature of the disease process and medical management requirements, the homebound ventilator-dependent patient may be leaving a large tertiary care institution or major referral center that is not always close to home. When the patient returns home, the family physician and respiratory therapy personnel at the local hospital should be informed of the patient's circumstances in case he or she needs immediate emergency attention.

FOLLOW-UP AND CONTINUING CARE

The actual follow-up and continued observance of the patient and caregivers begins before the patient is sent home. The equipment and supplies should be brought to the home a day or two before the patient is discharged. This practice will allow the family to organize the care area and devise a scheduled care routine. Once the equipment and supplies are in place, the family usually has additional questions regarding care practices and equipment operation.

The day the patient returns home, it is essential that personnel from the home care team be present; this usually includes the respiratory therapist or the nurse. The team member(s) present should stay until the patient and family feel comfortable, knowing that all systems are operating and the patient is safe. Apprehension on the part of the patient and family is usually visible at this time. Although the caregivers may have felt secure in their responsibilities within the confines of the hospital, it is a different atmosphere at home without dozens of trained personnel available when needed. The first week will usually require daily phone checks and possibly two to three visits until the family begins to become more independent.

In this author's experience, it has been found that sending a therapist to the patient's home for routine supply deliveries whenever possible can be advantageous in two respects: (1) the home is visited unannounced, providing a more realistic view of intrafamily relationships and general care conditions; and (2) visits by qualified personnel are more frequent, thereby improving accessibility to the home care team for the caregivers.

Formal monthly visits to the home are made to furnish records pertaining to the progression (or regression) of the patient's ventilatory status and overall physical condition, vital signs, and total care routine.

A ventilator flow sheet is also supplied for the patient. This flow sheet identifies each control on the ventilator. The patient or caregiver is instructed to observe each control setting and record this on the form at least once daily. This directs someone in the household to ensure that all ventilator controls are set properly each day. The flow sheet is also a reference for substitute home team members or on-call personnel who are not completely familiar with the prescribed settings. Recording of equipment cleaning dates, changes in secretion color and consistency, and airway pressure changes are also recorded on the flow sheet.

In the event the patient lives in an outlying area or a significant distance from the place from which he or she was discharged, it is advisable to acquire the services of a local therapist who will be available to the patient and family for emergencies.

The psychologic concerns that are often observed to be associated with ventilator-dependent patients and their families may be far more frequent and serious than any other problems. Denial and depression often displayed by the patient and feelings of despair, guilt, and resentment generated in the family may combine to create serious conflicts within the home. These should be noted by the home care therapist, nurse, or other outside caregivers and reported to the physician.

SUMMARY

Providing the opportunity for ventilator-dependent patients and their families to return home to live in warm and familiar surroundings can be an exhilarating and rewarding experience.

The ultimate goal when sending patients home under these circumstances is to *enhance* life, not simply to support or prolong it. However, as greater numbers of patients and their families continue to return home, it is extremely important that they realize the comprehensive responsibilities associated with this type of home care.

REFERENCES

Alexander MS, Johnson EW, Petty J et al: Mechanical ventilation of patients with late stage Duchenne muscular dystrophy: Management in the home. *Arch Phys Med Rehabil* 1979;*60*:289.

Assembly for Comprehensive Respiratory Care (ACRC): *Statement Regarding Cleaning of Home-Based Respiratory Therapy Equipment*. Calif, American Lung Association of Orange County.

Chatburn RL, Kallstrom TJ, Bajaksouzian S: A comparison of acetic acid with a quaternary ammonium compound for disinfection of hand-held nebulizers. *Respir Care* 1988;*33*:179.

Fleig CP: Double quats disinfectant alternative to vinegar. R_x *Home Care* 1982;*4*:37.

Goldberg AI: International exchange of experts and information in rehabilitation fellowship, Report #20. Home Care services for severely physically disabled people in England and France. *Case Example: The Ventilator Dependent Person*. New York, World Rehabilitation Fund, 1983.

Goldberg AI, Faure EA: Home care for life-supported persons in France: The regional association. *Rehabil Lit* 1986;*47*:60.

Holtackers TR, Loosbrock LM, Gracey DR: The use of the chest cuirass in respiratory failure of Neurologic origin. *Respir Care* 1982;*27*:271.

Kacmarek RM, Spearman CB: Equipment used for ventilatory support in the home. *Respir Care* 1986;*31*:311.

Lucas J: Home ventilator care: Reimbursement from the DME perspective. Read before the American Respiratory Care Foundation Meeting, Dallas, Tex, February, 1987.

O'Ryan JA, Burns DG: *Pulmonary Rehabilitation: From Hospital to Home*. Chicago, Year Book, 1984, pp 211–233.

Schraeder BD: A creative approach to caring for the ventilator dependent child. *Matern Child Nurs* 1979;*4*:165,

Simmons BP, Wong ES: *Guidelines for Prevention of Nosocomial Pneumonia and Guideline Ranking Scheme: Hospital Infections Program*. Atlanta, Center for Infectious Diseases, Centers for Disease Control, 1982.

II

THE PSYCHOSOCIAL ISSUES

9

Psychologic Aspects of Ventilator Dependence

W. TERRY GIPSON, MD

INTRODUCTION

The medical technology of assisted ventilation has advanced from the chest-wall manipulation devices of the 1930s (rocking bed and iron lung, or tank respirators) to the current microcircuitry of ventilators, which have given us a new wave of acronyms in medicine (PEEP, for positive end-expiratory pressure, CPAP for continuous positive airway pressure, etc). However, at the other end of these modern devices are the same critically ill human beings. Now it is not polio that threatens life, but rather an acute illness like adult respiratory distress syndrome, or even a chronic illness like amyotrophic lateral sclerosis. The ability to treat disorders that either primarily or secondarily affect the respiratory system has allowed a whole new field of medicine to evolve, with proliferation of intensive care units.

Where in this advancing technologic assault upon disease is the place for the psychiatrist? The answer is at the bedside with the patient, or at times with the treatment team, and frequently with the family. The author, while working as a consultation-liaison psychiatrist at the Cleveland Clinic Foundation, together with Edward D. Sivak, MD, Department of Pulmonary Medicine and Director of the Medical Intensive Care Unit, worked for over 4 years in an endeavor to meet the physical, psychologic, and to some extent, the social needs of patients who require mechanical ventilation for either acute or chronic respiratory insufficiency disorders. A team approach has been developed for support of the patients with disorders that have required assisted ventilation at home. The cost-effectiveness of such programs for adults (Sivak et al, 1983) and children (Burr et al, 1983) has been documented.

The intent of this article is to: (1) review the psychologic aspects of dyspnea and ventilator dependency, acute and chronic; (2) share some of our clinical experiences to highlight issues; and (3) briefly mention some of the complex social and ethical issues associated with the interface of medical technology and home care.

PSYCHOLOGIC ASPECTS OF DYSPNEA

Discussion of the psychologic aspects of ventilator dependency needs to be viewed first of all from the perspective of the psychologic aspects of dyspnea. Dyspnea is associated with threat to life in the mind of the patient more often than most other symptoms. There are some similarities to pain, since both dyspnea and pain involve a perceived sensation and a subsequent reaction to that sensation. In both, the clinician is dependent on the report of the patient. A communication about any distressing or threatening symptom will be influenced by at least three factors: the patient's past experiences; the patient's personality style; and the immediate context and meaning of the experience.

For example, someone who has had a prior experience of near-drowning may respond to dyspnea with an overwhelming autonomic discharge approaching panic, regardless of the cause of breathlessness. As an example of the influence of personality style, the person with histrionic personality traits may well embellish the report of dyspnea with flowery descriptions while maintaining an outward appearance of indifference. And as for the meaning of the experience, there will be quite a difference in the reporting of dyspnea by someone who has had repeated episodes of reversible bronchospasm as opposed to the patient with abrupt onset of dyspnea from an acute medical disorder.

Therefore, one has to assess the psychologic factors accompanying the symptom or the reaction to the symptom. Is the perception of the degree of respiratory impairment factual, or is the reaction to threatened or fantasized impairment creating a negative feedback on the system? We are all familiar with the hyperventilation syndrome in which the threatened or fantasized impairment of ventilation sets in motion a vicious cycle of events that produces additional symptoms. The separation of the perception of breathlessness from the reaction to the symptom is obviously an artificial one for purposes of our communicating about the subject, quite similar to our mental constructs of psyche and soma. Obviously, impairment of ventilation produces immediate concerns about the consequences of that impairment.

The psychobiology of respiration was well studied and reported in the late 1950s and early 1960s by Dudley, Martin, and Holmes (1964). They systematically studied psychologically induced ventilatory changes. Adverse life situations or even the suggestions of such situations could be associated with either hyperventilation or hypoventilation. The difference seemed to be whether the major component of the psychologic reaction was action-oriented (either action or the desire for action) versus whether the major component of the response was oriented toward non-action.

The behaviors and emotions associated with hyperventilation were tension, restlessness, irritability, desire to act, panic, hostility, anxiety, and anger. The behaviors and emotions associated with hypoventilation were withdrawal, despair, apathy, sadness, and hopelessness. These observations were demonstrated in subjects with normal pulmonary function as well as patients with pulmonary disease. It is easy enough to see that the individual with decreased oxygenation may become compromised by a stimulus producing either action-oriented or nonaction-oriented behaviors and emotions.

It is interesting that within the brain there are separate but very closely interrelated systems for regulation of metabolic factors of respiration as opposed to the regulation of behavioral factors of respiration. The forebrain tends to control the behavioral aspects of respiration, whereas the hindbrain controls the metabolic functions. While this may be an oversimplified account of a very complex central nervous system (CNS) function, this interrelatedness of the two systems partially accounts for the effects of biofeedback. One is impressed with this biofeedback system in the use of relaxation training, in which a patient can be assisted to relax by first becoming aware of the rate and depth of respiration. The voluntary control of breathing, which is the only autonomic function regulated by skeletal muscle, is one key to relaxation and subsequent control of tension and anxiety. The reduction of anxiety permits the development of confidence from the sense of mastery that is developed. The utilitarian value of biofeedback was demonstrated by Corson et al (1979) in the use of biofeedback techniques in weaning several patients from respirator dependency.

PSYCHOLOGIC ASPECTS OF VENTILATOR DEPENDENCY

What are the physical and psychologic stressors associated with intubation and mechanically assisted ventilation? First, there are the stressors created by illness that put the patient in the intensive care unit. That illness may be a major source of pain that requires a balance between the use of narcotics and respiratory depression. Usually in the early stages the patient is paralyzed with a depolarizing drug to minimize resistance to the machine. Adequate sedation needs to be given during this period ("Paralyzed," 1981). Confusion may be present also as a part of the original illness (e.g., head trauma or stroke).

With preservation of awareness, there may be emotional factors associated with the patient's knowledge about the illness. The immediate fear is for one's life. The types of illness and injury that necessitate mechanical ventilation are obviously life threatening. Standing at the bedside of a person who has been denied the opportunity to communicate verbally, one can nevertheless see the nonverbal cues of fear. The panic is communicated by the wild stare with dilated pupils and the frequent glances, as if scanning the environment with expectations of further hurt. If awareness is preserved, the patient may have pain that is caused by the treatment of the medical condition. Other sources for pain include the laryngeal pain from the endotracheal tube, multiple venipunctures for intravenous fluids and laboratory determinations, arterial and venous devices for monitoring, bladder catheters, nasogastric tubes, and chest tubes.

In attempting to comprehend the patient's distress, we may be denied an understanding of the meaning of the illness because of the limitations of communication. The meaning of the illness to the patient frequently establishes the course of that individual's coping with the illness. As consultation-liaison psychiatrists attempting to support the patient and staff, we are at a disadvantage when the understanding of the meaning of illness is unavailable.

Many of the patients who require mechanical assistance for ventilation do not have primary lung disease. The CNS drive for respiration has been affected and ventilatory support is initiated to correct the secondary effects of the primary disorder (e.g., head injury, metabolic acidosis, etc). Many of the patients lose consciousness as a result of the physical distress of intubation and ventilation in the earliest stage. While delirium is an ominous complication (Rabins & Folstein, 1982), it may also produce amnesia for the more unpleasant experiences if the illness is acute and the ventilator support required only for a brief period.

PSYCHIATRIC CONSULTATION IN THE INTENSIVE CARE SETTING

The psychiatrist's approach to the patient experiencing severe dyspnea, or one who already has been intubated, will obviously have to be tailored or modified to the situation. These types of consultations can be the most exasperating of all of those in consultative psychiatry. One has to be prepared to spend a lot of time at the bedside. The initial goal is to facilitate communication, and it has to be established under very difficult circumstances. Written answers may well be the only response beyond affirmative or negative nods of the head. The technique of interviewing in which open-ended questions are asked frequently cannot be used, and one has to settle for questions with yes–no answers. Observation of nonverbal behaviors is crucial. While one has to be cautious about the inferences regarding nonverbal behaviors in these patients, the psychiatrist gathers all the value possible from every bit of data. Touching is not only allowed but is essential as a means of establishing contact under such restrictions of verbal communication.

As with all psychiatric consultation, mental status evaluation is essential. The major points of appearance, behavior, thought content, stream of thought, mood, and affect need to be assessed. Granted, the data base for these parameters may be abbreviated. The patient's orientation, cognition, insight, and judgment are essential for deciding whether or not the patient is delirious. Delirium represents acute brain failure, and it is still poorly understood by many clinicians. In delirium, there is a clouding of consciousness with impairment of cognitive processes including thinking, perceiving, and remembering. There are three aspects of this reversible syndrome: (1) the patient is awake and usually capable of responding verbally; (2) the impairment of the attention, thinking, and memory tends to fluctuate over time; and (3) there is defective reality testing, so that the patient's ability to integrate cues from the internal and external environment with past knowledge and experience is impaired.

Regardless of the brevity of the interview, one needs to have enough data to answer three questions:

1. Is the patient delirious?
2. What is the patient's mood?
3. What is the reaction of the individual to the illness and to the environment, especially when the environment is an intensive care setting and a ventilator as well?

The ventilator-dependent patient is usually able to communicate by writing. The characteristics of the responses when writing may well give an early cue to the presence of delirium. Dysgraphia seems to be the most sensitive indicator of delirium. Motor impairment of writing is manifested by reduplication of strokes in letters and inability to orient lines up and down. Spelling errors are common and are out of proportion to the patient's educational level. In the course of evaluating the patient's mood, one can ascertain to some degree the psychologic defenses of the patient. Certain psychologic defenses are adaptive and useful in combating overwhelming threats to life, while others may be maladaptive and hinder recovery. Obviously, the initial emotional response to life-threatening illness is anxiety. In the early stages of illness, the anxiety is global and focused on sheer survival. Hackett and Cassem (1971) documented a sequence of responses in patients with myocardial infarction. The early global anxiety was followed within 48 to 72 hours by denial, and depression was present by the third or fourth day.

The psychiatrist can assist both the ventilator-dependent patient and the staff in the intensive care setting with making such judgments as:

- Is the level of anxiety appropriate to the individual in the context of the illness?

- Is the denial reasonable and adaptive to the task of organizing coping skills, or is the denial maladaptive and thereby preventing the best care?
- Is the depression simply a symptom, or is it part of a syndrome that carries a graver prognosis and may require medication in addition to psychologic support?
- Is the regression of the patient to a necessary level of dependency, or has it progressed to a state of helplessness unsuitable for adaptation to the illness?

The answers to these questions help the staff to adjust their expectations of the patient based on a better understanding of the patient's needs as well as an understanding of their own reactions to these patients.

Occasionally, the psychiatrist will be consulted regarding concern that psychologic issues are impairing the success of weaning from mechanical ventilation. A study of such patients (Mendel & Kohn, 1980) has pointed out some frequent issues. The fear of sudden death once the patient is off ventilatory support is perhaps the most common. Secondary depression resulting from chronic illness may impair motivation to return to spontaneous breathing. Occasionally, interpersonal conflict and anger at either staff members or family members is found to be a factor in weaning difficulties.

CLINICAL EXPERIENCES

The author interviewed patients and family members in the medical intensive care unit. In addition, home visits were made. Several of the patients were already at home when the interviews began, so they were not seen by the liaison psychiatrists in the intensive care setting. The interviews were standard psychiatric interviews to assess mental status, present and past coping, and presence of psychopathology. Special attention was paid to the issues of chronic illness and machine dependency. The following brief clinical descriptions will illustrate the variability of response.

Patient One
Mrs T was 58 years old when initially seen in the medical intensive care unit. Psychiatric consultation was requested because the physicians and nurses were aware that the patient was depressed out of proportion to her state of illness. There were clear-cut indications of improvement from the medical standpoint. She had been found to have central alveolar hypoventilation of uncertain etiology. Mrs T had undergone elective tracheostomy and was being taught the technique of using a portable volume ventilator at home during the night.

During the psychiatric interview, the patient admitted that her depression was not because of her illness. She actually felt better with the nighttime ventilation; however, she was very concerned about her family. Her husband was a binge drinker, and with the stress of her hospitalization, he had had a weekend of heavy alcohol intake after having previously maintained sobriety for several months. As a consequence, there had been a fight between him and the two sons, aged 17 and 19. In addition, a 15-year-old daughter was severely depressed and suicidal. These events occurred while Mrs T was in the intensive care unit.

Arrangements for a family meeting were made and measures were taken toward management of what proved to be preexistent, long-term family conflict. The daughter was referred to their local community mental health agency for individual supportive therapy. During the meeting, family members were able to discuss their concerns about Mrs T's illness as well as their fears for her long-term survival.

Mrs T functioned satisfactorily for the first year and a half of home ventilator support at night. The family conflict was not totally resolved, but it seemed to settle back into the preillness patterns of interaction. Unfortunately, Mrs T later developed progressive deterioration of speech and dysphagia. Diagnostic studies confirmed amyotrophic lateral sclerosis. Currently, she is markedly depressed and beginning to attempt to struggle with the issues of how much medical technology she will accept and for how long.

Patient Two

Mr G retired in 1977 at the age of 56 because of progressive weakness of obscure origin. Thirteen months later he developed respiratory failure and a diagnosis of amyotrophic lateral sclerosis was made.

This man had been trained as an engineer and worked as an executive with a large corporation. He incorporated his mechanical skills into coping with his disability. He accepted the illness as a challenge, much as he would have taken on an assignment of problem solving in the corporation.

When Mr G and his wife were initially interviewed in their home, he immediately displayed both his mechanical and psychologic skills of coping. He sat in a mechanized wheelchair, the design of which he had modified to hold his portable oxygen supply and his portable volume ventilator. His immediate response to the opening question of "What has it been like to be dependent on a respirator?" was to point to the ventilator and respond with gasping speech, "It has been a friend. It has given me some extra years of life."

Mrs G was having difficulty coping because of some resentment and hostility. They had had a good marriage of many years. However, now that Mr G was dependent upon her, a role reversal, she had difficulty tolerating his demands. He used the same executive manner toward her that he would have used with one of his employees in his former times on the job. Mrs G was able to ask for sanction for her feelings from the visiting psychiatrist by asking in the presence of her husband, "Doctor, is it all right for a wife to be angry at her husband when he is sick?"

With gradual deterioration in Mr G's already severely compromised functioning, it has been a strain on the couple to maintain their faith in God, which had been a source of strength to them. Unanswered prayers have caused them to question their belief system.

Patient Three

At the age of 62, Mr C developed respiratory failure just 3 months after the diagnosis of amyotrophic lateral sclerosis had been made. For over a year before that he had had dysarthria.

The first home visit indicated an immediate state of tension manifested by Mrs C and her two daughters. There was a quick ushering of the psychiatrist to a room sufficiently distant from the patient so he would not hear the conversation. As the interview progressed further, manifestations of the denial in this family became obvious. The wife denied any stress currently on herself and displaced her concerns onto the younger daughter: "It's Mary that I am concerned about." Indeed, the 22-year-old daughter was stressed. She was chronically depressed and now would not go into the room with her father. If he were brought into the room she would immediately leave. The 40-year-old married daughter was a very assertive woman who was overinvested in the care of her father as a displacement from her own chronic marital discord.

Mr C behaved as if there were no family conflict. He had been able to maintain some mobility with a mechanical wheelchair and the use of a golf cart on his grounds and around the neighborhood.

Patient Four

Mr B was a 69-year-old retired automechanic who developed acute respiratory failure. Several days after initiation of diagnostic tests a diagnosis of amyotrophic lateral sclerosis was made.

The patient was initially seen in the medical intensive care unit for anxiety that was inhibiting his recovery. Upon evaluation of the patient, his wife, and their married daughter, the source of his anxiety was discovered. Mrs B had a long history of dependence upon her husband and had a history strongly suggesting hypochondriasis. With the role reversal necessitated by Mr B's illness, he was frightened at the prospect of being dependent upon his wife.

Fortunately, the daughter was an aggressive person, who took charge of her father's care. She and her mother had conflict because of the mother's anxiety at having to learn the operation of the ventilator as well as respiratory care. When Mr B left the intensive care unit after 2½ months to be on continuous ventilator support at home, the entire staff was concerned about his wife's anxiety, even though it had diminished considerably. To their surprise, on a home visit a few months later, it was observed that Mrs B had assumed complete control of her husband's care, and the patient was quite content with it. The daughter was not being used for caregiving at all.

Some 15 months later the patient developed peritonitis from volvulus of the sigmoid colon. He required surgical resection with colostomy and was able to return home but died 12 days later. At the time of his death, his life could have been extended, but he chose not to return to the hospital. This was a decision mutually agreed upon by the patient and his wife.

Patient Five

Mr S was aged 61 when he had to retire as a commercial laundry salesman because of weakness. Six months after his retirement the diagnosis of amyotrophic lateral sclerosis was made, and 6 months after that, respiratory failure developed. The patient and his wife elected to have mechanical ventilation and began training for home care ventilation.

This couple had had over the years a relationship in which Mr S was the more passive and dependent member. The life-support measures were dealt with by an even greater degree of regression on his part. This fostered hostility on the part of the wife when she realized that Mr S could actually do more than he was attempting for himself.

During the home visit, Mrs S displaced her hostility on all sorts of substitutes other than her husband: the insurance companies, the equipment servicemen, the visiting nurse, and had the two physicians making the home visit not been present, they would have undoubtedly been the target for some of her displaced hostility. While discussing whether or not the right decision had been made regarding the use of home ventilation, Mrs S was openly ambivalent about the decision. She discussed that ambivalence in the presence of the husband. He felt positive about the decision to be on the ventilator.

Discussion

These brief clinical vignettes illustrate that the response to respiratory failure and mechanical support at home are as varied as the individuals who experience the disorders. And they should be. Illness, as opposed to disease, is a very subjective experience. The following observations represent some of our impressions developed during this multidisciplinary effort to support patients who are treated with the technology of modern medicine.

One of the most interesting observations was the difference in the attitudes of the patient and family members when we, the physicians, were on their territory as opposed to their attitudinal set when they were in our "domain." Because of our familiarity with the intensive care setting, few of us realize how threatening it is to the patients, and even more so to families. Many times we learned much more about the family dynamics when visiting in the home than we had learned in the hospital. With respect to the reactions of the patients to their illness, as a group they displayed the same transition from fear and anxiety to despondency in the earliest stages of their disease. As a group they tended then to settle into a style of coping that was usually a further elaboration of a combination of individual personality traits and coping styles. Denial, displacement, projection, and sublimation were present in all to some degree. The maladaptive use of such defense mechanisms was consistent with the unconscious needs of the individual to maintain a preillness image of themselves.

What about the reactions of the families? Basically, the same observation can be extended from the individual styles to the family style of coping. That is to say, families who previously coped well made adjustments to even such great demands as home ventilator support requires. Families with preexisting conflict often became more embroiled in an exacerbation of issues for which the patient's illness was a scapegoat. Obviously, when this happened, the patient's care was compromised. In this regard, previous family behaviors tended to predict adaptive or maladaptive adjustment to the technology in the home. By being involved with the entire family, we were able to make some interventions that seemed to help restore balance and induce a lessening of tension.

The issues of machine dependency and body image for these patients was qualitatively similar to our experiences with renal failure patients requiring home dialysis and patients on home parenteral nutrition (Gulledge et al, 1980). A similar multidisciplinary approach has been developed for support of patients using these technologies. Quantitatively, however, it appears that the issues of machine dependency and body image are greater for the patients on home ventilation. These patients spend more time being dependent on the machine and the caregivers. Their mobility is much more restricted. Similar to patients in other investigators' reports, patients who were able to incorporate the machine into their lives in an ego-syntonic fashion fared much better.

The ethical issues of home care ventilation are complex. The advances in medical technology have given us the power to sustain life indefinitely in some cases. With this power, however, we need to exercise responsibility. We are aware of the ethical issues involved in initiating ventilator support for patients who have progressively incapacitating illness such as amyotrophic lateral sclerosis. The ethicists tell us that physicians are the best judges of the efficacy of treatment and that patients alone are the best judges of desirability. But how does one communicate to a person with such diseases what the late stages of the illness will be like? And how does one communicate that information in a way that does not bias the patient? Difficult as it may be, we have to do it. The hope is that we might afford better day-by-day functioning in exchange for a gradual death by incessant respiratory failure.

The bioethical literature is not helpful in addressing the issue of using mechanical support systems in disorders for which the support system does not replace the diseased organ. The model of renal dialysis does not apply, because the diseased organ (the kidney) is replaced by the function of a machine. In patients who have their lungs affected by neurologic disease, the ventilator assists an organ system (the lungs) that is not primarily diseased.

At the time of the initial interviews with these patients, the issue of termination of ventilatory support, if initiated, is discussed. The patients are aware of the inevitable course of deterioration in the context of this discussion. Several patients have declined the initiation of the support with mechanical ventilation. The most desirable situation is for the patient's autonomy to be preserved throughout the course of the illness.

A realistic concern with the effects of mechanical support technology on the cost of medical care is an issue that has to be confronted. It is hoped that the practical concerns of this matter will not supercede the need to relieve suffering.

CONCLUSION

In summary, home ventilator support is a treatment modality that offers improved quality of life for some people with chronic respiratory failure. A treatment approach has been described for both the intensive care setting and for home follow-up. This is done in the context of a team approach, which obviously involves nurses, respiratory therapists, and social workers as well.

The effort to meet the psychologic needs of patients, their families, and the staff in the critical care units represents a challenge to all of us who work in these areas. Unfortunately, there are occasions when our technologic support systems are too far ahead of our psychologic support systems. By our sharing information through reports such as this, it is to be hoped that the gap between the two systems can be narrowed.

REFERENCES

Burr BH, Guyer B, Todres ID, et al: Home care for children on respirators. *N Engl J Med* 1983;*309*:1319.

Cassem NH, Hackett TP: Psychiatric consultation in a coronary care unit. *Ann Intern Med* 1971;75:9.

Corson JA, Grant JL, Moulton DP, et al: Use of biofeedback in weaning paralyzed patients from respirators. *Chest* 1979;*76*:543.

Dudley DL, Martin CJ, Holmes TH: Psychophysiologic studies of pulmonary ventilation. *Psychosom Med* 1964;*26*:645.

Gulledge AD, Gipson WT, Steiger E, et al: Home parenteral nutrition for the short bowel syndrome: Psychological issues. *Gen Hosp Psychiatry* 1980;*2*:271.

Mendel JG, Khan FA: Psychological aspects of weaning from mechanical ventilation. *Psychosomatics* 1980;*21*:465.

Paralyzed with fear, editorial. *Lancet* 1981;*1*:427.

Rabins PV, Folstein MF: Delirium and dementia: Diagnostic criteria and fatality rates. *Brit J Psychiatry* 1982;*140*:149.

Sivak ED, Cordasco EM, Gipson WT: Pulmonary mechanical ventilation at home; a reasonable and less expensive alternative. *Respir Care* 1983;*28*:42.

10

Psychosocial Readjustment and Community Services

LINDA E. SINNWELL, ACSW

INTRODUCTION

Chronic obstructive pulmonary disease (COPD) is one of the nation's fastest growing health problems. Nearly 15 million people are affected with some form of COPD (American Lung Association, 1981). Recent statistics indicate that it may be the third leading cause of disability among Americans receiving social security disability payments. It is exceeded only by heart disease in economic cost to our society (American Lung Association, 1981).

Like other chronic illnesses, the general course of COPD is one of steady degeneration, marked by frequent exacerbations that usually require hospitalization. Early detection of this disease is difficult because of its insidious nature. Often, afflicted individuals are unable to recognize the development and progression of this disorder. They do not seek medical treatment until the symptoms are sharply pronounced and they no longer have adequate cardiopulmonary reserve to meet their physical needs.

A chronic illness such as COPD necessitates many alterations in an individual's life style. The extensive impact of this chronic condition affects an individual's emotional stability, social role, occupational status, body image, and sexuality (Lambert & Lambert, 1979). The remainder of this chapter will focus upon each of these areas of concern, the means by which health-care professionals can facilitate adjustment, and finally upon a compendium of resources specific to the unique needs of the COPD patient.

ALTERATIONS IN LIFE STYLE WITH COPD

Emotional Impact
Anger, anxiety, and euphoria are active psychologic states that have been associated with an increase in energy expenditure, elevated ventilation, high oxygen consumption, and skeletal muscle tension. Nonactive psychologic variables such as apathy, depression, and deep relaxation are associated with a decrease in energy expenditure, decreased ventilation, low oxygen consumption, and skeletal muscle relaxation (Dudley et al, 1980). Because individuals with COPD have a compromised respiratory system, it is difficult for them to supply the air exchange necessary to meet the metabolic demands required by psychologic states of action. A decrease in ventilation resulting from nonactive psychologic variables adds further insult to an already inefficient respiratory system (Dudley et al, 1980).

Both the active and nonactive emotional states may increase symptom development in the COPD patient, creating a vicious cycle of emotion-related shortness of breath. When individuals with COPD experience an emotion such as anger, happiness, or depression, they may experience breathlessness. This in turn may result in fear and an increase in breathlessness, which subsequently increases fear (Fig 10–1).

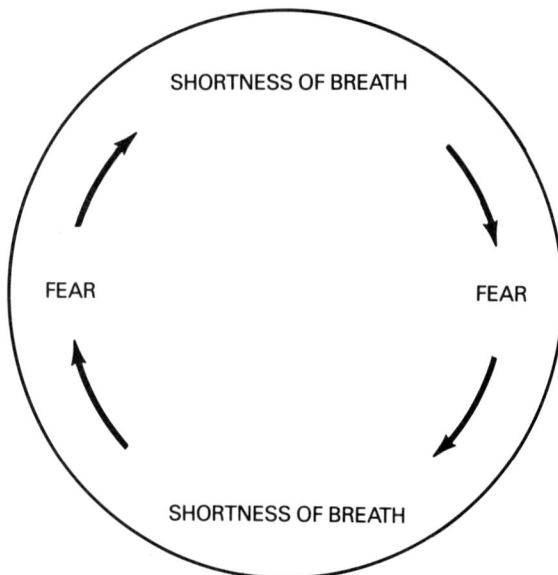

Figure 10–1. Both the action and nonaction emotional states may increase symptom development in the COPD patient creating a vicious cycle of emotion-related shortness of breath. *(Adapted from* Living with Lung Disease. *Phoenix, St. Luke's Heart Lung Center, 1983.)*

As individuals with COPD begin to realize that changes in their emotional status increase their incapacity and disability, they may protect themselves from emotionally charged situations through isolation, denial, and repression. Often they believe they cannot face their feelings, life events, or significance of their disease without risking an exacerbation. As a result, they isolate themselves from others to avoid emotional stimulation (Rowlett & Dudley, 1978). Avoidance of emotional change perpetuates emotional and interpersonal problems, which in turn increases frustration, anger, and despair. Because of the silent nature of COPD and its insidious onset, individuals may deny their own symptoms for fear of being regarded as a hypochondriac or malingerer (Dudley et al, 1980). As the disease progresses, the need for medical treatment increases. Individuals with COPD become fearful of alienating those people upon whom they depend for medical care and therefore may repress feelings of anger and frustration (Dudley, Wermuth, & Hague, 1973).

The isolation, denial, and repression that characterize COPD patients are often seen as a means to maintain comfort and at times survival. Unfortunately these defense mechanisms will not prevent pulmonary decompensation or alleviate symptom development. Various health-care professionals can be of great assistance in helping COPD patients develop the skills needed to effectively cope with changes in emotional status. They can encourage the patients to ventilate their feelings and concerns about the disease process. By doing so, situations that provoke an emotional response can be more easily identified. Once identified, these situations must be avoided if at all possible, especially during times of acute exacerbation when they can be life threatening. Verbalizing fears and concerns can also be an effective technique for breaking the emotion-related shortness of breath cycle previously mentioned. Once a fear has been identified and discussed, one has a much better chance of controlling it. Unless individuals with COPD can learn such techniques to cope with changes in their emotional status, they will not be able to maintain the necessary therapeutic regimen. The chances for long-term survival will then be significantly decreased.

Social Impact
COPD patients are among the most isolated of those individuals with a chronic illness or disability. As the disease progresses, there is a continuing reduction of social contacts and activities. Withdrawal from social activities is often one of the first major life style alterations noted (Lambert & Lambert, 1979). Individuals with COPD simply may not have the energy to socialize or participate in physical activities. Even talking can prove to be too exhausting. As a result, COPD patients often withdraw from social interaction and experience loneliness, boredom, and depression.

As social outlets decrease, the caregiving family of the COPD patient becomes the major social field. This degree of dependence upon the caregiver can become a source of stress and tension within the family. Spouses feel overwhelmed with the responsibility of meeting numerous care needs. The responsibility of assuming roles that individuals with COPD can no longer fulfill and financial concerns also contribute to family dissension.

Social activities must be planned around good and bad breathing days. Given the uncertainty of the disease, this can be extremely difficult. COPD patients and their families are frequently disappointed with their inability to participate in an activity to which they had been looking forward for quite some time. Those activities that elicit strong emotional responses such as laughter, excitement, or anger can exacerbate respiratory difficulties and must be avoided on days when symptoms are more pronounced. Large crowds and areas with high concentrations of air pollutants can increase the patient's susceptibility to respiratory infections and irritants. These situations therefore must be avoided.

Encouraging the COPD patients to pursue only those activities that are within their physical capabilities can enhance their ability to cope with the uncertainty of their disease. Planning activities that are conducive to rest periods can prevent physical exhaustion that may result in respiratory distress. Reinforcing the need to follow prescribed pulmonary regimens for clearing airways before the social engagement can prevent respiratory difficulties during the social interaction. Finally, making use of nonsmoking sections in public facilities can reduce exposure to air pollutants.

With adequate preparation, traveling can be a therapeutic means to expand the COPD patient's social field. Before planning a vacation, it is important that travel plans be discussed with the physician. It may be suggested that visiting areas with extreme temperature changes be avoided. Extremely high temperatures increase metabolism, which in turn increases oxygen consumption. Exposure to cold weather can irritate the respiratory tract, which subsequently can lead to respiratory distress (Lambert & Lambert, 1979). If temperature extremes are unavoidable, preheating and precooling automobiles is important. Obtaining accommodations with air-conditioning in warm climates and heat in cooler climates can minimize the stress placed on the respiratory system.

Depending upon the extent of the disease, the physician may recommend that areas of higher altitude be avoided. Less oxygen is available at higher altitudes, which may necessitate supplemental oxygen for an individual who does not usually require oxygen. Liter flow may need to be increased for those persons who use it on a continuous basis.

Allergies can produce respiratory difficulties in COPD patients. If allergies exacerbate the patient's condition, areas with high pollen counts should be avoided if at all possible.

In the event medical help may be required while on vacation, it is helpful to have the name and telephone number of a local physician. Often physicians will have a contact in the area to be visited. If not, one can be obtained by contacting the local medical society, which will provide a referral to a specialist in the area that one will be visiting. For extended vacations it is recommended that COPD patients obtain a copy of their medical record. If medical treatment is required, past medical history will be readily available.

Before departure the COPD patients must obtain an adequate supply of medication. Most pharmacies are unable to fill out-of-state prescriptions. Medications should not all be packed in one place in case baggage is lost or stolen. A time schedule for taking medications and breathing treatments should be written out. Time-zone changes and excitement can result in deviation from prescribed medication regimens. If traveling to a foreign country, adapters are required for electrical outlets. Automobile cigarette-lighter adapters are available if breathing treatments are required while traveling by car.

Traveling by air requires additional preparation. Airlines must be notified well in advance if an individual requires any special services such as oxygen, diet, or wheelchair. Some airlines are not equipped to accommodate oxygen. If oxygen is required in flight, documentation from a physician as to diagnosis, ability to fly on a commercial flight, and prescribed liter flow is required. Additional charges are incurred for oxygen use in flight. Scheduling a direct flight is recommended as airlines are only equipped to deliver oxygen when the plane is airborne. Coordinating oxygen delivery to the destination point can be complicated. Many home care companies have branches throughout the country and are willing to assist with this task.

Smoking is a principal cause of the majority of respiratory disorders, specifically chronic bronchitis, emphysema, and lung cancer (Kent & Smith, 1977). It is always an issue in the lives of COPD patients and often contributes to their isolation. Because smoke acts as an irritant to the respiratory tract, it is not uncommon to find pulmonary patients avoiding any situation where people may be smoking. Phobic reactions to smoke are not unusual in this population. Given the overwhelming evidence implicating smoking as a major health hazard, all pulmonary patients are encouraged to stop. Unfortunately, many cigarette-related diseases are diagnosed too late to be reversed by smoking cessation. Research does, however, indicate improvement in most conditions once the patient has quit smoking (Schwartz, 1983).

Health-care professionals can offer support and encouragement to COPD patients in their smoking cessation efforts. Reinforcement as to the health hazards of smoking is crucial. Approximately one half of all individuals currently smoking have not accepted the fact that cigarette smoking is dangerous to their health and could lead to lung cancer. There is even less acceptance of the significant relationship between smoking and specific health consequences such as emphysema and chronic bronchitis (Schwartz, 1983).

Suggestions as to how smoking habits can be altered may be beneficial. Disposing of smoking paraphernalia, buying cigarettes one pack at a time, and placing cigarettes in an inconvenient location are a few examples. Preparing the patient for possible short term side-effects such as headaches, nervousness, irritability, drowsiness, insomnia, and coughing is necessary. Patients will find it reassuring to know that their symptoms are a normal part of the quitting process.

Finally, the health-care professional must not smoke in the presence of individuals with COPD. Smoke is an irritant to their respiratory tract. Also, having a smoker present may increase the COPD patient's desire to smoke.

If individuals have been smoking for a number of years, they may experience difficulty when they attempt to quit. There is no particular method or technique that works best. Of those people who quit smoking, 95% do so on their own (Schwartz, 1983). Instructional materials are available to assist people with their efforts to stop. These materials can be obtained by contacting the American Cancer Society at 777 Third Avenue, New York, NY 10017, or the American Lung Association at 8 Mountainview Avenue, Albany, NY 12205.

For those individuals who have not been successful on their own, there are a wide variety of smoking cessation methods and programs available. Educational lectures, small group discussions, nicotine gum, individual counseling, hypnosis, and behavior modification classes are some of these. Although a few methods have been reported to produce better results, most methods achieve approximately the same results after one year (Schwartz, 1983). Local hospitals and chapters of the American Lung Association and the American Cancer Society can identify programs available in a particular area.

Occupational Impact

Because COPD generally affects middle-aged individuals at a time when they are at the peak of their careers, the occupational impact of COPD can be devastating. With the physiologic consequences of COPD producing a decrease in energy level, the afflicted individual may be forced to make changes in occupation. Depending upon the disease, these changes may have a significant impact upon the person's standard of living.

Earlier in the disease process, an individual may be able to fulfill job responsibilities with minimal alterations in the work environment. By eliciting support from the employer, work schedules and routines can be rearranged to maximize productivity. Beginning the work day later in the morning when the patient is breathing better or scheduling more frequent and shorter breaks can be helpful. Avoidance of substances and temperatures that can be irritating to the respiratory system will be beneficial in alleviating symptom development. For example, relocating to a non-smoking area or a project that does not involve work with irritating fumes can be of help. Avoiding drafts from air-conditioners and wearing a mask or scarf over the mouth and nose when going out into cold weather may also be of benefit.

If the work environment cannot be modified or the disease process has progressed to the point where the person cannot meet the physical and emotional demands, the COPD patient may be forced to change careers completely. Often, obtaining another job is very difficult. Potential employers may consider individuals with COPD an economic risk and refuse to hire them. Letters of recommendation from previous employers may not be available because of absenteeism and use of insurance benefits. Vocational rehabilitation is available to assist with job retraining but programs may be reluctant to invest resources in individuals with a poor rehabilitation prognosis.

As the disease progresses, individuals with COPD are often unable to sustain any type of employment. They are forced into retirement much earlier than anticipated at the peak of their work productivity. Family economic responsibilities are high at this time because offspring are often attending colleges, marrying, or being assisted with the development of their careers (Lambert & Lambert, 1979). Medical expenses increase with the progression of COPD. Medications and health-care insurance can be very expensive. Government financial assistance is limited. Social security disability applications may take months to process, leaving an individual without an income for an extended period of time.

Health-care providers can be of assistance in helping COPD patients recognize potential problem areas in the work environment that may increase respiratory difficulties. They also may be of support in facilitating communication between the patients and their employer as to ways in which the work area can be modified to maximize functioning and productivity.

COPD patients must be encouraged to remain as active as possible. This is very important. Without physical activity, the respiratory patient may become physically and emotionally immobilized. This immobilization may contribute to the progression of their chronic condition. Respiratory secretions may become obstructed as a result of physical immobility and an increase in respiratory symptoms may be noted. Emotional immobility results in boredom, which leads to physical immobility and subsequent respiratory complications (Lambert & Lambert, 1979). Encouraging participation in a pulmonary rehabilitation program may be a means to increase physical activity and also reinforce the need for breathing retraining, physical conditioning, and energy conservation. Exploring volunteer opportunities available in the community may also decrease physical and emotional immobility.

Health-care providers, specifically social workers, can assist COPD patients in identifying and mobilizing those resources that may be of benefit. COPD patients may qualify for social security benefits, state financial assistance programs, food stamps, vocational rehabilitation, and government-subsidized health-care programs, all of which may lessen the financial strain precipitated by their illness. These resources and criteria for eligibility are discussed in more depth later in this chapter.

Somatic Impact

Changes in body image have also been associated with COPD. A barrel-shaped chest, increased sputum production, altered breathing patterns, coughing, wheezing, and skin pallor are common physical changes experienced by individuals with COPD. Reliance on respiratory equipment and oxygen can be embarrassing and for some creates a sense of being unattractive. For others, the changes in body conformation resulting from steroid therapy can be discomforting. Often, these changes result in feelings of hopelessness, self-consciousness, and frustration. These stressful feelings may trigger emotional responses that may increase symptom development.

To cope with these changes in body image, an individual requires a great deal of personal strength and social support. Health-care providers can educate COPD patients to better cope with these changes and mobilize the necessary supports. The patient should be encouraged to follow the physician's recommended medical regimen for clearing airways, which will reduce sputum production as well as coughing and wheezing. Education as to the importance of oxygen and prescribed medications and treatments may help increase compliance. Suggesting that the patient avoid tapered and form-fitting clothing will help to deemphasize the barrel-shaped chest. The patient should be encouraged to experiment with different colors of clothing to find those that do not accentuate the ashen skin color.

Health-care providers need to be aware of the possibility that the COPD patients may harbor concerns about their physical appearance and how others perceive them. The patients need encouragement to verbalize these feelings concerning the somatic impact of their illness. Openly airing these concerns better allows both the family and the health-care team to engage in mutual problem solving. Ways in which the patients might better cope with these changes can be identified through this process.

Sexual Impact

A chronic illness such as COPD also affects an individual's ability to function sexually. Sexual activity increases energy expenditure, elevates ventilatory rate, and increases oxygen consumption. COPD patients with an impaired respiratory system may have difficulty supplying the air exchange necessary to meet the metabolic demands created by intercourse (Lambert & Lambert, 1979). With adequate information, creativity, and adaptation, individuals with COPD can have a satisfying sex life.

COPD is a chronic condition with physiologic changes that tend to occur over a period of time. COPD patients may gradually withdraw from intimate relationships. Depression, fear of suffocation, rejection, and failure have all been attributed to this decrease in sexual activity. Many COPD patients are fearful of any activity that may induce dyspnea. Therefore, they will avoid even realistic physical activity such as intercourse. Their partners often reinforce this behavior by avoiding sexual intercourse in an effort to avoid placing undue stress upon the COPD patients. Humiliation occurs if individuals fail in their attempt to complete intercourse. Depression, which is common among COPD patients, decreases libido. Somatic changes such as a barrel-shaped chest, increased sputum production, coughing, wheezing, and skin pallor may leave the COPD patients feeling unattractive and fearful of losing their partner.

Sexual functioning of COPD patients must be addressed. Providing correct information and reassurance to the patients and their sexual partners is the responsibility of the health-care professional. Patients must be informed that intercourse is not extremely stressful and requires about the same amount of energy as walking 3 miles an hour or climbing two flights of stairs (Conine & Evans, 1981). Documented cases of death during lovemaking are rare.

One of the most disruptive effects of COPD is dyspnea during sexual intercourse. Patients should be told that shortness of breath during intercourse is natural and can be tolerated within limits. Both the patients and their partners should be reminded that becoming anxious or fearful will increase shortness of breath.

Patients should be encouraged to discuss with their physicians the effects prescribed medications will have on their sexual performance. Drugs prescribed for treatment of pulmonary conditions such as steroids and theophylline will have little effect on sexual performance. Sexual functioning may be impaired by drugs prescribed for management of other conditions. Antihypertensive drugs depress sexual functioning, as do narcotics, ethyl alcohol, cholinergic blockers, monoanine oxidase (MAO) inhibitors, tricyclic antidepressants, phenothiazines, thioxanthines, haloperidol, and benzodiazepines (Kravitz, 1982).

An explanation as to effects the aging process has on sexual functioning may be helpful since COPD patients may blame such changes on their disease. Erections may take longer and may be less powerful in older men, and it may take longer to achieve an erection after ejaculation. Many women experience a delay in or lack of lubrication in later years that is easy to rectify by using a lubricant. This is not related to the disease process, and the patient should be made aware of this. Intercourse may differ from earlier days but need not be less satisfying (Kravitz, 1982).

Health-care providers, depending upon background and professional expertise, may offer specific suggestions that address the patients' sexual concerns. Some possibilities are as follows:

1. Use diaphragmatic and pursed-lip breathing techniques during intercourse.
2. Consult with the physician as to the possibility of using a bronchodilator or supplemental oxygen 10 to 15 minutes before intercourse to reduce dyspnea.
3. Plan for a good sexual experience. Rest before sexual activity. Avoid excessive alcohol and heavy meals before coitus.
4. Avoid coital positions that place pressure on the chest. Attempt to use those positions that take less physical work. For males, the female superior position is recommended since the lateral position reduces exertion for both men and women.
5. Consider the use of a water bed because it reduces the amount of physical exertion required during sex.
6. Encourage the sex partner to avoid using scents, powders, or aerosol products that might elicit symptom development.

COPD patients must be encouraged to share both their breathing and sexual needs with their partner. Likes and dislikes need to be communicated. If individuals with COPD are unable to tolerate sexual intercourse, alternative forms of pleasuring can be explored. Touching, oral-genital sex, and mutual masturbation can enhance intimacy.

If patients' sexual difficulties are unresponsive to intervention by their physician or health-care professionals, referral to a competent sex therapist is indicated. If problems can be attributed to a dysfunctional marriage, either individual or marital counseling may be recommended.

RESOURCES

A broad range of patient care services are available to the chronically ill population in the United States. Medical social workers can be of assistance with identification of resources that may meet the specific needs of the COPD patients. Assisting patients and their families with resource mobilization also falls within the province of the social worker. The services to be discussed in this chapter can be divided into the following categories: government agencies, disease-related foundations, home-health-care agencies, home-care companies, and miscellaneous support services.

Government Agencies

The federal government offers health insurance to persons 65 years old and older and to the disabled through Title 18, or the Medicare program. The program consists of two basic components. Part A is a compulsory hospital plan that covers hospitalization, skilled nursing facilities, and home health care under certain predetermined conditions. This program is financed by employer and employee contributions and through a tax on the self-employed. Part B represents a voluntary program of supplemental medical insurance that pays a percentage of approved physicians' services, outpatient services, and home health care in addition to certain medical services and supplies. Financing is achieved through monthly premiums paid by enrollees and matching funds by the federal government.

Individuals are eligible for Medicare part A benefits on their 65th birthday or after they have been receiving Social Security Disability benefits for 2 years. Those persons requiring dialysis or a transplant for chronic kidney disease are also eligible for Medicare. When individuals become entitled to part A benefits, they are automatically enrolled in part B benefits unless they indicate they do not wish to participate in the voluntary medical insurance program. Local social security offices should be contacted to initiate the enrollment process.

Hospital benefits (part A) are measured by increments of time known as benefit periods. A benefit period begins with hospitalization and ends when the patient has been discharged from the hospital or skilled nursing facility for at least 60 days. If individuals are able to remain out of an institution for 60 days, they begin a new benefit period with a full 60 days of coverage. If readmission to an institution occurs within 60 days, the patient remains on the same benefit period and is covered for only the number of days not used during the first admission. For example, if a patient used ten days during the first hospitalization, then returned to the hospital within 60 days, only 50 days would remain for the second hospitalization.

If an enrollee meets admission criteria and the deductible has been met, Medicare will pay 100% of the hospitalization. If hospitalization extends beyond 60 days, the enrollee becomes responsible for copayment for the next 30 days. Should the patient require hospitalization beyond 90 days, an increased copayment is required, in association with lifetime reserve days. Each individual has 60 lifetime reserve days. Once these days have been used, they cannot be recaptured.

Part A benefits cover 100% of the first 20 days in a skilled nursing facility, providing admission criteria have been met. If skilled care is required beyond 20 days, a daily copayment becomes necessary and the patient can be covered for an additional 80 days.

Home health care is also covered under part A benefits. Providing a patient meets Medicare criteria and receives service from an approved agency, Medicare will cover 100% of home health care visits.

Physicians' services, home health care, outpatient hospital services, and other medical services and supplies are covered under part B benefits. Medicare will pay 80% of reasonable charges, as determined by the Social Security Administration.

Out-of-pocket payments for Medicare benefits, deductibles, copayments, and limitations increase significantly each year. Many recipients are finding it necessary to supplement their benefits with private insurance plans. Unfortunately, for those on a fixed income, additional insurance premiums are not a solution to the limited coverage.

Medicaid, or Title 19, is a program to provide health-care benefits to the indigent. Depending upon state wealth, the federal government contributes 50% to 83% of the funds to state programs. Eligibility for the program varies from state to state. Medicaid is designed to pay for medical expenses not covered by Medicare. Unfortunately, most persons are not eligible for Medicaid reimbursement until all personal resources are exhausted. Application can be made at local state offices to determine eligibility.

In addition to Medicaid, state and local governments provide cash grants to the indigent through federally subsidized programs including Aid to Families with Dependent Children, Food Stamps, and General Assistance. State programs typically provide rehabilitation services through vocational rehabilitation programs that offer counseling, guidance, medical assistance, and job training and placement. Application for these services can be made at local state offices.

The Social Security Administration provides financial assistance to the disabled through Social Security Disability and Supplemental Security Income benefits. Providing disabled individuals meet the strict guidelines, they will receive a monthly Social Security Disability check. To qualify, the person must have a physical or mental condition expected to last at least 12 months and prevent substantial gainful employment. Sufficient contribution through previous employment is also required. Generally, the individual must have worked at least 5 of the past 10 years. If individuals do not meet Social Security Disability criteria, they may qualify for Supplemental Security Income. This is a program that pays monthly benefits to those who are disabled, blind, or at least 65 years of age and in financial need.

Applications for both Social Security Disability and Supplemental Security Income are filed at local Social Security offices. Individuals are encouraged to file an application as soon as it appears their condition will prevent them from working. Claims take approximately 2 to 3 months to process. In determining disability for those with impaired ventilation, pulmonary function studies appear to be the single most important factor.

Disease-Related Foundations

For those with impaired ventilation, the American Lung Association provides the most common source for patient assistance out of the disease-related foundations. The American Cancer Society, the American Heart Association, and others are also potential sources of information and support. Health education through pamphlets, films, speakers, workshops, loan equipment, self-help groups, and clubs, and information and referral are typical services. Limited financial aid for grants and scholarships is occasionally available. One must realize that the focus of these foundations is research, with education and patient care as secondary goals. Local chapters can be contacted to determine availability of support.

Home Health Care Agencies

Home health care agencies provide continuity of care to patients making the transition from the hospital to a home setting or to patients homebound because of illness or injury. Many home health services are covered by Medicare and private insurance companies. A broad complement of services are available including skilled nursing care, physical, speech, and occupational therapy, home health aides, social services, nutrition counseling, respiratory therapy, and clinical laboratory services.

In general, reimbursement for home health services is limited to intermittent skilled care. Often home health care agencies offer nonskilled care such as homemaking and home health aid services. Fees for these services are based on an hourly rate and are not reimbursed by insurance carriers. A written order from a physician is required for home health care. Evaluation for service can be initiated by the physician, various health-care providers, or by the patient contacting the agency directly.

Home Care Companies

Home care companies or medical supply companies offer a full range of services, medical equipment, and supplies to patients in the comfort of their own homes. Through the creation of new, compact, computer-assisted, safe products, these suppliers make care at home much simpler and more sophisticated. Portable volume ventilators have allowed many ventilator-dependent persons to live at home. Liquid oxygen systems make travel and ambulation more practical for those with impaired ventilation.

A number of products offered by home care companies are reimbursed by Medicare and private insurance companies. Many medical supply companies are willing to accept insurance assignment. Some sponsor educational workshops and scholarships. Access to these companies is gained through referral from physicians and health-care professionals or by the patient contacting the company directly.

Miscellaneous Support Services

A plethora of other programs are of potential benefit to the ventilation-impaired person. Home delivered meal service programs are available in many communities. Regular and special diets are provided to the elderly and disabled in their homes. Persons may pay a minimal fee or use food stamps for this service. Special transportation services are also available to the elderly and disabled. The American Red Cross provides transportation to medical appointments. Local governments also offer transportation to this population at a minimal fee. Case management services, also offered by local governments, coordinate programs such as homemaking and cleaning services, home health aides, meals, and adult day care for the patient in his or her home. Availability and eligibility criteria vary from state to state. Information concerning these services can be obtained by contacting a local hospital or home health social worker, or a United Way information and referral service.

Counseling, another support service, can assist COPD patients and their families in coping with the many losses associated with their chronic illness. Services are available through family service and mental health agencies as well as through psychiatrists, psychologists, and social workers in private practice. While these counselors may not be familiar with the medical aspects of pulmonary disease, they can effectively treat personal or family problems precipitated by illness. Hospital-based psychiatrists, psychologists, and social workers are more likely to have an awareness of issues specific to chronic illness. Some patients may prefer the medical setting for intervention because of its familiarity.

Reimbursement by Medicare and private insurance companies is often limited. There are agencies available that offer services on the basis of a sliding fee scale, according to the patient's ability to pay. Physicians, local hospitals, and various health-care professionals can be of assistance in providing the patient with information on the availability of counseling services.

Pulmonary rehabilitation aims at restoring patients with COPD to their fullest possible medical, mental, emotional, social, and vocational potential. A structured program of education, progressive exercise, physical conditioning and relaxation, and group support affords COPD patients the opportunity to better control symptom development and acquire the skills needed to maximize their quality of life. Medicare and private insurance companies often will cover participation in a rehabilitation program. Hospitals, chapters of the American Lung Association, and various health-care providers may be of assistance in identifying availability of rehabilitation programs in a particular area.

Support groups are recognized as a valuable resource for helping people cope with a variety of human problems. These groups are composed of peers with a common experience or problem. Support groups for the pulmonary patient offer an opportunity for individuals to learn more about their disease and how to cope with it. Peer support is also helpful in minimizing the isolation that individuals with COPD often experience. Local chapters of the American Lung Association and hospital social workers may be of assistance in identifying availability of such groups.

In conclusion, there is a spectrum of community resources available to the person with impaired ventilation. While there remain gaps in services and many unmet needs, recent trends are encouraging. The increasing development of resources that promote patient care in the home has the potential of affording the COPD patient a greater freedom of choice and maximizing overall quality of life.

SUMMARY

Care of the COPD patient is often a complex, challenging, and energy-intensive task for the health-care professional. Appreciation of the psychosocial impact upon this patient's emotional stability, social role, occupational status, body image, and sexuality is crucial. Not only must health-care providers possess skills to help facilitate adjustment to these life style alterations, they must also be familiar with patient help services appropriate to meet the unique needs of the COPD patient.

REFERENCES

American Lung Association: *Chronic Obstructive Pulmonary Disease: A Manual For Physicians*. New York, Author, 1973.

American Lung Association, Epidemiology and Statistics Unit: *Magnitude of Chronic Respiratory Disease in America*, Fact Sheet. New York, Author, December 7, 1981.

Conine, TA, Evans JH: Sexual adjustment in chronic obstructive pulmonary disease. *Respy Care* 1981; 26:871.

Dudley DL, Glaser EM, Jorgenson BN, et al: Psychosocial concomitants to rehabilitation in chronic obstructive pulmonary disease: I. Psychosocial and psychological considerations. *Chest* 1980; 77:413.

Dudley DL, Wermuth C, Hague W: Psychosocial aspects of care in the chronic obstructive pulmonary disease patient. *Heart and Lung* 1973; 2:389.

Kent DC, Smith, JK: Psychological implications of pulmonary disease. *Clin Notes Resp Dis*. Winter 1977, 3.

Kravitz M: Sexual counseling for the COPD patient. *Clin Challenge in Cardiopulm Med*. 1982; 4:1.

Lambert VA, Lambert CE: Alteration in respiratory function, *The Impact of Physical Illness and Related Mental Health Concepts*. Englewood Cliffs, NJ, Prentice-Hall, 1979.

Rowlett DB, Dudley DL: COPD: psychosocial and psychophysiological issues. *Psychosomatics* May 1978; 19:273.

Schwartz JL: Myths and realities of smoking cessation. *NY State J Med*. 1983; 83:1355.

11

Discharge Planning for the Respiratory Patient

JERRY O'RYAN, RRT

The intent of this chapter on discharge planning for the patient with pulmonary impairment who requires respiratory care in the home or extended-care facility is to introduce the various socioeconomic, government-regulated, and related factors that directly and indirectly affect plans for an effective, safe, expedient, and comprehensive discharge. This information is important because home care planning begins the moment the patient is admitted to the hospital, not when the patient is being wheeled out through the lobby doors on his or her way home. Home care planning begins even before a needs assessment is made by the responsible discharge planning parties. Indeed, it begins, with the help of computers and relevant stored data, while the patient is sitting in the admissions office of the hospital, waiting to be admitted to the hospital.

The preliminary information given in this chapter will define terms and apprise the reader of the many socioeconomic and medical factors that affect the discharge planning process. This information should serve to augment the practical aspects of home care planning, i.e., the selection of the needed respiratory and related durable medical equipment.

The recent changes in our health-care system's methods of reimbursement for hospital and home care costs necessitate an understanding of the forces affecting alternate-site therapies and long-term care. Alternate-site care is defined as any medical or paramedical care taking place outside the traditional hospital setting. The patient's personal residence or that of a relative, or a skilled extended-care facility are the more common alternate-site places of care. Nonskilled nursing facilities, boarding houses, retirement villages, hotels for the elderly on limited or fixed incomes, etc, also fall into the definition of alternate-site care, although they do not constitute the majority of the conventional home care sites.

The remainder of the chapter will contrast past and current discharge planning practices and suggest future practices that need to be adopted in toto or adapted into current plans to effectively and efficiently meet the needs of the patient and the health-care industry as a whole.

WHAT IS DISCHARGE PLANNING AND WHO ARE DISCHARGE PLANNERS?

There are several definitions of discharge planning, depending on which academic approach one chooses to use. Table 11–1 lists the common definitions, as offered by academic groups with an expressed interest in discharge planning. Regardless of the definition, the planning process may be said to start at or even prior to the patient's admission to the hospital. Termed "day-one" home care planning, this approach has, in this author's experience, been most successful, whether the patient enters

TABLE 11–1. DEFINITIONS OF DISCHARGE PLANNING

Organization	Definition
American Association for Continuity of Care	Continuity of care is an essential component of the health-care delivery system. Every patient has the right to quality coordinated discharge planning, which is an integral part of total patient care. Discharge planning is a holistic health approach that is centered on the patient and family.
American Nurses' Association	Discharge planning is the part of continuity of care process that is designed to prepare patient or client for the next phase of care and to assist in making any necessary arrangements for that phase of care, whether it be self-care, care by family members, or care by an organized health-care provider.
Amerian Hospital Association	Successful discharge planning is a centralized, coordinated, interdisciplinary process that ensures a plan of continuing care for each patient. It reflects both the patient's and family's internal and external social, emotional, medical, and psychological needs and assets.
	It recognizes that the transition from the hospital is often more threatening than the actual hospitalization and that a plan must be developed to both provide for a continuum of care and address the patient's immediate needs following discharge.
	It is the clinical process by which health-care professionals, patients, and families collaborate to ensure patients have access to services that enable them to regain, maintain, and even improve the level of functioning achieved in the hospital.

through the admissions office or via the trauma room of the emergency room.

Profile of the Discharge Planner

Discharge planners (DPs) are individuals who bridge the gap between acute care and long-term care (Nichols & Feather, 1984). They are important for the facility because they facilitate patients' leaving the hospital. They are also a critical link for home care, since they find, coordinate, and direct patients to specific services and agencies: respiratory home care companies, nursing home health care agencies, and public agencies such as the United Way.

Discharge planners are most often female (75%) and typically have other duties in addition to discharge planning. For some DPs, discharge planning may not even be an official part of their job description (nurse DPs are a good example), or they have other duties that would usually be assumed by a full-time person such as a utilization review officer.

The social services worker is an excellent example of one professional whose training qualifies him or her to deal with most of the varied needs of the patient, whether the diagnosis of respiratory disease is primary or secondary, and thus this professional is well suited for discharge planning. A respiratory patient about to be discharged requires more than just oxygen; the services of multiple community agencies are also needed, and this is where the talents of the social services worker excel. His or her background makes the social services worker an excellent coordinator of the other health professionals' services needed in the discharge planning effort.

Some hospitals use the professional nurse as a DP as part of an overall coordinating effort. She or he may work out of an office separate from the Social Services Department or work out of the same location. This approach is often used when there are two types of discharge planning professions involved, i.e., nurse and social services worker; the nurse takes responsibility for the patient's medical-related home needs and the social services worker tends to the psychosocial and financial concerns of the patient.

The Hospital Respiratory Therapist in Discharge Planning. One might think that respiratory patients requiring ongoing home care services, chiefly oxygen and related respiratory equipment and supplies, would naturally be put into the hands of the hospital-based professional knowing the most about oxygen, respiratory equipment, and related supplies: the respiratory therapist. After all, this is a person trained in the anatomy and physiology of the pulmonary system, with didactic and clinical training that includes oxygen therapeutics, principles, and mechanics of respiratory therapy devices. Countless clinical hours, both in training and in actual practice, are spent analyzing, monitoring, and attending to the various oxygen-administering devices used in respiratory care. Added to this is the physician-supervised judgmental capacity in which today's respiratory practitioner often finds her or himself employed.

In actual practice, the credentialed respiratory therapist usually functions as a consultant to the traditional discharge planning department staff of his or her hospital, i.e., the social services worker or registered nurse, because total discharge planning involves more than just attention to one organ system (in this case, the lungs) and concerns the patient as a whole, including mental, emotional, and social aspects. Although nurses and social workers working together possess the most nearly complete abilities to tend to the patient's *total* discharge needs, this does not preclude the involvement of a professional respiratory therapist who has been properly trained and is actively involved in the respiratory care plans of the home-bound patient. Responsibility for determining the oxygen and related respiratory needs of the patient about to be discharged should rest with the respiratory therapist and the supervising physician trained in pulmonology. However, it is up to the traditional DPs with their diversified knowledge, to supervise the patient's overall home care needs.

The Home Care Respiratory Therapist in Discharge Planning. The professional home care company, although not an official part of the hospital structure, actually has a most important long-standing health-care role. After all, the patient who has spent 2 or 4 weeks in the hospital being cared for by one team of health-care professionals is now being turned over to the next set of professionals, the home care respiratory therapist and home care company staff, who will take on the patient for months or years.

The long-term relationships that usually develop between the patient and the home care respiratory therapist and those behind the scenes, i.e., the home care company's billing department, insurance reimbursement specialist, and driver-delivery employees, are usually only second to the one the patient has with his or her personal physician. The trust and dependency the liquid oxygen using patient, for example, places on the liquid oxygen service specialist is usually a sacred one, for the patient's life may literally depend on prompt, uninterrupted service by the liquid oxygen service specialist. Likewise, the patient's or caregivers' dependence on high-technology home care equipment such as ventilators or apnea monitors will require the same prompt service by and trust in the professional home care respiratory therapist.

The role of the home care respiratory therapist is one that has only evolved over the past few years. Virtually all large national chains and local independent home care companies employ full time credentialed respiratory therapists. The national chains may employ the therapist to see that the proper equipment is selected and delivered to the patient's home. He or she then may personally do the setup and instruction in the use of the equipment, especially if the equipment consists of ventilators or apnea monitors or similar sophisticated high-technology equipment that requires much patient education. The local independent firm may use the therapist in a similar fashion and include some selling, marketing, and public relations activities as additional duties.

It is important, especially for those involved in discharge planning and working with outside vendors and home health-care professionals, to be aware of the essential role this professional plays in the patient's discharge plan. The home care respiratory therapist needs to have the *earliest* opportunity to participate in and plan for the patient's discharge while the patient is still in the hospital—and *not* at the last moment when the patient is being wheeled out the lobby doors.

The earlier the home care therapist is given the opportunity to participate, the sooner he or she can make the DP's job easier. The home care therapist needs to be utilized by the DP and other hospital-based personnel for just what he or she is, an outside professional consultant. The home care therapist should be invited to the hospital to participate in all discharge conferences involving the patient. Because the respiratory therapist's company has been selected to provide service to the patient at home, the therapist should have the earliest opportunity to get acquainted with the new patient, for whom he or she will be responsible for the rest of the patient's natural life.

The home care therapist has the same background, training, and capabilities as the hospital-based respiratory therapist. In fact, the home care therapist may at one time have been employed by the very hospital at which he or she has been asked to consult. Furthermore, the therapist may be a board member of the local lung association, a respiratory therapy association, or may possess additional education and skills in community health matters. Thus, the DP is often obtaining the assistance of an outside professional who has more than just clinical experience to offer the patient and DP.

Table 11–2 outlines the various duties and activities the home care respiratory therapists will have in participating in hospital discharge planning and in home care services provided to the patient in need of long-term ventilator care, as one example. It is important to note the home care therapist's role is *not* to provide hands-on medical care in the home but to be an assessor, educator, facilitator, and communicator between the patient, family members, caregivers, and physician.

The discharge planning process requires a multidisciplinary approach. All professionals who might be directly or casually involved in the discharge planning process are listed in Table 11–3.

TABLE 11-2. HOME CARE THERAPIST'S ROLE IN DISCHARGE PLANNING FOR A VENTILATOR-DEPENDENT PATIENT

Extra-Step Assurance

Only credentialed respiratory therapists will be used
Staff will be thoroughly trained
Equipment will function properly
Response to emergencies will be prompt

Step 1: Help Select Acceptable Patients	Step 2: Prepare for Discharge	Step 3: Discharge and Transfer	Step 4: Follow-Up Care
Identify stable patient	Work with hospital discharge planner to coordinate staff training	Assist in initial transfer	Visit on regular schedule and prn
Assess equipment requirements	Train staff using formal instructional materials	Answer questions: review equipment operation	Update referring physician
Review long term care facility prescription	Evaluate long term care facility and provide equipment required	Support adjustment	Provide ongoing service as needed
Complete preliminary assessment			Evaluate staff compliance
			Perform routine maintenance
			Ensure emergency response via 24-hr service

TABLE 11–3. DISCHARGE PLANNING DUTIES OF PULMONARY REHABILITATION TEAM

Team Member	Duties
Physician	Does final assessment of patient, writes all drug and equipment prescriptions
Respiratory therapist	Evaluates all facets of patient's respiratory status, reviews equipment and supplies needs
Nurse	Assesses all bodily needs, individually and as a whole, and writes initial home care plan
Physical therapist	Evaluates patient's current musculoskeletal status, reviews all self-care patient must perform with self and family
Dietician	Writes home nutrition plan, makes sure patient will have adequate nutritive intake or makes alternate plans (e.g., Meals on Wheels)
Occupational therapist	Reassesses patient's gains since occupational therapy began in hospital and informs home care team of strengths and weaknesses
Psychiatrist/psychologist	Writes patient profile summary and shares *allowable* areas with home care team
Social worker	Checks and double-checks to make certain all outside agencies involved with patient's home care are ready to assist and have all red tape out of way
Pastoral member	Makes arrangements to see patient on regular basis once patient is home or sees as needed

Reproduced with permission from: O'Ryan J, & Burns DG: Pulmonary Rehabilitation: From Hospital to Home. *Chicago, Year Book, 1984, p 200.*

FACTORS CAUSING THE NEED FOR BETTER AND QUICKER DISCHARGE PLANNING OF THE RESPIRATORY PATIENT

Two factors have created the major pressure on DPs for better, quicker, and more thorough discharge care plans for the patient with pulmonary impairment and the ill population in general. These factors are:

1. The increased population of the elderly.
2. The implementation of Medicare's prospective payment system (PPS).

The first factor is a naturally occurring exponential growth caused by a combination of the total increase in the elderly population since the early 1900s and at the same time, the attainment of a sophisticated level of health care. In 1900 only 1 in every 25 Americans was 65 years old or older; today that number is 1 in 10, a 250% increase. Fig 11–1 shows that by the year 2030 20% of the United States population will be aged 65 or older.

The second factor, the implementation of the federal government's

By the year 2030, an estimated 21 percent of all Americans will be over the age of 65, and nearly one-seventh of these senior citizens will be over 85. In light of the complicated financial and emotional burdens inherent in caring for parents, experts on aging are troubled by the prospect of a society in which the old will be looking after the very old.

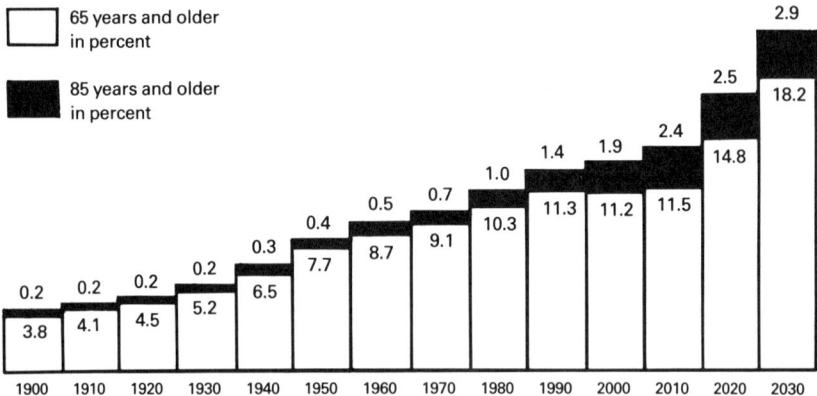

Figure 11–1. America's aged: longer lives, heavier burdens.

PPS for health-care reimbursement of its Medicare patients, has caused an almost immediate impact on patients, health-care institutions, society, and finally the home health care industry.

Health-care workers, at all administrative and patient-care levels, must deal with both medical and financial responsibilities if they are to function effectively. In essence, we must now deliver the same range and quality of health care, but within the confines of financial boundaries, which was never required under the old cost-plus method of health-care reimbursement. And, depending on the diagnostic-related group (DRG) the patient with pulmonary impairment falls into, we must also do it in less time and with less money.

MEDICAL AND SOCIOECONOMIC DISADVANTAGES AND ADVANTAGES OF A PROSPECTIVE PAYMENT SYSTEM

For the chronic obstructive pulmonary disease (COPD) patient, there can be inherent disadvantages and advantages to the PPS of health-care reimbursement. These need to be examined from both the patient's and the medical-care provider's point of view.

Disadvantages
The disadvantages, which in reality affect both the patient and the hos-

pital, are that the various categories of respiratory disease inherently involve multifaceted problems that may only be revealed clinically at various and inopportune times during the patient's hospital stay. A classic example would be the patient admitted as an emergency whose primary complaint appears to be acute dyspnea stemming from hypoxia resulting from pneumonia. Several days' stay in the hospital, however, shows the underlying cause to be the clinical onset of COPD, necessitating further workup and treatment.

Sad as this observation may be, chronically ill patients occasionally exhibit a reluctance to leave the hospital. Social workers, nurse discharge planners, staff psychologists, and respiratory therapists have all encountered patients who are often repeat users and abusers of the health-care system. One study showed the disinclination of blue-collar workers over white-collar workers, both groups postpneumonectomy, to return to work after discharge from the hospital and a home convalescence. Only 20% of the laboring patients returned to work; in contrast, 70% to 89% of the white-collar workers returned to their jobs. (Morgan, 1982) Furthermore, a family support system may not be available for the patient going home after a lengthy illness. Formerly, hospitals had the economically feasible option (on the cost-plus basis) to allow the patient a few extra days of hospital-based convalescence that was paid for by insurance.

The disadvantages of the PPS for this type of patient may thus be twofold:

1. Medically, the sudden onset and eventual course of the respiratory patient's disease, both the acute and chronic aspects of it, may not conveniently allow for a treatment regimen that falls into the predetermined DRG category the patient's diagnosis is supposed to most nearly match.
2. Socioeconomically, the patient's psychosocial environment, coupled with economic disincentives, may not produce a natural willingness in the patient to return home at the first opportunity.

Regardless of the reasons for delayed discharges, whether medical or socioeconomic, the costs to the hospital can be significant. The costs do not stop here though; they go on to be borne both financially and socially by the patient, family members, and society as a whole.

These problems do not conveniently fit into the health-care system's new PPS. Incentives may need to be presented to flagrant abusers to alter the second problem. One incentive might be reduced insurance premiums to the employer, who in turn would allow the employee to pocket the savings. On the other hand, such incentives obviously do not address the problem of the legitimately ill patient who requires continued care beyond what the DRG category may allow, thus the reason for the development of "outliers," or special DRG categories that do allow for these extenuating circumstances.

Advantages

Let us now turn to the advantages of the health-care system that we have been working under.

1. One of the medical advantages of working under our health-care system is that it has the potential for freeing needed beds for the more seriously ill, whose care is the most intensive and costly. An excellent example of this practice in action is the increasingly prevalent practice of sending medically stable but otherwise un-weanable patients home on ventilators.
2. Socioeconomic advantages should be apparent: most patients wish to be home.

Regardless of advantages or disadvantages, PPSs are in practice. Health maintenance organizations (HMOs) and preferred provider organizations (PPOs) also promote reducing unnecessary hospitalizations, shortening length of stays, and even offering alternative health-care measures, such as an increased focus on outpatient testing and physician office visits in lieu of admission to the hospital. Today's health-care worker, whether hospital or home care based, must learn to work within these confines, both from a medical and financial perspective.

CURRENT PRACTICES IN DISCHARGE PLANNING FOR THE RESPIRATORY PATIENT

A review of the literature yields a moderate number of general articles dealing with discharge planning. Unfortunately, these are articles often dealing with the subject in a generic sense and not often with any specific patient type or disease entity in mind. Except for a few instances (O'Ryan & Burns, 1984; O'Ryan, 1986), the patient with pulmonary impairment also falls into this literally neglected category.

Social workers and nurse DPs do not learn respiratory care discharge planning procedures so much as they find it a part of a total integration of discharge planning in general. In the profession of respiratory care, academic attention to pulmonary rehabilitation and home care practices is just beginning, with only a few respiratory therapy school programs teaching the subject. However, interest in this area of care is burgeoning. It is also expected that other home health care disciplines will focus more attention on and develop standards and guidelines for this area of discharge planning as it pertains to them. Nursing programs, for example, usually include general community nursing principles as an integral part of their curriculum.

Currently discharge planning practices for the patient with pulmonary impairment vary from institution to institution. The level of preplanning, autonomy of discharge planning intervention by the DPs themselves, and the level (or lack) of a formal program vary according to institution, its size, and leadership in the hospital.

Current overall approaches to the specific discharge planning process may fall into the following general patterns:

1. The discharge planning department has a current set of general policies and guidelines on discharge practices, some of which may concern respiratory patients.
2. Some type of interaction occurs with other departments (e.g., the respiratory care department), which may be used for consultative purposes to help round out total discharge planning for a patient with pulmonary impairment.
3. The hospital has a good medical director in the respiratory care department who takes active part in patient's care up to the time of discharge.

In summary, certainly some attention is being paid to the fact that the pulmonary patient does require a little more forethought and consultative direction from other health professionals. However, in view of the health-care system under which the pulmonary patient's hospital admission takes place, an approach that is more carefully thought out, more thorough, and more prospective needs to be used if this type of patient's discharge plan is to be effective, efficient, and timely.

A COMPREHENSIVE PLANNING APPROACH

A comprehensive discharge plan integrating the abilities of the available personnel can yield a highly effective, efficient, timely, and cost-saving discharge plan. The following sections consider the desirable characteristics, activities, and structures found within a comprehensive discharge planning program. Regardless of the institution's size, all or part of these ideas can be used.

The author suggests a linear joint effort, starting with the reader, then her or his subordinates, superiors, and finally administration, to carefully review these ideas and implement those that can be put into effect immediately. Those that cannot be put to immediate use should be at least trial-tested and implemented at a later date if found feasible.

Suitable Patients and Selection Criteria

It is fairly easy to identify those respiratory patients who would normally *not* require any discharge planning. Young and relatively healthy patients usually fall into this category; their very age and relative state of good health usually precludes the necessity for any assistance in home-going matters. In addition, there is usually parental support. Exceptions would be the mentally deficient, emotionally unstable, or otherwise noncompliant patient. Another noted exception would be virtually any young patient who will require extensive multifaceted home care services. An excellent example is the high-spinal cord injury patient who will require continuous ventilatory assistance, tracheostomy care, and attention to bronchopulmonary and personal hygiene needs. Obviously, any patient fitting into this particular category, regardless of age and socioeconomic status (even those with good intended compliance and family support group), will find a comprehensive discharge plan an absolute necessity. The targets of discharge planning are usually elderly individuals with multiple problems who will more than likely not be able to return home easily. The most important criterion is the patient's social situation. The amount of support and assistance that can be provided by family and friends and the patient's living conditions are two major concerns of discharge planners. The determining criteria for respiratory patients who commonly are in need of discharge planning are listed in Table 11–4.

Day-One Home Care Planning

Discharge planning needs for the respiratory patient involve many dimensions. In actual practice, the individual patient must be assessed and the findings acted on. Information gathering (both documented and anecdotal) throughout the patient's hospital stay will provide a convenient chronological history that will permit estimations of the patient's eventual home care needs; even early estimations will prove to be fairly accurate and beneficial. *The sooner information gathering occurs, the sooner the eventual discharge occurs.* One need not be reminded of the cost efficacy of this in view of PPSs. This is the concept and practice called "day-one" home care planning.

It is desirable to begin developing discharge plans even before the patient is admitted, if a preliminary diagnosis is available. Otherwise, plans may be developed during the course of the patient's hospital stay if a prearranged, systematic approach is followed. Health-care professionals who used to balk at such a concept now find that this practice is widespread, and they have begun to accept and work with this system. Entrepreneurial health-care workers see it as an inevitable occurrence, prepare for it, and largely gain from it both financially and in terms of better patient care. The three examples below, drawn from the author's experience illustrate this pre-admission planning concept.

COMPUTER-ASSISTED DISCHARGE PLANNING

One of the primary tools that can assist in day-one home care planning is the use of the computer to gather, analyze, and even suggest the patients

TABLE 11–4. SCALE DETERMINING FACTORS FOR RESPIRATORY PATIENTS REQUIRING DISCHARGE PLANNING

How to Use Scale

Circle your assessment of each factor. Total up and then average out the scale. Patients should arbitrarily have a minimum of 0.75 (75%) or better score for safe, comprehensive home care. You can add other factors to this list for individual patients with specific other needs.

Goal	Rating Scale		
	(Circle one)		
	Good	*Fair*	*Poor*
1. Severity of patient's illness	2	1	0
2. Prognosis of disease	2	1	0
3. Patient's actual and potential compliance abilities	2	1	0
4. Patient's understanding (cognitive) of illness	2	1	0
5. Patient's attitude (affective) toward illness	2	1	0
6. Patient's abilities (psychomotor) to care for self and to care for any home care equipment	2	1	0
7. Judgmental abilities: knows when to call for help, order new supplies from home care vendor, make and keep doctor's appointments	2	1	0
8. Economic factors: patient's ability to afford home care equipment (e.g., out-of-pocket expenses, 20% copay), pay for home nursing assistance	2	1	0
9. Environmental factors: home conditions, clean, safe, conducive to long-term care of patient	2	1	0
TOTAL = _____	AVERAGE = _____		

Reproduced with permission from: O'Ryan J: O'Ryan Model for Comprehensive Home Care (OMCHC). Work in progress; copyright © 1985.

and case mixes that would benefit most from such early plans (Rossen, 1984). As time passes and experience in working with PPSs increase, one can expect this type of computer-assisted planning to be a basic feature of the patient's data file, valuable both in terms of medical and financial benefits. Numerical values can be assigned to patients admitted for the first time on the basis of previously collected data from patients with similar diagnostic and other assigned values. Data can then be gathered and extrapolated for clinical use in planning a more structured hospital stay.

At first glance, this concept may appear to be pigeonholing patients (which is exactly what the 467 categories for DRGs do). However, the intent is to provide a data base on which to draw to create a potentially more successful comprehensive discharge plan. Table 11–5 presents this concept hypothetically. In fact, the concept (called **ADAPT**), if expanded, could conceivably be used to plan the patient's regimen for the entire hospital stay.

Example One

Mr Smith is a 65-year-old male presenting with a diagnosis of gradual onset of amyotrophic lateral sclerosis. In fact, since his initial diagnosis, he has already begun to decline noticeably, ventilatory insufficiency being the more serious problem clinically.

He is to be admitted to the hospital for an extensive workup and tracheostomy, the latter for improved airway maintenance and eventual connection to a home-type ventilator. Mr Smith will have multiple needs for home care services and a professional support network once he is discharged. The discharge planning team has already met before Mr Smith's admission, at the physician's request, to compile a needs list based on the advice of the consulting pulmonary physician and respiratory therapist on this patient-type category. Although only a general list of needs can be established at this preliminary meeting, some specifics are known. The patient will require tracheostomy care and ancillary supplies, a ventilator, and a hospital-style bed for his home. All these preliminary items can be discussed at this meeting and the patient has not even been admitted to the hospital.

Comments

The advantages to this approach are manyfold:

1. The discharge planning team has time to assess the patient's basic needs in an unhurried manner, thus possibly avoiding overlooking important needs for this patient.
2. An atmosphere of cooperation among the discharge planning team members is developed, and equally important, the attention and input of the physicians are gained at the very beginning, thus avoiding a last-minute, hastily constructed discharge.
3. The home care company has the advantage of being called in ahead of time and thus gains lead time to assemble a list of required and suggested home care items. This also gives the home care company the time needed to check on payment source and get an early start on their assessment of the patient and education of the family.
4. There is greater likelihood of adhering to the DRG requirements in terms of allowable hospitalization days for the patient.
5. All of the above advantages reduce errors and thus liability risks for everyone.

TABLE 11–5. ADAPT* SCORE FOR COMPREHENSIVE DISCHARGE PLANNING

The higher the score, the more the patient will require in terms of comprehensive discharge planning in this hypothetical scoring mechanism.

How to Assess Value Numbers		
Area Analyzed	**How to Assign Value Number: For Area Number:**	**Point Value**
1. Age	1. Ages up to 30, assign 1; up to 40, assign 1.5; up to 60, 2.5; up to 70, 3.2; up to 75, 3.7; 75–80, 4.1; past 80, 5.	___
2. Current state of health on scale of 1–5 (1 = best)	2. Current health: 5 very poor; 4 poor; 3 fair; 2 good; 1 very good.	___
3. Total number of hospital admissions last 2 years	3. 1 point per admission	___
4. Number of hospital admissions last 2 years related to current problem	4. 2 points per admission	___
5. Average length of stay per admission (average of 3 and 4 above)	5. 1 point per each 3 days of stay	___
6. Number of exacerbations during current hospital stay	6. 2 points per exacerbation	___
7. Score on O'Ryan Model for Comprehensive Home Care (OMCHC)	7. Take number as scored and divide by 2	___
	Total Points	___

*Accomplishing Discharge through Analysis and Planning Techniques.
Reproduced with permission from: O'Ryan Model for Comprehensive Home Care (OMCHC). *Work in progress; copyright* © *1985.*

Example Two

Mrs Stewart is a 58-year-old female with an 8-year history of chronic pulmonary disease and associated right heart failure resulting from pulmonary hypertension. She lives alone and is visited twice weekly by her 32-year-old daughter. Mrs Stewart has a socioeconomic history of poor medical compliance and lives on a fixed income in a low-rent housing district. Her primary income is from her deceased husband's pension.

Two previous admissions over the past 6 months (she had three last year mainly for treatment of the pulmonary hypertension) have led to a third impending hospital stay, this time for acute congestive heart failure. Mrs Stewart has an H-cylinder of oxygen at home that her family physician ordered for "occasional nocturnal use when orthopneic and prn." She is being admitted this time to the pulmonary care services department of the hospital.

The hospital discharge planning team, consisting of a social services worker, nurse, and respiratory therapist, met on the day Mrs Stewart was admitted and devised a hospital stay and discharge care plan that included the following main points:

1. Improve compliance by teaching Mrs Stewart about the more important facets of her respiratory care. The respiratory therapist and a pulmonary nurse will work on this together.
2. The respiratory therapist will obtain an order for a liquid oxygen system so that the patient will be able to have a system encouraging and enabling ambulation.
3. The social services worker will meet with the patient and daughter to work out a schedule for a visiting nurse and a Meals on Wheels program.
4. Outpatient visits will be made by Mrs Stewart to check her progress and compliance.

Comments

The patient's previous health history and repeat hospital admissions show steadily increasing health problems related to her congestive heart failure and augmented by poor compliance. Intervention by development of an early, well-thought-out discharge program, with a heavy emphasis on support at home, should minimize future admissions.

Example Three

Bryan is a 17-year-old male who suffered a severe C-2 injury and subsequent quadriplegia while participating in a physical education event at school. The extent of disability or permanence of such "fresh" injury of this type, especially on young adults, cannot always be determined. However, the overall clinical signs were such that it was suggested to begin a preliminary team conference consisting of the social worker, floor nurse, physician, and the home care vendor selected to provide the products and services Bryan would need at home.

Since Bryan was already on a hospital ventilator, the first decision was to introduce him to the home-type ventilator provided by the vendor. The respiratory therapist from the home care company worked with the hospital respiratory therapist and pulmonary physician to do this. The occupational therapist suggested a power wheelchair with special features to enhance mobility and resocialization processes.

Due to the newness of the injury, coupled with the patient's total dependency on the ventilator for life support, it was suggested that the discharge planning process for Bryan be broken up into phases (called "life phases" or "needs phases"*). The discharge team would look at Bryan's need from the present up to the next 6 to 9 months and then examine the next 2 years in segments of 6-month periods. Such crystal ball gazing is of course not entirely accurate, but it provided greater economies in the type and amount of equipment the patient would need to just get home and begin a convalescence and physical rehabilitation program.

Thus, with the above perspective, the team came up with this initial "needs phase" chart:

Period	Equipment Needs	Other Needs
0–6 months	Ventilator and related supplies, power wheelchair with accessories	Physical therapy, home tutoring
6–15 months	Additional ventilator for outside excursions, wheelchair modifications as required.	Vocational rehabilitation counseling

Comments
The above approach had many benefits:

1. Early planning reduced hospitalization days.
2. Family members got a realistic view of what to expect.
3. The home care company's early and full involvement sped up the discharge process by avoiding last minute holdups often caused by the ordering of special wheelchairs, etc, that are custom-made and take time to produce and get delivered.
4. The patient's morale was kept up, since he could see concrete activities were being performed on his behalf.
5. The insurance company was more cooperative once they were made aware that expediency and economy were the results of this type of discharge process.

When expanded even further, this computer-assisted concept could help administrators plan week-to-week or day-to-day operations for the most cost-efficient medically efficacious management system. (Nursing de-

---

*Reproduced with permission from O'Ryan J: *O'Ryan Model for Comprehensive Home Care* (OMCHC). Work in progress; copyright © 1985.

partments in hospitals and nursing homes have used a rough, minor form of this concept for years to plan weekday and weekend staff scheduling rosters.)

FUTURE OF DISCHARGE PLANNING

Nichols and Feather (1984) observed that discharge planning "is a complex issue . . . , is not uniformly organized and is difficult to evaluate." In the past, discharge planning was partly seen to be a public service a hospital provided to its patients, usually the elderly and the indigent. It was, at times, a perfunctory service of the hospital, and under the golden years of health care was viewed as an afterthought by the physician. Indeed, the discharge planner or astute nursing staff in some cases had to remind the physician of the need for a discharge planning consultation.

Today under the supervision of cost-observant administrators *and* physicians, discharge planning ranks alongside the other traditional medical services. Hospitals and discharge planners know that timely and well-coordinated discharge planning activities not only reduce costs and improve patient care, but also make a favorable impression upon the patient and promote the desire to return to that same hospital for future health-care needs.

Some specific factors that will not only maintain but increase the need for and stature of discharge planning and planners are

1. Further tightening of the medical reimbursement policies of governmental and other thirdparty payers.
2. Trends that emulate or parallel the philosophy of the new health-management systems, such as the already widely accepted HMOs and PPOs. Attempts to avoid socialized medicine as practiced in Europe will create even further rein-tightening by both health-care workers and third-party payers. However, these methods will bring with them an even greater demand for cost-conscious yet medically sound hospital care with appropriate discharge planning measures.

Earlier observations in this chapter regarding computer-assisted discharge planning, coupled with entrepreneurship, can bring the complexities of the discharge planning process into a more easily managed system, thereby allowing a greater ease of hospital-to-home transition for the patient with pulmonary impairment. All patients with a medical or surgical problem, pulmonary or otherwise, can benefit from a conscientious discharge plan.

REFERENCES

Morgan WKC: Pulmonary disability and impairment: Can't work? Won't work? *Basics Resp Dis Am Lung Assoc* 1982;*10*:1.

Nichols L, & Feather J: Discharge planning. *Homecare Rental/Sales* April 1984, p 80.

O'Ryan JA, & Burns DG: *Pulmonary Rehabilitation: From Hospital to Home*. Chicago, Year Book, 1984.

O'Ryan JA: An overview of mechanical ventilation in the home and alternate-site facilities. *R_x Home Care* 1986;*8*:43.

Rossen S: Adapting discharge planning to prospective pricing. *Hospitals*, March 1984;71.

12

Federal Regulations and Home Care

PHILLIP PORTE

BACKGROUND

The impact of the Federal government on the delivery of health care in general has been dramatic, particularly since 1965 when the Congress adopted Titles 18 and 19 of the Social Security Act, commonly referred to as Medicare and Medicaid. The implementation of these two programs unquestionably has been the basis for this nation's national health policy for the past two decades, mandating a wide range of benefits for the nation's elderly and economically disadvantaged citizens. While private insurers have not always followed suit by developing identical benefit packages, there is no question that private insurers watch with great care the lead that Medicare takes in reimbursing new procedures. In the field of respiratory care, the role of Medicare has been somewhat tangential, primarily because the development of current levels of respiratory care postdates the advent of Medicare.

In 1965, as Congress debated the actual legislation and the Department of Health, Education, and Welfare (HEW, which became the Department of Health and Human Services in 1978) attempted to draft the implementing regulations, the field of respiratory care was not much more than a fledging practice known as inhalation therapy. There was no specific mention of this therapy in either the statutes or the regulations for 15 years. By association, inhalation therapy was lumped together with "other therapies" for the purpose of reimbursement, and this failure to establish true identity still haunts the profession and makes advances in the reimbursement area more difficult.

To make sure that the historical importance of this sequence of events is understood, let us go back in history to a time when inhalation therapy and oxygen jockeys were common, as were oxygen tents and iron lungs. Mechanical ventilators were surely not commonplace, and compact computer circuitry was a dream as yet unfulfilled in a California garage.

Congress was paying close attention to Vietnam, and the Great Society was well under way with the passage of Medicare and Medicaid, voting rights legislation, and fair housing laws. It was a time when special interests in Washington, DC, worked behind closed doors and almost without limitation.

Because it was a time when costs were not a major consideration (Medicare expenditures in its first year of operation were $3 billion; 1989 expenditures for Medicare may reach as high as $95 billion), cost consciousness was not yet a part of the manager's credo (Budget of the United States for Fiscal Year 1989). The failure of Congress to project more carefully the impact of these two programs is still being felt today as the government faces a deficit of $3 trillion.

In the area of home care, Congressional consideration was not very thorough. In fact, there is a fair amount of evidence that the home care statutes were added as an afterthought to the benefit package rather than considered as a well-developed, carefully analyzed policy decision. That afterthought now accounts for the most rapidly growing facet of Medicare expenditures, and this fact alone has the attention not only of health policymakers but of regulators such as the inspector general as well.

To appreciate the predicament of respiratory care in the 1980s one needs to understand not only a basic legislative history of the development of Medicare but also the changes that have been made in the program in the past 20 years. More importantly, one needs to understand the logic behind such decisions and the problems the solutions were meant to solve.

For example, by the early 1970s, it was becoming increasingly clear to hospital administrators that the cost-plus basis of reimbursement for hospital care could be manipulated in certain ways to increase revenues. Hospitals raised the per diem rates dramatically, especially after the termination of price controls in the mid 1970s. Understandably, the government responded by developing a watchdog organization, Professional Standard Review Organizations (PSROs), to monitor such things as hospital per diems and appropriateness of the length of stay. Many hospital administrators responded to this new scrutiny by keeping per diems artificially low and increasing the charges for ancillary services. In the early 1970s per diems accounted for roughly 65% of a hospital's costs, with 35% of the costs attributed to ancillaries. But by the late 1970s the ratio had changed, with ancillaries accounting for the larger share of costs (Bureau of Data Management, Health Care Financing Administration, Department of Health and Human Services).

Now, put yourself behind the hospital administrator's desk. The Federal government was clamping down on hospital costs, but they had not really begun to examine ancillary services carefully, particularly radiology, the laboratory, respiratory therapy, and a few other "money-makers."

Once again the government responded, and this time the solution was prospective payment, and the exact methodology was known as diagnosis related groups (DRGs). One day you generated profits for the hospital, and the next day you had to show evidence that you were cost-effective if you wanted to survive the DRG crunch.

Home care, for the most part, escaped the scrutiny that hospital care underwent, and that may have resulted in as much harm as good. Some say the last bastion of fraud and abuse in Medicare is found in home care, and a big chunk of home care is unquestionably in the field of respiratory care. But a look at the mechanics of respiratory home care, particularly from the reimbursement side, is worthwhile before we make a detailed examination of financial considerations surrounding home care.

In the eyes of the Federal government, at least for reimbursement purposes, there are two approaches to home care. The first, and more traditional approach, is through Medicare certified home-health agencies. These agencies, like hospitals and nursing homes, must adhere to conditions of participation if they wish to participate in the Medicare program. These conditions are designed to ensure that the patient is well cared for by competent and qualified individuals. For the most part, home-health agency costs are reimbursed after appropriate cost reports are filed with Medicare although prospective payment for home-health agencies may be on the horizon. Importantly, Congress outlined very specific services that would be available through home-health agencies, and in 1965, you remember, there was no real practice of respiratory home care. Sophistication and knowledge was yet to be developed, so it was logical that Congress identified only "physical, occupational, or speech therapy" as reimbursable therapy services. The doors are open, however, for home-health agencies to hire respiratory therapists for education and training purposes. Although such employees are not eligible for reimbursement on a cost-per-visit basis, their salaries are considered legitimate overhead of the home-health agency.

Whether by accident or design is unclear, but Congress did create another avenue for the respiratory care profession under the "durable medical equipment" (DME) benefit. That benefit includes no specific professional component but does reimburse for the costs related to lease or purchase of certain medical equipment. It is vitally important to note that approximately 65% of the entire DME benefit is attributable to oxygen and oxygen-related equipment. Costs for all durable medical equipment in 1985 ran to $739 million (Bureau of Data Management, Health Care Financing Administration, Department of Health and Human Services).

Therefore, when someone generally refers to "home care companies," it is difficult to determine exactly what kind of provider the person is specifying. In the eyes of Medicare, there are certified home-health agencies that provide direct patient care, some of whose employees' services are reimbursed on a per-visit basis; and there are DME providers, who are reimbursed for the provision of equipment but not for professional services. Home-health agencies go through a very rigorous certification process in order to deliver hands-on care. DME providers go through very limited scrutiny to provide equipment where appropriate.

The twist has come in the past several years when Congress began debate on the appropriateness of ventilator care in the home. This issue came to national attention when President Reagan, at a televised news conference, in November, 1981 cited the example of Katie Beckett, a young Iowa girl who was confined to a hospital even though home care was available and, in fact, significantly cheaper. The problem was Federal law and regulations: it was a situation where Medicaid would cover Katie's costs if she was in the hospital but would not pay the money for appropriate home care.

The dilemma continues today even though legislation has been adopted to authorize reimbursement for "Katie Becketts" across the country. The Omnibus Budget Reconciliation Act of 1986 includes modifications of the Medicaid statutes authorizing individual states to modify State plans authorizing reimbursement for respiratory care services for ventilator dependent individuals. As of early 1988, not a single state has applied to the Health Care Financing Administration for such a waiver.

FINANCIAL CONSIDERATIONS

The growth of home care has mushroomed dramatically in the 1980s. It appears to be one of the last areas of major growth in health care, and the reasons for such expansion are numerous. The simplest and most logical explanation is the shift in incentives: under a prospective payment system such as DRGs, hospitals have very strong financial incentives to discharge patients as quickly as possible. While much has been written about premature discharge, there appears to be little hard evidence that premature discharges are common. There is no doubt, however, that Medicare patients are being discharged from the hospital earlier than ever before. Just prior to implementation of DRGs, the average Medicare hospital length of stay was approximately 9.5 days. Only 2 years after the program has been in effect, the length of stay for prospective payment hospital stays had dropped 2 full days (Bureau of Data Management, Health Care Financing Administration, Department of Health and Human Services). That impact should not be minimized because it must be considered that a hospital's reimbursement was based only on a percentage formula relative to DRGs and that a hospital's historical costs played a larger role than DRGs in the hospital's actual reimbursement (this financial impact was true for the first 2 years of the DRG program).

Given that hospitals have a very clear financial incentive to discharge patients as soon as possible, one would expect that the need for home care would escalate. That expectation is unquestionably supported by the rapid growth in the number of home-health agencies. Between 1965 and 1982, the year prior to the implementation of DRGs, there were approximately 3000 Medicare-certified home-health agencies. The number is now just under 6000, a growth of close to 100% in 4 years (Bureau of Data Management, Health Care Financing Administration, Department of Health and Human Services).

One can also make some important assumptions about continued growth of home care. There is little doubt that baby boomers are growing older, and as they age they will put increasing demands not only on the hospital system but also on home care. Well into the twenty-first century we will likely see a major cultural change as a greater percentage of the population retires and leaves the work force and fewer and fewer younger citizens will be able to support a large elderly population.

Considering these demographics, it is not too difficult to make some intelligent assumptions about the growth of home care in the future. More and more hospitals are exploring joint ventures and other approaches to establish home health agencies and durable medical equipment companies to hold onto the captive patient. Large hospital chains will attempt to expand even further. Insurance companies, and perhaps Medicare, will begin to pay on a capitation payment system, an approach that could have an even more dramatic effect on the delivery of health care. If, for example, an insurance company such as Blue Cross or Prudential chose to pay one lump sum for the care of a patient through prehospital admission testing, hospital care, nursing home care, and home care, such a capitation payment would undoubtedly affect the attitude of providers of such diverse levels of care. If the hospital were to receive the lump sum, surely it would not be eager to part with the payment for nursing home or home care. If the attending physician were the recipient of such funds, new and testy relationships would unquestionably develop among family practitioners and internists on the one hand and surgeons and other specialists on the other hand. Simply stated, as the delivery system adjusts to changes in reimbursement methodologies, new providers arrive with innovations to maximize profits, thereby fueling growth.

FRAUD AND ABUSE

There is little question that home care opens a Pandora's box of puzzles in terms of what is acceptable behavior in the realm of referrals. Congress probably had a little less insight than we give them credit for on this issue because, despite the fairly strong statutes on the books since 1977, the intended targets of the fraud and abuse amendments were the clinical laboratories and physician referrals, not the area of respiratory therapists, DME providers, and home care companies. Congressional intent was to prevent kickbacks in these areas; that same law is now applied to home care referrals. Regardless, those statutes and accompanying regulations shape the behavior of respiratory therapists across the country who may question the appropriateness of certain referral situations.

Section 1877(b)(1) of the Social Security Act states:

> Whoever knowingly and willfully solicits or receives any remuneration (including any kickback, bribe or rebate) directly or indirectly, overtly or covertly, in cash or in kind—
>
> (A) in return for referring an individual to a person for the furnishing or arranging for the furnishing of any item or service for which payment may be made in whole or in part under this title, or
>
> (B) in return for purchasing, leasing, ordering, or arranging for or recommending purchasing, leasing, or ordering any good, facility, service or item for which payment may be made in whole or in part under this title, shall be guilty of a felony and upon conviction thereof, shall be fined not more than $25,000 or imprisoned for not more than five years, or both.
>
> (2) Whoever knowingly and willfully offers or pays any remuneration including any kickback, bribe or rebate, directly or indirectly, overtly or covertly, in cash or in kind to any person to induce such person—
>
> (A) to refer an individual to a person for the furnishing or arranging for the furnishing of any item or service for which payment may be made in whole or in part under this title, or
>
> (B) to purchase, lease, order, or arrange for or recommend purchasing, leasing, or ordering any good, facility, service or time for which payment may be made in whole or in part under this title, shall be guilty of a felony and upon conviction thereof, shall be fined not more than $25,000 or imprisoned for not more than five years, or both.

It is clear that the statutory intention of the law is to prohibit, at least in the field of respiratory home care, respiratory therapists from receiving fees or gifts for referrals of Medicare or Medicaid patients they may make to DME companies for the provision of certain services. Likewise, it is intended to prohibit DME providers from offering any kind of remuneration, cash or in kind, for referrals.

The area of questionable relationships is unfortunately much larger than the areas in which the situation is clearly legal or illegal. Consider the following examples:

Case One:

Helen is a respiratory therapist working at Memorial Hospital, which is located in a fairly large urban area. About 15 patients a week are discharged needing some level of respiratory care in the home. Helen, through her experience, knows that there are many suppliers who want the referrals, but only three have met the criteria established by the hospital's respiratory therapy department. Therefore Helen refers patients to the three providers on a rotating basis.

Analysis:
Helen does not benefit financially from making the referrals. She is acting in accordance with Federal law. It is a positive sign that the hospital has established objective criteria to identify acceptable home care companies.

Case Two:

Jeff is a therapist in a small hospital located in a rural area. There is only one DME supplier in the area that can provide satisfactory service. Jeff is short on cash because he wants to buy a new car, and the DME supplier has offered him a part-time job helping the DME company. What rules should Jeff follow?

Analysis:
It is perfectly legal for Jeff to work for the hospital and the DME company as long as he removes himself totally from the referral process. He must not benefit from any referral, and if he is making referrals to a company where he is employed, even if it is on a fee-for-service basis, there can be questions about legality.

In order to protect himself, Jeff does the right thing. He informs both the hospital and the DME supplier in writing of his intentions but goes the extra step and informs the local Medicare carrier and intermediary as well. In addition he insists that the hospital adopt a policy that requires patients who are being referred to a home care company sign a statement that clearly acknowledges that the family or the individual is making the choice of who shall provide the care, not a hospital employee.

Case Three:

Bob is the director of a medium-sized respiratory care department in an urban area. He refers most, but not all, of his patients to one company in particular. His rationale is solid in that it is documented that this one company provides superior service. Bob's wife owns the DME company.

Analysis:
A prosecutor could probably make a strong argument that Bob benefits financially from referrals he makes. It would be an extremely wise move for Bob to consult an attorney.

Case Four:

Deborah is employed by University Hospital, and DRGs have really taken their toll on the hospital. The institution is eager to find alternative sources of revenue and has established its own home-health agency and DME company. The hospital is asking Deborah to refer all the patients to the new hospital-owned companies, excluding other reputable providers. Deborah is not sure what to do.

Analysis:
Deborah has a strong obligation to show the Medicare law to her administrator. She can probably argue that her opinion is that the administrator may be asking her to violate the law. The administrator tells her that the hospital's attorneys have looked at the situation carefully and believe that everything is legal. Deborah asks for her new instructions in writing, and the administrator refuses.

There must be some reason why the administrator refuses to put the new components of Deborah's job description in writing. If the hospital eventually does put this new directive in writing, it goes a long way to relieving Deborah of any liability. The hospital may be guilty of restraint of trade if it excludes other providers from the marketplace, but Deborah has protected herself. If the administrator refuses to put the new assignment in writing, Deborah must ask herself the difficult question, "Why?"

It would appear that there are several ways respiratory therapists and suppliers can protect themselves. First, clearly a therapist who works for both a hospital and some sort of home care company must remove him- or herself from the referral process. That is a nonnegotiable; doing otherwise gives Medicare the opportunity to claim that the therapist benefits financially from the referral process. Suppliers should police themselves, and when questionable behavior arises, Medicare carriers should be notified immediately. Hospitals have an obligation to ensure continuity of care and should emphasize that to its discharged patients. Hospitals should develop objective criteria to determine what requirements a company must meet in order to receive referrals, and then stick to that policy. Ideally, all companies that are qualified and economically acceptable should have the opportunity to compete in the marketplace.

Interestingly, Medicare attempted through the regulatory process to apply strict guidelines on this issue. In Transmittal B–84–9 published in September, 1984, the Health Care Financing Administration (HCFA) stated,

The opportunity to generate a fee is itself a form of remuneration. The offer or receipt of such fee opportunities is illegal if intended to induce a patient referral. Thus a supplier who induces patient referrals by offering therapists fee generating opportunities is offering illegal remuneration, even if the therapist is paid no more than his or her usual fee.

Such a strong statement clearly prohibited therapists from working both sides of the aisle, even on a fee for service basis, if one could make the argument that the home care employment was based on the referrals. HCFA implied that the questions that needed to be asked by a therapist were, "Would I have this job in home care if I did not have the job in the hospital? What is inherent in my hospital job that makes it necessary for me to work in the hospital if I also want to work in home care?" After a fair amount of protest, HCFA repealed those three sentences in April of 1985 via Transmittal B–85–2. At that time HCFA stated, "We have received a number of inquiries regarding the meaning of those [three] sentences, and have concluded they unduly prejudged the legality of certain referral arrangements which cannot be determined without consideration of the relevant factors and practice patterns described [earlier]."

It is clear that, at best, the issue of referrals and conflict of interest in respiratory home care is not well-defined. What is legal and what is not can be very cloudy, and it is difficult to give generic directions to therapists and DME providers. For example, this author has been informed that in the state of Virginia, as recently as 1987, the going rate for referrals was $120. Some providers were willing to talk confidentially, citing competitors who were offering money for referrals. They felt very resentful not only of the therapists who accepted such remuneration but even more resentful that, in order to remain competitive in the marketplace, some felt they were being forced to make similar arrangements.

RESPONSIBILITY OF THE RESPIRATORY CARE PROFESSION

The respiratory care community must accept a major responsibility in home care. That responsibility encompasses cost containment, appropriateness of care, ethical considerations, and competitive issues. To shirk these responsibilities is to hand them over to others, perhaps government or private insurance companies. While government may have a level of obligation to listen, it certainly does not have an obligation to act to meet individual desires. Private companies do not have an obligation to even listen to an individual view. Simply put, if the respiratory care community does not assume the appropriate level of responsibility, someone else will assume it for them.

Cost containment is an area in which there is room for some improvement. There is little indication that the provider community has gone to great lengths to hold costs down, and there is some evidence that the opposite is true. Expenditures for respiratory home care have gone up dramatically in recent years, and the support for strong Federal guidelines was far from universal. The impact of recent Federal regulations that require certain medical documentation for use of oxygen in the home will go a long way to controlling costs, but the Federal government has a long memory and will recall the failure of certain elements of the respiratory care community to support its efforts to contain costs.

Linked to this issue, of course, is appropriateness of care. The stories of inappropriate oxygen-delivery systems are almost comical, yet tragic at the same time. Unless the respiratory care community establishes strong medical criteria for answering the following questions, it is unlikely that reimbursement and general attitudes of Federal health policymakers will improve:

- When is a concentrator appropriate, and when are other delivery mechanisms more appropriate?
- When is mechanical ventilation in the home appropriate? What other considerations are important when making the evaluation for such home care?
- Who is best qualified to deliver home care?
- What is appropriate home care?

If medical research needs to be conducted, then respiratory health care should be moving in that direction. If consensus is possible, it should be obtained. If certain modalities are questionable, ought we to hold off using them until there is definitive analysis of all the variables? And perhaps most importantly, what about the ethical considerations that face the patient and family?

The question of medical ethics is one that cannot be ignored by the respiratory care community. Physicians, therapists, and home care companies should work together to examine important issues and create an open forum for candid discussion. In the past few years, as technology has become more and more sophisticated, it has become clear that new technologies can prolong life for extended periods of time. Is this always desirable? If not, what are the limits that we should set for making such decisions? What role does cost play in such decision-making processes? Should all patients who are medically able to go home actually go home? What if the family is unwilling to accept responsibility? Should the government pay for care in such cases? Because the entire community is concerned with these issues, the discussions should emanate from within the community.

CONCLUSION

There is little doubt that Medicare, the Federal government's program of health care for the elderly, has had a major impact on the delivery not only of hospital care but of home care as well. Respiratory care lags behind some services from the perspective of reimbursement, primarily because historically the development of Medicare preceded the maturation of respiratory care from inhalation therapy. Unfortunately this has led to a game of catch-up for the respiratory care profession.

Respiratory home care has evolved primarily in one direction: a direct link with DME suppliers. Respiratory therapists really have not pursued direct employment with home-health agencies as other allied health professionals have because of the failure of Medicare to reimburse respiratory care on a per-visit basis. The relationship between respiratory therapists and equipment suppliers has become complicated in recent years because of the dramatic growth in home care and the potential referral of hospital patients to home care providers. As ventilators have become more commonplace in the home, a new thrust for respiratory home care has emerged. Despite cost savings associated with such care, it appears that political pressures related to the Federal deficit of $2 trillion will stop any legislative effort to change the reimbursement laws relative to respiratory home care.

The entire respiratory care community, including therapists, physicians, manufacturers, and DME providers have an obligation to assist one another in developing cohesive and coordinated strategies to meet these and other political pressures facing respiratory care. Issues such as conflict of interest, restraint of trade, competition, and appropriateness of care can only be addressed through cooperative efforts of all who have a vested interest in the outcome.

Index

Letters following page numbers indicate
tables (t) and figures (f).

Letters following page numbers indicate
tables (t) and figures (f).

Letters following page numbers indicate
tables (t) and figures (f).

Letters following page numbers indicate
tables (t) and figures (f).